Percentages in the English Population

	%
Fy(a+b−)	17
Fy(a+b+)	49
Fy(a−b+)	34
Jk(a+b−)	25
Jk(a+b+)	50
Jk(a−b+)	25
Lu(a+b−)	0·15
Lu(a+b+)	8
Lu(a−b+)	92
Le(a+b−)	23
Le(a−b+)	71
Le(a−b−)	6

	%
Haptoglobin 1	16
Haptoglobin 2–1	47
Haptoglobin 2	37
Gc 1	56
Gc 2–1	38
Gc 2	6
Gm^a(Gm(1))	60
Gm^b(Gm(5))	88

AN INTRODUCTION TO

BLOOD GROUP SEROLOGY

Schematic representation of the quantitatively dominating proteins ($\gtrsim$30 mg/100 ml) of fresh human plasma separated by electrophoresis in a Ca^{++}-containing buffer.

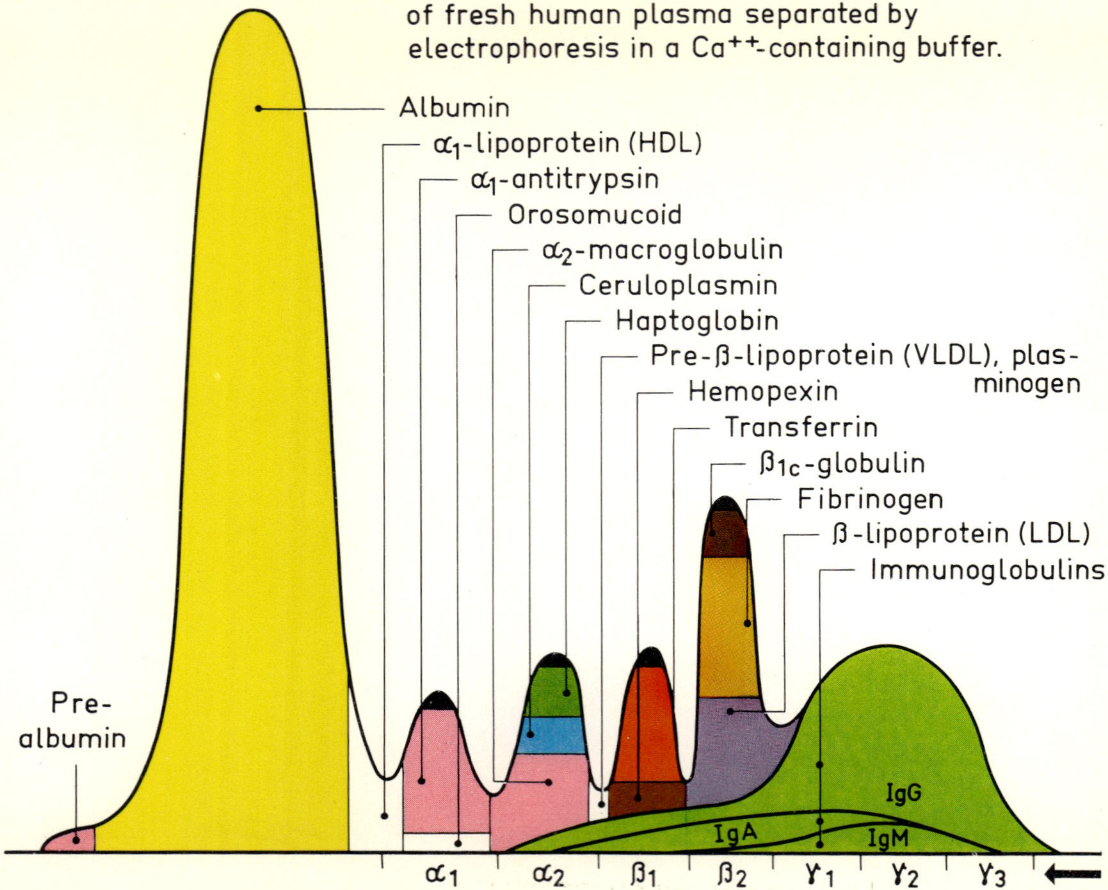

Frontispiece. Reproduced by kind permission of A. B. KABI

AN INTRODUCTION TO
BLOOD GROUP SEROLOGY

Theory, Techniques, Practical Applications

by

KATHLEEN E. BOORMAN

Principal Scientific Officer, South London Blood Transfusion Centre, Sutton, Surrey

and

BARBARA E. DODD

M.Sc. (Lond.), Ph.D. (Lond.)

Senior Lecturer in Forensic Medicine, Department of Forensic Medicine
The London Hospital Medical College

FOURTH EDITION

with 14 plates and 18 text figures

J. & A. CHURCHILL

104 GLOUCESTER PLACE, LONDON

1970

First Edition 1957
Second Edition 1961
Third Edition 1966
Fourth Edition 1970

International Standard Book Number
0 7000 1438 1

Made in Great Britain at the Pitman Press, Bath

PREFACE TO THE FOURTH EDITION

As is to be expected there has been a great quantity of original work published since the last edition; some of it has modified the work of the routine laboratory and where this is so we have dealt with it in the appropriate section. Many of the new discoveries however are rare alleles or unusual forms produced by the action of modifying genes and much of the new thought (*e.g.* modern ideas as to the complex pathways of inheritance) is mainly of theoretical interest. We have dealt with these subjects in Section VII. This is in line with our policy of putting the main emphasis on the knowledge necessary for the safe and efficient working of the routine laboratory. We hope however that the routine worker will appreciate the glimpses of the more exotic world of the specialist. It is also important that when one of the rarer sub-types is encountered that it is recognised as being unusual and sent to the appropriate reference laboratory for identification and study.

We have expanded the section on non-red cell blood group systems. While they still remain the province of the specialist to a large extent, they are beginning to infiltrate the routine laboratory and will do so even more in the future.

Two appendices have been added; the first a description of the glass-rubber transfusion apparatus (reprinted from the first edition) for the benefit of those who still use it, the second an account of well tried methods of preparing IgG, IgA and IgM fractions from whole serum by column chromatography.

There are, of course, additions throughout the book; in particular we have included 20 new techniques covering subjects as varied as serum typing for Gc, V.D.R.L. testing and antibody elution.

We are continually encouraged to hear from those who have found this book readable and helpful and we hope that the alterations we have made in this edition will make it more useful to all who work in this field.

KATHLEEN E. BOORMAN
BARBARA E. DODD

PREFACE TO FIRST EDITION

SEVERAL books have been written relating to blood group serology. Each has had its own emphasis; in one, technical methods, in another, the clinical importance, in another, racial distribution, etc. In this book our aim has been to deal with all aspects of the subject in such a way as to give a general picture but concentrating on those which relate to the working of a serological laboratory. The approach, therefore, is threefold, firstly theory, secondly technique, and thirdly laboratory and bench organisation. It is intended as a reference book suitable for all engaged in routine blood group serology, whether in the large transfusion centres, in specialised or in general pathological laboratories. For the benefit of those who do not specialise in blood group serology a table of contents of a "shortened version"* which will meet almost all their needs is included. Technicians will also, it is hoped, find that this book covers all the aspects of the subject needed for the final examination in blood transfusion techniques of the Institute of Medical Laboratory Technology. There are some deliberate omissions, mainly in highly specialised fields. In short, we are concerned not so much with the "peaks" dear to the heart of the research worker but with the "plains" of the safe and competent handling of the larger volume of routine work.

The ABO blood groups are studied first and in considerable detail because these, the first human blood groups to be discovered, are still the most important. Moreover, the techniques involved in their determination form the basis of almost all blood grouping methods, those used for other blood group systems being to a large extent modifications using different reagents, media and temperatures of reaction.

We are much indebted to Dr. R. A. Zeitlin, Director of the South London Blood Transfusion Centre, at which so much of the experience necessary for the writing of this book was gained. We are grateful also for his helpful criticism of many of the chapters and his permission to publish the method of preparation of dried Anti-A slides, including figure.

We should like to acknowledge the kindness of Professor F. E. Camps, Director of the Department of Forensic Medicine, The

* This "shortened version" is now published separately under the title *Basic Essentials of Blood Group Theory and Practice.*

London Hospital Medical College, in granting facilities which have greatly expedited the writing of the book.

Dr. S. R. M. Bushby and Miss E. W. Ikin have patiently read much of the first draft of the text. We are most grateful for their many useful suggestions. We should like to thank Dr. M. E. Mackay for valuable help.

We have been fortunate in having help from Miss E. M. Brooks and Miss D. A. Eeles in various ways, not least in the tedious task of reading proofs. All the photographs, including the photomicrographs, are the work of Mr. A. E. Densham, and the black-and-white figures were drawn by Mr. W. T. J. McRae. We much appreciate the endless pains that they have taken. We should like to thank those who typed and re-typed the manuscript, and particularly Mrs. L. Joiner for the tables and some of the more complicated parts of the text.

We are indebted to Drs. R. R. Race and A. E. Mourant and to Blackwell Scientific Publications for permission to quote figures for various gene and blood group frequencies from their books, and to Dr. J. V. Dacie for allowing us to reproduce his scheme for the serological investigation of auto-antibody types of hæmolytic anæmia.

There are many others whose work has contributed either directly or indirectly to this book; we appreciate, although we cannot enumerate, all that they have done.

The literature on blood group serology is so extensive that we have not attempted a comprehensive bibliography. We have, in the main, concentrated upon those papers in which new discoveries are described and those which themselves contain extensive references which the interested reader can consult. At points in the text we have mentioned standard works which deal more fully with particular aspects of the subject; to these we continually refer, since they are not only excellent in themselves but contain extensive references to original work.

KATHLEEN E. BOORMAN
BARBARA E. DODD

LIST OF PLATES

CONTENTS

AN INTRODUCTION TO

BLOOD GROUP SEROLOGY

Section I—Introduction

"*Let me introduce you . . . said the Red Queen, Alice—Mutton; Mutton—Alice.*"

Lewis Carroll, THROUGH THE LOOKING GLASS

CHAPTER 1

HUMAN BLOOD GROUPS—WHAT ARE THEY?

BLOOD groups are inherited characters which give rise to antigen-antibody systems. A short résumé therefore of the relevant theory both of antigens and antibodies and of genetics, is a useful starting point for an introduction to human blood group serology.

Blood Groups as Antigen-antibody Systems

The classical definitions of antigen and antibody are as follows:

1. An antigen is any substance which, when introduced parenterally into an individual who himself lacks that substance, stimulates the production of an antibody, and which, when mixed with the antibody, reacts specifically with it in some observable way.
2. An antibody is a substance which appears in the plasma or body fluids as a result of stimulation by an antigen and which reacts specifically with that antigen in some observable way.

Although these definitions are not perfect in that antigens and antibodies are found which do not (or do not appear to) conform strictly to them, they are still the most useful definitions and remain valuable criteria by which this class of substances may be recognised.

Antigens

Antigens are substances of large molecular size, usually protein, sometimes having a polysaccharide component which determines the specificity while the amino acid component determines the antigenicity (*i.e.* the ability to stimulate the production of antibodies). While this is broadly true, some polysaccharides of large molecular size are in themselves weakly antigenic. Moreover, recent work has shown that the amino acids may contribute in some measure to the specificity (*see also* Chapter 32).

Substances which possess specificity but little or no antigenicity are called haptens. The blood group substances which are secreted in saliva are examples of haptens. However, the distinction between haptenic and antigenic blood group substances is not very clear-cut and whereas purified substances (haptens) are not strongly antigenic in rabbits unless previously combined with a protein, they do cause considerable antibody production when injected into man. Blood group antigens, especially those of the ABO system, are probably present in all cells of the body but have been most carefully studied in the red cell. There is evidence that they are situated at varying depths in the cell envelope. Any individual red cell carries a large number and variety of blood group antigen molecules.

Antibodies

Antibodies are immunoglobulins and form part of the serum globulin; they are also found in other body fluids, *e.g.* saliva and urine. The immunoglobulins are subdivided into three main classes IgG, IgA and IgM. These are clearly seen in the Frontispiece where they have been separated by electrophoresis.

These three classes can be differentiated in a number of ways. While some antibody activity is associated with IgA, most blood group antibodies are either IgG or IgM. IgG has a smaller molecule than IgM, molecular weight 150,000 as opposed to 900,000. IgM antibodies are usually agglutinins causing red cells which contain the corresponding antigen to agglutinate in saline while IgG antibodies are mainly the so-called incomplete antibody which attaches itself to red cells of the appropriate type but does not cause them to agglutinate in saline. IgA antibodies when they occur can either be saline agglutinins or incomplete antibodies. IgG antibodies have the most important property of being able to cross the placenta freely from mother to infant, while it is most unusual for IgA or IgM antibodies to do so. This means that when we are considering the possible effect of a maternal antibody on the fœtus in utero it is the presence and strength of the IgG antibodies that we must determine.

However, it is important to realise that not all IgG antibodies are incomplete, some can cause agglutination of red cells suspended in saline and not all IgM antibodies are agglutinins, some are incomplete. IgG agglutinins are found in many immune group O sera and examples of IgM incomplete antibodies are not infrequently found in the Rh system.

The specificity of an antibody is not necessarily related to whether the antibody is IgG or IgM. In fact antibodies of most specificities can be either IgG or IgM or both. When we deal with the separate blood group systems we shall indicate whether the antibodies are likely to be IgG or IgM and where they are mixtures how to show this and to reveal the presence of IgG antibodies in a mixture of IgM or IgG. As a broad distinction IgM antibodies are often naturally occurring while IgG antibodies are usually the result of a known antigenic stimulus.

Naturally Occurring Antibodies

Naturally occurring antibodies are those found in a serum when no specific antigenic stimulus causing them to be present can be traced. They usually develop during infancy at about 4–8 months and in late childhood attain a level which is maintained with very little variation throughout life, tending to decrease again in old age. These antibodies can belong to many blood group systems, but their frequency of occurrence is very variable. In the ABO blood group system, for instance, they are regularly present in the serum of individuals who lack the corresponding antigen, in the P system the antibody anti-P_1 is common in P_1 negative persons, while the sera of the very rare persons who are truly P negative always contain antibodies against all the P antigens, and are thus a mixture of anti-P, anti-P_1 and anti-P^k. Other naturally occurring antibodies are found in only a few persons who lack the corresponding antigen, for instance, nearly all persons are Wr^a negative and yet only one per cent of all sera contain anti-Wr^a.

Immune Antibodies

In contrast to naturally occurring antibodies, those that are formed in response to a traceable stimulation by the corresponding antigen are termed immune antibodies. The process of formation of immune antibodies is called immunisation. If the process is brought about by the introduction of an antigen from another member of the same species it is called iso-immunisation and the antibodies formed, iso-antibodies. This production and increase of antibody in a serum is known as an immune response. Usually the peak of an immune response occurs 10–20 days after the injection of the antigen (*see* Chapter 5). In the process of immunisation there is a wide spectrum of antibody production and antibodies are formed from the stimulation of a single antigen differing from one another in physical and chemical properties and even to a certain extent in specificity.

Immune antibodies can be IgM, IgA or most commonly IgG. Some of the blood group systems in which antibodies are naturally occurring, can also form immune antibodies of the same specificity if there is stimulation by the corresponding antigen. For instance, a serum may contain naturally occurring anti-A and immune anti-A, most of the former will be IgM while the latter will often be a mixture of IgM and IgG. In some systems, such as Rh in which naturally occurring antibodies are rare, the immune antibody produced often follows the usual pattern of antibody production, in which IgM is produced first, followed by IgG as the immunisation continues so that many anti-Rh sera eventually contain mostly IgG antibodies. It is as well, however, to remember that the whole process is exceedingly complicated and influenced by many factors which we do not understand. In some sera, almost all the Rh antibody is IgM. It will be seen later that these can either be sera with a high titre of saline agglutinin or of the "papain-type" antibody only detected by enzyme techniques.

Identification of IgG and IgM Antibodies

On account of their difference in reaction and ability to cross the placenta and possibly damage the fœtus in utero, it may sometimes be important to know whether a given antibody is IgG or IgM or even IgA. Now these immunoglobulins can be distinguished in many ways. Precipitation in agar and immunoelectrophoresis will both show if IgG, IgA and IgM are present in a serum. For our present purpose, however, these techniques are not particularly helpful (although modifications can be devised) as they will only show whether the serum contains the usual amounts of IgG, IgA and IgM and not in which immunoglobulin fraction, the antibody in which we are interested, occurs as, strangely enough, the total quantity of IgG, IgA or IgM is not significantly altered by antibody production; there are not, for instance, more IgG molecules after an immune response to, for example, the Rh antigen, merely more of them are anti-Rh in specificity. The cells producing IgG have produced the same amount of IgG, but its configuration is altered so that it can react with the stimulating antigen.

Techniques which actually separate the sera into fractions separating IgG from IgM are more useful because then the fractions can be tested individually for their antibody content. Such techniques are fractionation by means of DEAE cellulose or sephadex

G200 or ultra-centrifugation. These techniques are still mainly confined to specialist and research laboratories and will not be described in detail, though a simple modification of the first (the DEAE fractionation) is given in the chapter on hæmolytic disease of the fœtus, as it is a quick and useful method by which the specific antibody content of the IgG constituent of any serum can be determined. (For the conventional DEAE fractionation technique *see* Appendix 6.)

Suffice it for the moment to state the general theory of these three techniques without going into practical details. When serum is allowed to pass down a column of diethylamino-ethyl cellulose (DEAE) which has been equilibriated with a buffer of pH 8·0 and molarity 0·02 (pH and molarity can be slightly varied, Mollison recommends 7·6 and 0·01) only the IgG passes down the column. the other immunoglobulins (and indeed other proteins) being absorbed onto the column. These immunoglobulins can be successively eluted by increasing the molarity and decreasing the pH. The fractions can be concentrated to the original volume of the serum and the antibody content of each estimated.

In the separation using sephadex, serum is washed through a column of this material and the larger molecules come through faster than the smaller ones. The IgM fraction is thus obtained first and the IgG later (together with the IgA). While being quite a good method for obtaining IgM, it is not as useful as DEAE for preparing IgG fractions.

Ultracentrifugation also does not separate IgG satisfactorily from IgA; moreover, the IgM which is spun down to the bottom is not completely free of the other immunoglobulins.

A third type of technique is one which alters the IgM or IgG molecules so that they are inactivated. If a serum is treated with sulphydryl compounds, the usual one being 2-mercapto-ethanol, the IgM molecules split and are no longer capable of agglutinating red cells although they are still able to sensitise the cells as can be shown by performing an indirect anti-human globulin test. IgG molecules on the other hand are not inactivated by 2-mercapto-ethanol.

IgM molecules can also be inactivated by heat. In early work serum was diluted one in two and heated at 75°C for 20 minutes—this treatment was too drastic and destroyed some of the IgG molecules also. A better method is to heat the serum at 56°C for 3 hours. This inactivates some IgM molecules, *e.g.* anti-P_1, but is less satisfactory for anti-A or anti-B.

Immunisation

This is the process by which an individual produces antibodies in response to an antigen which he himself lacks. When the process is brought about by the introduction of an antigen from another member of the same species, it is known as iso-immunisation and the antibodies formed are termed iso-antibodies.

The process of immunisation has been studied in great detail. We will confine ourselves to mentioning a few of the known facts which have a direct bearing on iso-immunisation to blood group antigens in man.

The ability of an antigen to stimulate antibody production depends both on the intrinsic antigenicity (*e.g.* B is a good antigen in all group O and A persons, while P_1 is a comparatively poor antigen in most persons who lack P_1) and partly on individual variation between individuals of the same blood type receiving the same dose of antigen (*e.g.* while some group A persons may have a fourfold increase in anti-B activity when stimulated by a small injection of group B cells, others will respond to the same small dose by a hundred-fold or greater increase. It is obvious that blood group antigens which are strongly antigenic and to which the majority of suitable individuals respond will be of greater clinical importance than those which are weakly antigenic.

The response to an antigen is also influenced by whether or not the individual concerned has previously had an injection of the antigen. The first "dose" of antigen is known as the primary or sensitising dose—the response to it is slow and usually very weak. The secondary dose, on the other hand, usually elicits a strong response, with large amounts of antibody being rapidly produced. This is of importance, both with regard to immunisation by transfusions—immune blood group antibodies will more often be found among persons who have already had previous transfusions and to immunisation by pregnancy, where antibodies are comparatively rarely produced during a first pregnancy. In some cases of course the primary stimulus may be a pregnancy and the secondary a blood transfusion, or vice versa. This means that obstetric history is important when considering transfusion and transfusion history important when dealing with pregnant women.

Antibodies once produced may remain in the circulation for many years. As a general rule IgM antibodies disappear more quickly than IgG. On the whole, individuals in which the antibodies persist are less at risk when a further transfusion is contemplated as these antibodies are detected at the time of the direct match and suitable compatible blood can be selected. When an antibody has almost or entirely disappeared, blood containing the same antigen may well appear compatible at direct match, but will act as a secondary stimulus, the antibody being restimulated and possibly destroying the transfused cells within a few days or even hours. If the former, it may seem clinically to be merely a failure to obtain the expected Hb level after transfusion—if the latter there may well be all the classical symptoms of a hæmolytic transfusion reaction.

The plasma cells of the body are largely the sites of antibody formation. There is a multiplication of these following immunisation. By means of the fluorescent antibody technique the cells producing antibody can be identified and even in some cases the technique can be adapted to show which plasma cells are producing which of two antibodies being formed at the same time by the same individual.

The spleen is also thought to play a part in antibody production, although its exact role is not clear. Certainly, post-splenectomy patients can and do respond to immunisation and produce immune antibodies.

Antigen-antibody Reaction

Much has been written about the nature of antigen-antibody reaction, but the modern outlook may be stated briefly as follows. Certain chemical groupings called "determinants" on the large molecule which is behaving like an antigen combine with certain other groupings on the molecule of globulin which is the corresponding antibody. These groupings have been variously named "receptors," "combining sites" or "active patches." The combination is specific in that a given antigen will react only with its corresponding antibody and not with others. However, specificity is not always absolute as, particularly after prolonged stimulation, antibodies may be produced which will react, albeit not so strongly, with related antigens. The reason for this is probably that there are many different chemical groupings on the large antigenic macromolecule which vary individually both in their ability to stimulate antibody production and in the quality of the antibody which they cause to be produced. Some of these chemical groupings will be possessed in common by a number of related antigens. In blood grouping, cross reactions are occasionally encountered but the worker is more usually impressed by the high degree of specificity of reaction displayed.

The combination of antigen with antibody gives rise to the

"observable" ways of reaction to which reference was made in the definition. In blood grouping three "observable ways" are relevant, namely precipitation, agglutination and hæmolysis.

(a) **Precipitation**

When the antigen is soluble then mixture with its corresponding antibody often causes precipitation of the antigen-antibody complex provided certain conditions, in particular the correct proportion of antigen to antibody, are fulfilled. Such a soluble antigen is known as a precipitinogen and the corresponding antibody, a precipitin. In blood grouping the precipitin reaction is not used routinely although valuable research work has been carried out in the ABO system using this technique with purified A and B substances.

(b) **Agglutination**

This is by far the most important and most widely observed phenomenon in blood grouping.

If the antigens are cellular, as in blood cells or bacteria, mixture with their corresponding antibodies may cause a clumping or agglutination of the cells containing the antigen. Hence the term agglutinogen for the antigen, and agglutinin for the antibody.

Thus in blood grouping, clumping or agglutination of red cells is the observable result of mixing cells containing a particular antigen (agglutinogen) with a serum containing the corresponding antibody (agglutinin).*

The agglutination of red cells takes place in two stages. In the first stage the serum agglutinins become attached to agglutinogens on the red cell surface. A red cell which has thus taken up agglutinins is said to be sensitised. In the second stage the actual agglutination or clumping of the sensitised red cells takes place. The cells form aggregates which, if large enough, are visible to the naked eye (*see* Plate 3). There are degrees of agglutination which cannot be seen without the aid of a microscope (*see* Plates 6 and 7). If the agglutinins are potent, the agglutinating stage of the process may, under certain conditions, follow the sensitisation of the red cells within a few seconds of mixing the red cells and the antiserum together. As the potency of the agglutinins diminishes more time is required to develop the agglutination fully.

* Even for the detection and measurement of the group specific substances in soluble form the phenomenon of agglutination of red cells is used. The agglutinin is reduced in strength, or even completely neutralised by the corresponding soluble antigen. This is shown by its inability to agglutinate red cells to the same degree as before the addition of the antigen.

The red cells which form the clumps or aggregates are distorted in shape, and sometimes the red cell membranes break and liberate hæmoglobin. However, unless the cells are hæmolysed the reaction is in some measure a reversible one. Agglutinated cells can be partially and often completely dispersed and the attached agglutinin recovered from them by alteration of temperature. In most blood group systems a good deal of attached agglutinin can be recovered from agglutinated cells and collected in a small quantity of saline by raising the temperature of agglutinated cells to 56°C for a few minutes. The antibody solution is called an eluate.

Eluates are of value in proving that certain red cells have in fact taken up antibody. Moreover, information about the specificity of each component of a mixture of antibodies can often be obtained by an elution technique.

It might be considered that the mere agglutination of red cells is sufficient proof that they have become sensitised. This would indeed be true if it were not for the existence of factors which occasionally cause pseudo-agglutination; in appearance this is sometimes difficult to distinguish from true agglutination (*see* Plate 5 (a) and (b)). For example, an alteration in serum proteins (*e.g.* as occurs in multiple myelomatosis) will bring about a pseudo-agglutination of red cells which has no antigen-antibody basis. No eluate containing antibodies can be prepared from pseudo-agglutinated cells.

It is equally true that cells which are not agglutinated cannot *ipso facto* be considered to be unsensitised. There are three reasons for this. Firstly, the amount of antibody taken up by each red cell may not be sufficient to bring about actual agglutination of the cells. Secondly, the red cells may be subjected to such a temperature as will allow sensitisation of the cells but not their agglutination after sensitisation. Thirdly, the red cells may be sensitised by a kind of antibody which by itself is not capable of causing the cells to agglutinate. These antibodies, which in turn have been called blocking, or incomplete antibodies, or agglutinoids, play an important role in blood group serology. They were first discovered in the Rh system but by now have been found for practically all the known blood group antigens. They are able to sensitise red cells suspended in saline but are incapable of bringing about agglutination in this medium. Much of the research work connected with blood groups has been in devising and improving the sensitivity of techniques which would induce incomplete antibodies to agglutinate red cells. At the present time three methods are used routinely, usually in parallel. (i) A substance of high molecular weight is introduced into the system. This is commonly bovine albumin and it has the effect of causing red cells sensitised with incomplete antibody to agglutinate. (ii) Another antibody is made by injecting human globulin into rabbits or other domestic animals. The globulin, as might be expected, considering its protein nature, stimulates the production of anti-human globulin antibodies. Treatment of red cells sensitised by antibody globulin, with anti-globulin, brings about agglutination. (iii) Various enzymes are used, notably trypsin, papain and ficin. Treatment of red cells with one of these enzymes renders them susceptible to agglutination by incomplete antibodies.

The blocking nature of the incomplete antibody can be demonstrated by a simple experiment. A saline suspension of red cells of appropriate specificity is exposed to a serum containing incomplete antibodies. After the red cells have had time to become sensitised there is added to them agglutinins of the same specificity. These would normally cause agglutination, but if the cells are already sensitised by incomplete antibodies they fail to do so. The agglutinogen of the red cells has been coated by the incomplete antibody and is, therefore, not available to react with an agglutinin of the same specificity.

The practice of employing a variety of techniques in parallel for the detection of incomplete antibodies has led to the finding of antibodies which will react better by one technique than another or which will even fail entirely to react by one method although detectable by another. These differences are not satisfactorily explained by variations in sensitivity of the methods used but almost certainly reflect differences in quality between antibodies which, however, are identical in specificity. For example, a type of incomplete antibody has been described which fails to give a positive blocking test, although it is revealed by anti-human globulin technique and very often by the use of high protein media such as bovine albumin. This antibody has been termed crypt-agglutinoid.

The name "incomplete" given to a class of antibodies merely reflects the fact that these antibodies sensitise red cells but do not cause them to agglutinate in a saline medium, it does not imply that these antibodies are defective. They were also sometimes called "univalent" antibodies; it is almost certain that this name was based on a misapprehension and that they are bi-valent.

Some incomplete antibodies only sensitise cells in the presence of fresh serum (provided either by using a freshly taken sample containing the antibodies or by adding fresh human serum of the same ABO group).

The factor in the fresh human serum is a fraction of complement.

(c) **Hæmolysis**

Sometimes, when cellular antigens are concerned, the corresponding antibody may cause a breaking up or lysis of the cells. In this case the antigen is known as a lysinogen, and the corresponding antibody a lysin, or if red cells are involved the antigen is called a hæmolysinogen, and the antibody a hæmolysin.

Some hæmolysins are of blood group specificity. When these react with red cells containing the corresponding antigen hæmolysis occurs, hæmoglobin is liberated from the red cells and can readily be observed staining the supernatant fluid. The red cell envelopes remain undissolved but distorted in shape. The appearance of hæmolysed red cells as viewed by means of the electron microscope suggests that a series of small round holes have been made all over the surface of the red cell. It has been found that hæmolysins need an additional factor to enable them to lyse red cells. This factor, which is present in all human sera, irrespective of blood group, is called complement. Complement deteriorates upon storage. It is, therefore, essential to use fresh serum* as a source of complement for hæmolysin tests. Complement is inactivated by heating the serum at 56°C for 30 minutes. In fact, it was through its thermolabile property that complement came to be discovered. Further investigation revealed that complement consisted of a number of fractions, all necessary for hæmolysis.

Experiment has shown that it is the complement rather than the specific hæmolysin that actually lyses the red cell. The hæmolysin sensitises the red cell and conditions it for the hæmolytic action of complement. Red cells cannot be lysed by complement in the absence of the specific hæmolysin, nor will their mixture with, followed by removal of, complement-containing serum permit subsequently added hæmolysin to act. Complement, therefore, does not attach itself to the red cell in the absence of the specific hæmolysin.

The nature of hæmolysis of red cells by the action of hæmolytic antibodies has been dealt with in a series of classic experiments, and those interested should consult appropriate textbooks.

The specificity of hæmolysins is often the same as that of

* Fresh serum that has been "freeze-dried" is a good source of complement provided it is used immediately upon reconstitution.

agglutinins and incomplete antibodies, which has suggested that the hæmolysin may be the agglutinin or incomplete antibody producing a different effect under different conditions. This point is still controversial but all would agree that whatever the type of observable reaction between blood group antigen and its corresponding antibody *in vitro*, the evidence is in favour of a reaction which is largely hæmolytic when it occurs *in vivo*.

Blood Groups as Inherited Characters

(a) General theory of inheritance.

The nucleus of each cell of the body contains thread-like structures called chromosomes. These chromosomes are divided along their length into more or less discrete regions each of which has distinct genetical properties. These divisions are called genes and a large number of them are present on each chromosome. They are arranged in a characteristic order along its length so that each gene always occupies its own special position (or locus) on a particular chromosome. In man, it is now known that there are 46 chromosomes in 23 pairs. Each member of a pair contains the same number of genes and the gene loci are arranged in the same order. (The sex chromosomes are the only known exceptions to this rule.) The significance of the paired chromosomes can be seen in consideration of the gametes. In the sperm and ova there are only 23 chromosomes in each nucleus. This position is reached by special cell divisions (called meiosis) in which the homologous paired chromosomes part, one going into each of two gametes. Thus sex cells are produced which contain exactly half of the chromosome material of the body cells. When fusion of the male and female gametes occurs, the chromosome material doubles up again, each chromosome finding its homologue among chromosomes derived from the opposite sex, subsequent divisions giving rise to body cells containing 46 chromosomes in 23 pairs. Thus, every body cell (as opposed to sex cell) contains the same genes in its nucleus as every other body cell. Moreover, half of them had been derived from the male parent and half from the female.

A gene is usually extremely stable and its replication at cell division is complete. Occasionally, however, it may undergo a change, called a mutation, the new form of the gene being reproduced at each further cell division so that the mutant form persists. A number of alternative genes (possibly derived from a single gene by past mutations) occur at a particular locus. These are called alleles or allelomorphic genes. It will be realised that the same locus will be represented twice in a fertilised ovum, once on each member of a pair of homologous chromosomes. Therefore, an individual possesses two and only two alleles for that locus, one from each parent. If the same allele is derived from each parent, the individual is said to be homozygous for the particular gene and if different, heterozygous. It follows, therefore, that if two alleles which can be designated L and l exist at a particular locus, three genetically different types of individual can occur, LL, Ll and ll. Sometimes it is possible to distinguish clearly each of these from the other but often only two classes can be recognised, one which may be called "L" comprising LL and Ll and the other "l" corresponding to the genotype ll. In such circumstances L is said to be dominant to l and l recessive to L. The class "L" is called the phenotype and contains the two genotypes LL and Ll.

With increased knowledge and improved techniques, geneticists are finding that truly recessive genes are becoming fewer or, in other words, in the heterozygote Ll characteristics differentiating Ll from LL and ll can be distinguished. In blood groups, with few exceptions, it is possible to distinguish the heterozygote from the homozygote, although a gene when present in single dose in the heterozygote may not express itself so strongly as when in double dose in the homozygote form. This dosage effect is sometimes so marked that it can be used to differentiate between the homo- and heterozygote. If, for example, L and l were blood group antigens and anti-L was available but not anti-l, it might be possible on the results of titrations to say that titres over a certain figure indicated two doses of L (*i.e.* genotype LL) and titres below that figure one dose (*i.e.* genotype Ll).

Genes carried on the same chromosome are said to be linked. Sometimes linked genes become separated by the occurrence of crossing over at meiosis. Crossing over involves the exchange of material between two homologous chromosomes. By and large, the further apart the linked genes are on the chromosome the more likely they are to be separated by crossing over and conversely, closely linked genes will travel together through many generations before separation occurs.

Linkage and crossing over may be illustrated by supposing a gene O and its allele o carried on the same pair of chromosomes as the Ll genes discussed above. The possible gene arrangements are L with O, L with o, l with O and l with o and therefore, for example, people who are Lo/lO will hand on to their children Lo or lO; occasionally, however, due to crossing over they will hand on LO or lo.

When genes are more than a certain distance apart they cross over sufficiently often that they appear to segregate independently and it is not obvious that they are in fact in the same chromosome.

Linkage has been demonstrated between the Rh blood group systems and oval cells, also between ABO and nail-patella syndrome.

The Xg blood group system is sex-linked, being carried on the X chromosome. The study of this system has opened up a whole new chapter in the genetics of linkage and has helped in the "mapping" of the X chromosome (*i.e.* in saying whereabouts in relation to each other some of the sex-linked genes are carried on the X chromosome).

A good deal of biochemical evidence has led geneticists to the conclusion that many genes control inherited characteristics by controlling the synthesis of specific enzymes. It is indeed suggested that in most cases genes bear a simple one-to-one relationship with enzymes. Moreover, any mutation that occurs in a gene may cause complete or partial failure in the synthesis of a particular enzyme, or alternatively a qualitatively different enzyme may be produced although its activity may not always be apparent. This subject of genes and enzymes will be briefly discussed again in relation to the most recent advances made in our knowledge of the ABO blood group system (*see* Chapter 2).

It is probable that instead of thinking of a single gene we should think of a section of chromosome with a large number of genes all acting and interacting to produce their effect. Such a section of chromosome is called a cistron—two genes belonging to one cistron would produce effects when on the same chromosome which might differ from those produced if they were one on each chromosome of a pair. Two genes which belong to the same cistron and are on the same chromosome are said to be in cis position, while two genes which are on opposite chromosomes are said to be in trans position.

(b) The inheritance of blood groups

Every individual receives from each parent a gene or possibly, a linked combination of genes (*see* Rh factor) relating to each of the blood group systems. Fig. 1.1 shows the inheritance of an imaginary blood group system YZ in which Y and Z are allelomorphic genes so that either Y or Z occupies the particular chromosomal locus for this system, never both.

It is customary to give the genes the same designation as the antigen whose development it controls. Gene Y gives rise to antigen Y, and gene Z to antigen Z. This is unfortunate in some respects as it tends to lead to confusion of thought and gives the erroneous impression that genes and antigens are identical.

In this hypothetical blood group system, three types of individual are possible, YY, YZ and ZZ. Fig. 1.1*b* shows the mating of a group Y male with a group YZ female. It is clear the male of group Y

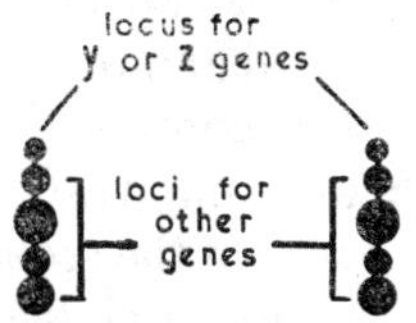

FIG. 1.1*a*. Diagrammatic representation of a pair of chromosomes.

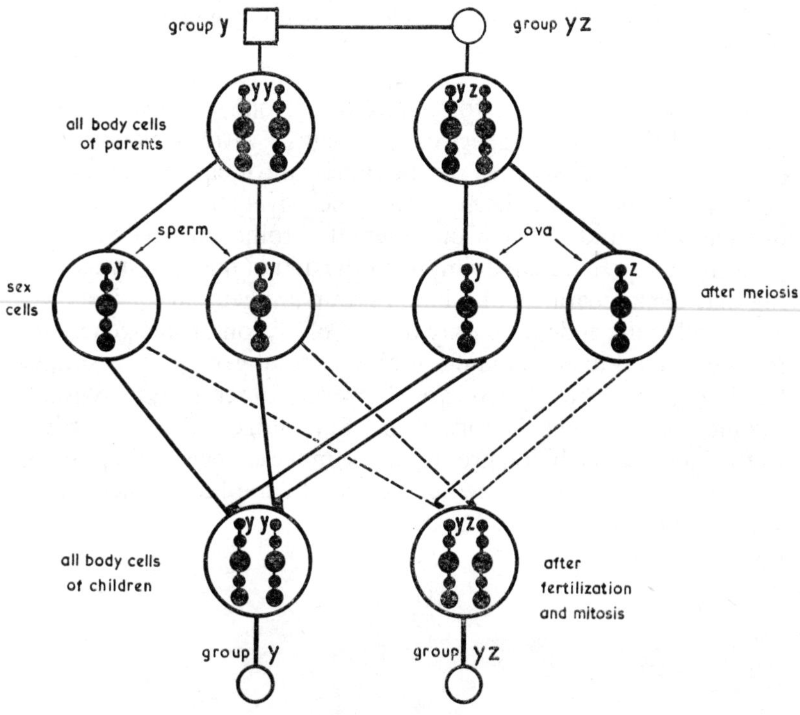

FIG. 1.1*b*. The inheritance of the blood group system YZ, showing the segregation of the genes in the sperm and ova.

must have received Y from each parent and so is of genotype YY, whereas the female has received Y from one parent and Z from the other and so is of genotype YZ.

In each body or somatic cell of the male each member of the relevant pair of chromosomes possesses Y one of which has been derived from one parent and one from the other. The female has one chromosome of type Y inherited from one parent and one of type Z from the other. Her body cells, therefore, contain chromosomes of two kinds with respect to the YZ system in question. After meiosis, the sperm cells are all alike and each possesses one chromosome having Y. Half the ova, however, have Y and half Z so that there are two kinds of ova. When fertilisation takes place the chromatin material is doubled and the body cells of the children from this mating (*see* diagram) contain either two chromosomes each with Y or one with Y and one with Z. Children of the first type belong to group Y, children of the second type to group YZ.

All known blood group systems are inherited along similar lines to the hypothetical case described above, the chief differences being in the number of allelomorphs controlling a particular system and the way in which they are designated.

It should, of course, be realised that in each body cell in the human species there are forty-six chromosomes in twenty-three pairs, and the different genes controlling the various blood group systems are not all situated on the same pair of chromosomes. In fact, most of them have been shown conclusively to be independent of each other and to occur on different chromosome pairs.

In this chapter we have simplified the actual position by assuming that the appearance of a blood group antigen, on for instance, a red cell is dependent on only one set of allelomorphic genes and for the general understanding of blood group genetics this simplification is justified. There are, however, other genes involved. Should these prevent the formation of an antigen which according to the individual's blood group genetic make-up he should possess, they are known as suppressor genes. Examples of such genes will be found in Chapter 32.

CHAPTER 2

THE SEROLOGICAL LABORATORY AND GENERAL BLOOD GROUPING PROCEDURE

THE subject of human blood groups is a large one and there are many, some would say a bewildering number, of techniques. In spite of the variety it is true, however, that the chief manipulation in a blood grouping laboratory is the mixing together of extremely small quantities of red cells and serum and afterwards observing whether or not the red cells have been agglutinated or sensitised by an antibody in the serum. The mixing is effected most accurately and conveniently by delivering small volumes with a graduated Pasteur pipette into precipitin tubes, or in some circumstances on to slides or opalescent tiles.

Alternatively, blood grouping may be performed by a multichannel modification of the auto-analyser. This is described at the end of the chapter.

Serological Apparatus

Tubes

These are made in hard glass in two main sizes.

(1) *The* 50 *mm.* (*Length*) × 11 *mm.* (*Internal Diameter*) *Cell Suspension Tube*. This will be found to be of convenient size for:

(*a*) Red cell suspensions.
(*b*) Anti-human globulin (Coombs) tests—there is room for an adequate volume of saline at the washing stage.
(*c*) Storage of typing serum of various kinds.
(*d*) The serial dilutions of "master" titres, dilutions of saliva, etc.

(2) *The* 50 *mm.* (*Length*) × 5·5 *mm.* (*Internal Diameter*) *Precipitin Tube*. This tube is used for almost all serological tests with the exception of the anti-human globulin technique. In a busy laboratory it is, therefore, required in large numbers.

Alternatively plastic tubes can be used. The most usual sizes are:

(3) 60 *mm.* × 8 *mm.* (*Internal Diameter*). This takes the place of the larger glass tube and is used for the same purpose.

(4) *Plastic tubes of* 35 *mm.* (*Length*) *and* 5 *mm.* (*Internal Diameter*).

These tubes which replace the precipitin tubes are shorter, to keep the cost low. This is a slight disadvantage but they are satisfactory albeit slightly more tedious to use.

Cleansing of Tubes

The adequate cleaning of tubes presents a considerable problem. The least trace of particulate dirt, of previously used potent anti-serum, or of alkali or acid, may be fatal to the subsequent tests. Dirty tubes should be covered with cold water, as soon as possible after the tests are read, and left to soak.

There are a variety of ways of cleaning the tubes. A machine which sprays jets of fluid into the tubes can be used, a satisfactory sequence is tap water, detergent, two rinses with tap water and then steam under pressure. If a machine fitted with jets is not available the tubes must be held under a fast-running tap, thoroughly shaken, boiled in detergent, rinsed in hot and then cold tap water and finally with distilled water. For the rinsing process the tubes are held upright in handfuls so that each tube is filled completely with the rinsing fluid. After each rinse they are vigorously shaken. They are dried quickly in a hot air oven.

The importance of an efficient cleaning process for tubes cannot be over-emphasised; without it first-class work may be ruined.

Racks for Holding Tubes

The small wooden blocks as shown in Plate 1 have been found to be satisfactory for holding the small precipitin tubes. A counter-part in perspex is an excellent alternative but is more expensive. Light aluminium racks will not withstand bench wear and tear but are used for storage of serum at low temperatures. Large wooden racks (*see also* Plate 1) are convenient for holding sample tubes.

Pasteur or Capillary Pipettes

These are the serologist's chief tool.

In Fig. 2.1 eight different Pasteur pipettes are depicted each designed for a different purpose. The first of these (A), is a general purpose pipette graduated to deliver two unit volumes 0·03 ml. each; the graduation marks both come well within the straight part of the stem. This is essential for accuracy. If the size of the bore and the required unit volume are such that it is necessary to make a graduation where the stem is starting to widen, the pipette is unsuitable as any slight inaccuracy that may occur in measuring a volume results in a larger error than when the volume is confined to the straight part of the stem. If the bore is such that the unit volume marking is less than 1 in. from the tip, the pipette is less accurate than one with the marking situated at the optimum distance of approximately 1½ in. up the stem. The overall length of the pipette, excluding the rubber teat is 5½–6 in. This is a comfortable length for the average hand but there will naturally be slight variations (of not more than ½ in.) according to personal preference. The graduation must be a fine line (not a grease pencilled blob!) which can be made with a mapping pen using either Gurr's glass ink or Chinese lacquer.

The second pipette, (B) in Fig. 2.1, requires little additional comment. It is essentially similar except that it is graduated to deliver three unit volumes instead of two. It is included to emphasise the point that even if further unit volume markings are needed they must all remain within the confines of the narrow part of the stem.

The third pipette shown (C) is designed solely for titration and should be reserved for this purpose. It bears a single graduation situated approximately two inches from its tip.

The fourth pipette (D) is for the delivery of micro-volumes (0·01 ml. or less). The bore of this pipette has to be very fine to allow the small unit volume to occupy a reasonable length of the stem (*i.e.* approximately 1–1½ in.). It is not advisable to mark such pipettes to deliver more than one unit volume.

The fifth pipette (E) is not graduated since it is used solely for the preparation of smears. It can with advantage be of slightly wider bore than the general purpose pipette.

The sixth pipette (F) shown is designed for the transfer of large quantities, *i.e.* several millilitres of any liquid, such as serum, from one container to another. Thus, the wide end of the pipette is increased to 5 in. and the narrow end reduced to ½ in.

The seventh pipette (G) is for the making of "master" dilutions. The bulge in the stem allows for a large unit volume (up to 0·3 ml. to 0·5 ml.) while maintaining both the fine point which reduces carry-over to a minimum and a graduation mark made in a narrow region of the stem so that accuracy in actual measurement of the volume is comparable with that of the other pipettes described.

The eighth pipette (H) is designed for use by the dropping technique. The aperture of a dropping pipette must be of standard bore and a gauge is used to ensure that the pipette delivers a drop of the correct size.

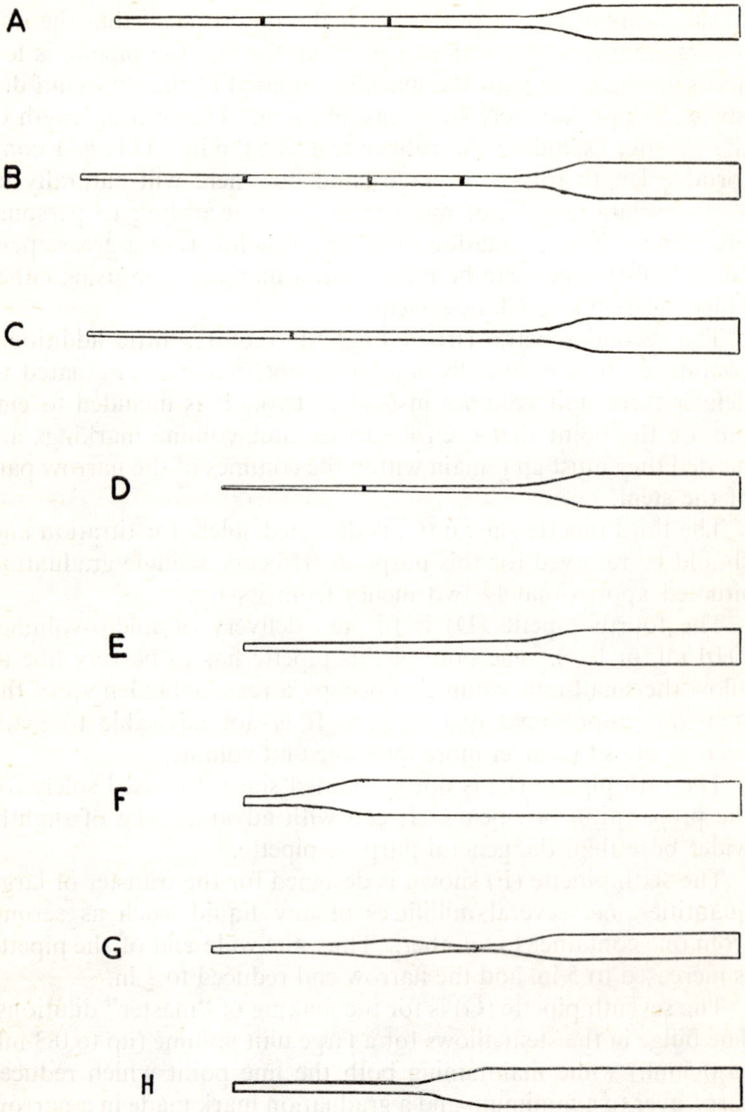

FIG. 2.1. The Pasteur pipettes used for blood group serology.

A. General purpose.
B. Three unit volume.
C. Titration.
D. Micro-volume.
E. Reading.
F. Transfer.
G. Master dilution.
H. Dropping pipette

Handling of Pasteur Pipettes

For blood grouping techniques Pasteur pipettes are used in a specialised way; the handling of them in other kinds of laboratory does not give the worker experience of their use for serological manipulations.

The measurement and delivery into precipitin tubes of small volumes of fluid requires a delicate touch and much practice, but an amazing degree of accuracy coupled with speed can be attained by the practised worker. The pipettes should be held at an angle, the glass stem just below the teat being gripped between the third and fourth fingers while the thumb and first finger rest gently on the rubber teat (cf. Plate 1). The weight of the pipette is supported by the third and fourth fingers, while the thumb and first finger are used entirely for controlling the measurement of the required volume. The next step is to exert very slight pressure on the teat with the thumb and first finger. The exact amount of pressure required must be learnt by experience but let it be said that it is far less than is usually imagined by the novice. The tip of the pipette is dipped just under the surface of the fluid which is to be measured and the pressure gradually released until the fluid is drawn up exactly to the mark. This is a simple procedure providing the preliminary pressure on the teat has been gauged correctly. The optimum pressure is such that the fluid within the stem just manages to reach the mark with little or no suction left over to raise it any further. If too great a pressure is exerted it will be found that the column of fluid fluctuates wildly, is difficult to control and will not come to rest at the desired spot.

Having obtained an accurately measured volume it is next delivered into a small precipitin tube; this also requires knack. The tip of the pipette is placed just overlapping the edge of the tube and pressure is again exerted with the thumb and forefinger, this time fairly sharply. It is released when the whole volume has been delivered. This method of delivery is slightly modified for micro-volumes since these are placed on the bottom of the tube which is taken out of the rack and held in the left hand. Lest it is thought that the foregoing description suggests a process which is cumbersome and lengthy, it should be recorded that the experienced worker would be capable of delivering several hundred accurately measured volumes in the time taken to read and digest the above description.

The technique of handling the dropping pipette is entirely different. The teat is squeezed and released sufficiently to allow liquid to enter to about two-thirds of the way up the stem. The pipette is then held vertically and one drop of fluid allowed to fall into each precipitin tube. This procedure is slightly faster than delivering unit volumes of fluid and slightly more inaccurate as the size of the drop is not only dependent on the aperture of the pipette but also on the viscosity of the fluid used, so that drops of,

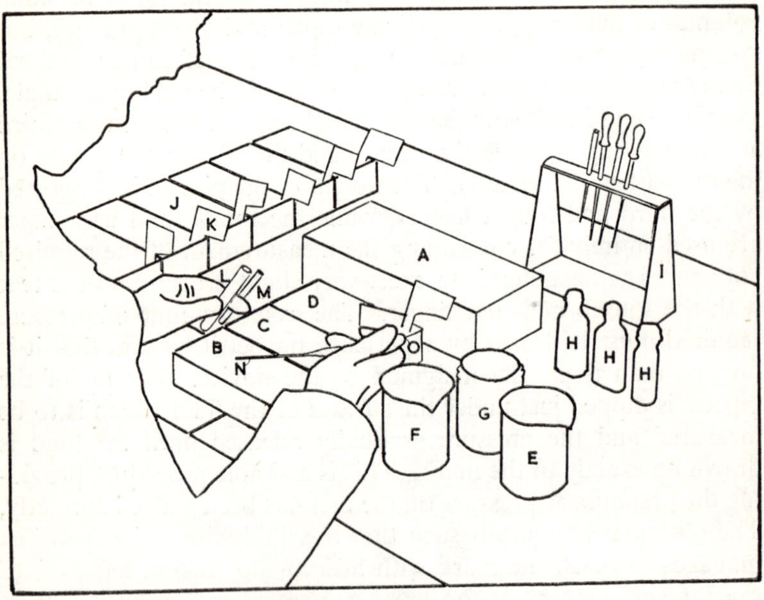

FIG. 2.2. Key to Plate 1.

A = Large block containing 37 unknown samples and A, B and O controls in positions 38, 39 and 40. B = Block for serum-grouping with standard A and B red cells. C = Block for cell-grouping with anti-A and anti-B sera. D = Block for testing with O serum ($\alpha\beta$). E = Beaker containing clean saline. F = Beaker containing saline used for rinsing pipette. G = Discard. H = Bottles containing anti-sera. I = Pipette rack. J = Blocks for the samples 11–40. K = Label. L = Sample tube. M = Cell suspension tube. N = Pipette. O = Teat of pipette.

e.g. saline, serum and bovine albumen will not all be exactly equal. For many purposes this is immaterial and provided the pipette is held upright and the fluid allowed to drop (not squirted) into the tube, a dropping technique is adequate for most typing techniques, except when very small quantities of fluid are to be delivered. In our opinion, however, a measuring technique as described above is to be preferred both for its additional accuracy and because the manipulator gains dexterity which stands him in good stead for techniques where it is essential that a measured volume is used.

Alternatively there are several automatic devices on the market. These can save time when large numbers of tests are set up at one

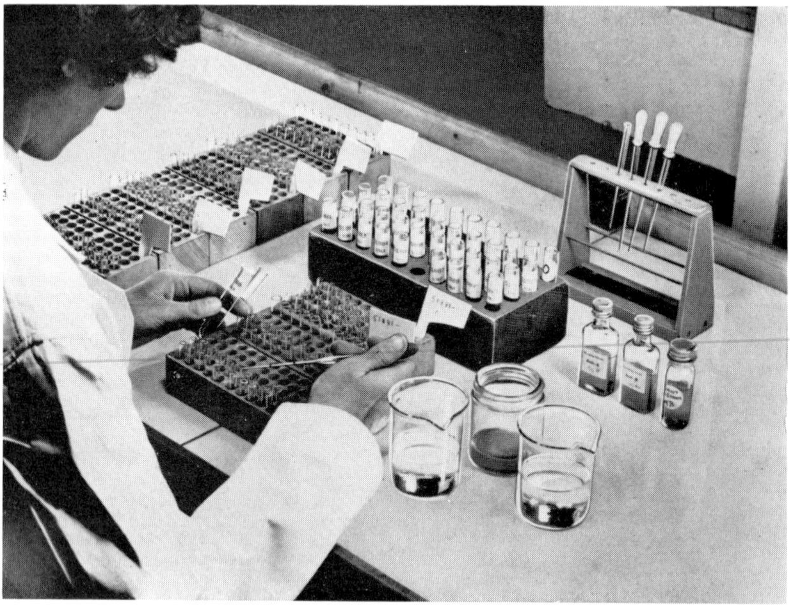

PLATE 1. Typical bench layout; (*a*) setting-up tests.

Comment on Plate 1

1. Note that the general layout is convenient, everything needed being within arm's reach, also that the beakers and jar are close to the worker's hand.

2. Note the strict alignment of the blocks, a precaution against placing volumes of red cell suspension or serum from the unknown samples into the wrong tubes.

3. The blood sample and the corresponding cell suspension tube are both held in the left hand throughout the whole running out process and then exchanged simultaneously for the next tubes in the row, the right hand being used to exchange the cell suspension tube while the left is exchanging the blood sample tube.

4. The serial number or name on the first tube of the row is written on to the label immediately after the tube has been taken from its position on the large block. Before the last tube is replaced, the number or name on this is also written on the label. This labelling is adequate if, and only if, the procedure described above (3) is adopted.

5. Note the handling of the pipette, especially the way it is supported by the second and third fingers, and there is no great pressure being exerted on the teat.

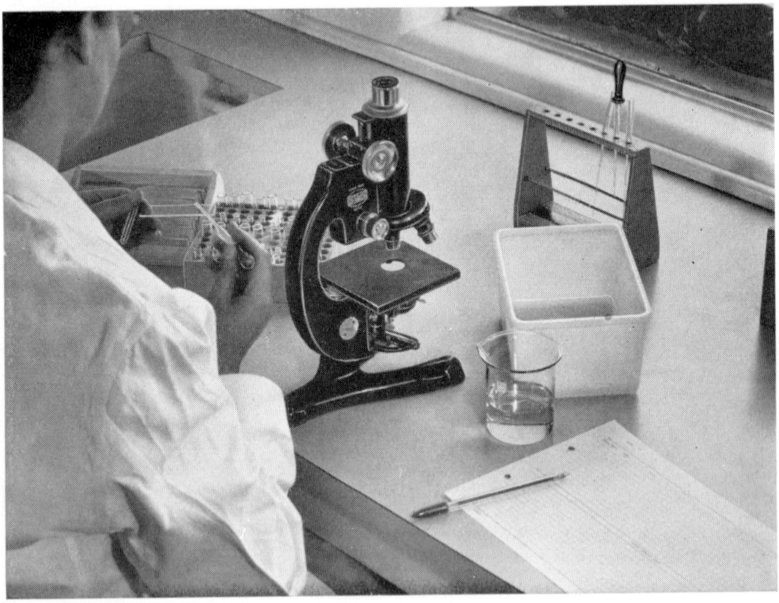

PLATE 2. Typical bench layout; (*b*) reading tests.

Comment on Plate 2

Note convenient arrangement of bench to facilitate the reading of many tests. The worker is at the final stage of preparing a smear. The liquid has been drawn along the slide from left to right behind the Pasteur pipette to which it adheres by surface tension. Note the position of the small precipitin tube A, the content of which has been placed on the slide; the tube is held in the left hand throughout the reading and discarding of the slide and is then exchanged for the next tube to be read. This is a way of marking position in a row of tubes.

time. For example, in one laboratory where we need anti-A, anti-B and group O sera for some 700–1,000 tests daily, these sera are run out by means of an automatic syringe graduated to deliver 0·02 ml. into each tube.

When using the pipette for preparing smears, it must be remembered that most cell sediments require gentle handling while they

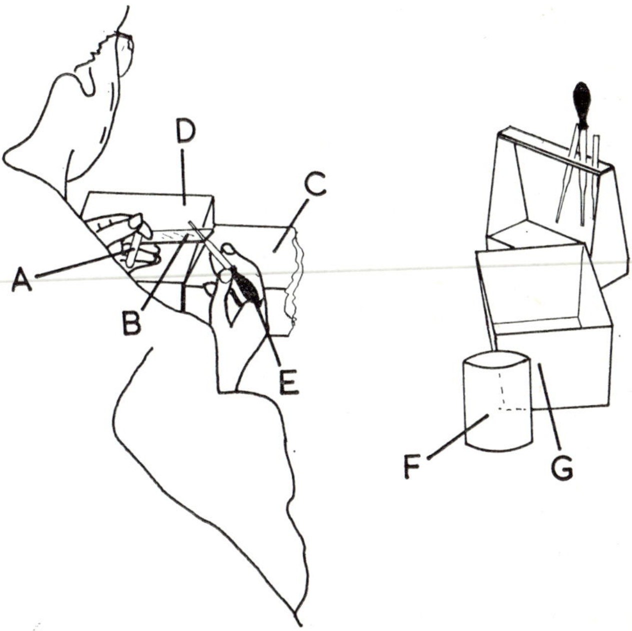

FIG. 2.3. Key to Plate 2.

A = Tube containing test to be examined. B = Microscope slide. C = Block containing tests to be read. D = Special rack for microscope slides. E = Smearing pipette (*see* Fig. 2.1. E). F = Beaker of saline. G = Container for used slides.

are being removed from a tube and spread on a microscope slide. The teat of the smearing pipette, therefore, must be squeezed before dipping the end into the liquid. If the pressure is not applied till after the end of the pipette is under the surface of the fluid, air will be blown on to the sediment and fragile agglutinates may be dispersed.

The cells are drawn gently into the pipette, care being taken that they do not rise as high as the wide portion. They are then pipetted on to a microscope slide and spread. Spreading is accomplished by first holding the pipette in a horizontal position, just touching the right-hand end of the drop of fluid on the slide; the fluid adheres to the pipette by surface tension and can be spread by moving the pipette to the right. If further spreading is required, it can be effected by gentle tilting of the slide. It should never be done by rubbing the pipette backwards and forwards over the surface.

When handling any of the described pipettes fluid should not enter the teat. Indeed for most manipulations it is entirely unnecessary to allow fluid to reach the wide part of the stem at all. In making serial dilutions the fluid must not be allowed to rise above the graduation as this could introduce a large error. Even when making 2 per cent red cell suspensions from samples of whole blood the fluid need not rise beyond the shoulder. If, inadvertently, it is allowed to get inside the teat, the pipette must be rinsed throughout its entire length, including the inside of the teat, at least six times with saline.

Pipettes are fragile and their tips are easily chipped which makes them unfit for use. They should, therefore, be kept either in special racks or in boxes lined with cotton wool.

Microscope Slides

These are used in large quantities since it is recommended that not more than two smears are made on any one slide. Although in serological work slides are used only for wet preparations which are discarded in a very short time they should be of good quality and should always be of the same thickness so that continual refocusing of the microscope is reduced to a minimum. This may seem at first sight an unimportant detail but for those who read many smears in a normal working day, the use of slides of all makes and thicknesses may become a major trial. As soon as the reactions are recorded the dirty slides are placed in a dish containing enough water to cover them. They should be washed in warm soapy water (detergent can be used if preferred), rinsed in cold water and in hot distilled water. They are then polished with a clean dry cloth, and care is taken not to finger the polished slides. Some kind of slide holder set at an angle of about 45° to the bench is an asset (*see* Plate 2).

"Long Slides"

For slide techniques individual microscope slides are obviously inconvenient. A slide, of glass or perspex, of about 8 in. × 2 in. divided lengthwise into two and cross-wise into 10 divisions is suitable for such methods. The divisions can either be shallow depressions or can be painted on; the latter is very successful, provided the painted lines are at least 0·1 cm. wide (*see* Plate 3).

Moist Chamber (Plate 3)

This is a box where slides can be kept in a moist atmosphere to prevent drying up of the test during incubation. It can be entirely of glass or perspex but in any case should have a transparent lid so that the tests can be watched without removing it. When results have been recorded the long slides are removed from the box and the negative reactions checked microscopically. The box shown is 9 in. × 11 in. and will hold 5 long slides, a total of 100 individual tests.

Opalescent Glass Tiles and Viewing Box

Squares and strips of white opalescent glass are invaluable for anti-human globulin (Coombs) tests and for any grouping test such as MN that may be done on tiles rather than in tubes. They should be thin enough to allow light to pass through when they are held over a lamp. Alternatively, it is useful to be able to use them in conjunction with a viewing box particularly for Coombs test. The tiles are placed on top of a box with an opalescent glass lid. Inside the box is a strip light which gives good luminosity with little heat.

Incidentally it is advisable to keep tiles used for anti-human globulin separate from those used for any other purpose. In this way no human serum ever comes into contact with these tiles.

Equipment for Temperature Control

Incubators and Water Baths

(*a*) 56°C. This is commonly required for the inactivation of complement and for the preparation of eluates.

In laboratories where a large number of Price Precipitation or VDRL tests are carried out, a 56°C water bath which will carry at least 250 samples at one time is convenient.

(*b*) 37°C. For this temperature either a water bath, an air incubator or hot room is needed. With a water bath the required temperature is reached more quickly than with an air incubator but for large-scale work water baths are not practicable because of the space required. Most serological laboratories use air incubators of various sizes to give them a temperature of 37°C. For large-scale work an actual room, the temperature of which can be controlled at 37°C, is ideal but rarely available. This hot room has the added advantage of usually being large enough to accommodate a bench with microscope and centrifuge so that manipulations and readings can actually be carried out at 37°C if desired.

(*c*) 18°C. This is the average temperature of the laboratory and most tests that require incubation at "room temperature" are left on the bench. However, it is convenient when studying the behaviour of those antibodies which are particularly sensitive to small temperature changes to use a water bath maintained at 18°C.

(*d*) 15°C, 12°C *and* 10°C. With the practice of hypothermia during operation becoming more common, water baths to give these temperatures are becoming part of the standard equipment of the serology laboratory. They incorporate a cooling coil and fan so that they can be quickly brought to and maintained at the required temperature.

Refrigerators

The optimum storage temperature for red cells is 4°C. A large blood bank will require at least one cold room at this temperature, but for small-scale work a domestic refrigerator is satisfactory. A precautionary measure if this is used, is the checking of the temperature in the various parts of the interior. An unevenness of temperature may sometimes be observed which may lead to over-cooling and, therefore, hæmolysis of red cells.

Typing sera of all kinds including anti-human globulin serum is best stored at −20°C, therefore, some kind of deep freeze capable of maintaining this temperature is essential.

A cabinet containing carbon dioxide snow can be used but its limitations should be realised. The temperature inside the container will vary widely according to proximity to the snow. In addition the atmosphere within becomes saturated with carbon dioxide which may have serious effects on the contents unless strictly air-tight containers are used throughout.

Any laboratory which stores rare cells may well find it best to keep them in liquid nitrogen. This entails special precautions and will be dealt with in connection with red cell storage (Appendix 1).

Centrifuges

The blood grouping laboratory requires a number of centrifuges of varying capacities. In a large laboratory, it is useful to have a centrifuge to hold a large number of test tubes or universal containers at a time. Angle centrifuges are indispensable for quick spinning and washing of Coombs tests. The heads of these should be chosen for their capacity to hold as many tubes as possible of the sizes most in use in the laboratory.

A useful centrifuge is one which will spin 50 holed plastic blocks. This is useful in those techniques where it is wished to speed or improve agglutination by centrifugation.

It is also valuable where large numbers of anti-human globulin tests are performed.

General Routine Procedure for all Serological Investigations

A pre-determined bench "lay-out" and pattern for each kind of serological procedure is a great time-saver and encourages a higher degree of accuracy in testing.

The first step is to assemble all apparatus needed, including blocks filled with tubes in the pattern required for each test. Plate 1 shows a convenient bench arrangement for the ABO grouping of 37 unknown samples. It is, however, of equal if not greater importance to adhere to a standard procedure even when only one or two samples are to be tested. After putting out the required rows of tubes the blocks are clearly labelled with the name of the test and the name or serial number of the first sample of the row. Flag labels, as shown in the photograph are convenient. Then all diluent fluids and standard anti-sera are run into the appropriate rows, rinsing the pipette very carefully 3 or 4 times between each fluid. It is essential to have a rule about which position a particular serum occupies. In the set-up shown, anti-A serum is always run into the front row of a block and anti-B into the second. Similarly, for serum-grouping A cells go into the front row and B cells into the second. This routine is never varied.

Next, the unknown sera are pipetted into all serum-grouping, and/or antibody detection tests; the pipette must, of course, be rinsed carefully between the delivery of each unknown serum. Before the appropriate red cells are added, the tubes are checked for their serum content. This is an extremely important step in the general procedure, which, if omitted, might have serious consequences. If perspex racks are used a glance will show whether all the tubes have their proper serum content, but with wooden blocks the tubes will have to be picked up.

Red cell suspensions, which are usually required to be 2–5 per cent in saline (as judged by eye), are made from the first unknown sample and without rinsing the pipette they are measured into the appropriate tubes. Note the strict alignment of the blocks, a precaution against placing volumes of red cells or serum into the wrong tubes. The sample to be tested and the corresponding cell suspension tubes are both held in the left hand throughout the whole procedure and then exchanged simultaneously for the next tubes in the row, the right hand being used to exchange the cell suspension tube, while the left is exchanging the blood sample tube. The serial number or name on the first tube of the row is written on the label immediately after the tube has been taken from its position on the large block. Before the last tube is replaced, the number or name on this is also written on the flag label. Standard cells are then run into the appropriate tests and into the controls of the cell typing tests. A known positive and known negative control is included for each anti-serum used and the controls are repeated for each batch of tests set up. The tubes are tapped to ensure good mixing of the contents,* then incubated for the required time at the appropriate temperature, after which the controls are read first and then the actual tests. Smears are made as described above. Results are entered as they are obtained although it is permissible to memorise consecutive identical results.

If this basic procedure is followed, each reagent or unknown serum or red cell suspension is handled only once in the whole manipulation, thereby reducing to a minimum the time taken and the risk of errors.

Automation

For many years now adaptations to the Auto-Analyser for antibody detection and for blood grouping and Rh typing have been available, The antibody detection machine is capable of detecting very weak antibodies sometimes before these are detectable by manual methods (*e.g.* in women early in pregnancy who are later shown by routine methods to have an antibody developing). The machine is basically simple; serum, test cells and enzyme (usually bromelin) are mixed together and pass through plastic tubing in a coil kept at 37°C (or any other temperature depending on the optimum for the antibodies expected), the reagents are thus continually gently mixed for a period of about ten minutes—the sample then passes on, is diluted with saline, the agglutinates settle as the sample goes slowly on its way to a decant "T" bored in a transparent plastic block—the agglutinates and a portion of unagglutinated cells are decanted while the supernatant travels on. The cells in the supernatant are lysed and the degree of lysis measured photometrically and recorded on a rotating drum. A low reading indicates that most of the cells have been removed as agglutinates and thus denotes a positive reaction. Samples showing such positive reaction are then further investigated either manually or by running several cells against the one serum in the auto analyser.

* There are a few techniques where "layering" is preferable to mixing; this detail is clearly indicated where such techniques are described.

The machine for blood typing is a fifteen channel model. It will take serum and cell samples from a single citrated sample using a double probe and can be programmed to test serum with A_1, A_2, B and O cells at room temperature, OR_1R_2 cells and for example OrrK+Fy^a+ cells at 37°C, and cells with anti-A, anti-B, anti-AB (O serum) anti-D, anti-CD and anti-DE, two more sera and a negative control *e.g.* AB serum. The process is similar to the antibody machine until the decant stage, at which with this machine the whole contents of each test are deposited on blotting paper and the reaction read by a technician. This is not entirely satisfactory although the reactions are usually quite easily read. One grave disadvantage is that occasionally the fifteen lines can get out of step and the results on one sample may not all be presented in a straight line. It is suggested that the paper is photocopied and stored as a permanent record.

This is a very expensive machine but may be worth using where it is difficult to get technical staff. The staff who control and service the machine and interpret the results have of course, to be highly skilled.

Section 2—The ABO Blood Group System

"*. . ., now let us begin. When we have got to the end of the story we shall know more than we do at present. . . .*"

Hans Christian Andersen, THE SNOW QUEEN

CHAPTER 3

THE ABO BLOOD GROUPS AND GROUPING METHODS

LANDSTEINER discovered the phenomenon of iso-agglutination in 1900. In 1901 he published the results of experiments which made it possible to divide the population into three groups, which he called A, B, and O. A year later the existence of a fourth, less common group, AB, was established. This marked the beginning of the whole subject of Blood Group Serology and made blood transfusion practicable.

The four groups are determined by the presence or absence in the red blood cells of the blood group antigens A and B, and, therefore, the blood group of the individual is either A, B, AB, or O (O denoting the absence of A and B).

In addition, it has been shown that corresponding to the antigens A and B there are antibodies anti-A (α) and anti-B (β), which occur as agglutinins in the sera of individuals whose red cells lack the corresponding agglutinogen. The agglutinogen and agglutinin content of the red cells and serum of the four blood groups are shown in Table 3.1.

Table 3.1

Agglutinogen and Agglutinin Content of the Red Cells and Serum of the Four Blood Groups

Blood group	Agglutinogen in red cells	Agglutinin in serum	Frequency in English population
A	A	Anti-B	41·7
B	B	Anti-A	8·6
AB	A and B	Neither	3·0
O	Neither	Both Anti-A and Anti-B	46·7

Although all individuals of the same blood group have the same kind of agglutinogen in their red cells, the sensitivity of the cells to agglutination varies from individual to individual. Moreover, there are very wide variations in the amount of agglutinin in the serum of different individuals belonging to the same blood group.

Table 3.2

ABO Grouping, Using Standard Sera and Standard Red Cells

Blood group	Reactions of red cells with standard sera		Reactions of sera with standard cells	
	Anti-A	Anti-B	A cells	B cells
A	C	—	—	C
B	—	C	C	—
AB	C	C	—	—
O	—	—	C	C

Key: C = clumping (complete agglutination)
— = no reaction

It is by means of the agglutination reaction of red cells that the blood group of an individual is determined. This can be effected either by testing the individual's red cells with standard anti-A and anti-B sera (for selection and method of preparation of standard sera *see* Chapter 4) or by testing his serum with standard red cells of groups A and B. The most reliable grouping is achieved if both these methods are used, so that they form a check on each other. The pattern of reactions obtained for each blood group by these two methods is shown in Table 3.2.

It is very important to distinguish between true agglutination and rouleaux formation. This latter phenomenon is a running together of the red cells to form aggregates, like piles of coins (Plate 4*a* and *b*). It is often well marked in the blood of patients suffering from acute infection, in conditions where the albumin-globulin serum protein balance is disturbed, and even in normal blood when a smear is beginning to dry or when a too concentrated cell suspension is used. When rouleaux formation is very heavy it is sometimes difficult even for an experienced worker to distinguish it from true agglutination, as the piles form compact masses very similar to the appearance given by true agglutination (Plate 5*a*). Usually, rouleaux formation can be dispersed readily by adding a drop of saline to the slide and gently rubbing. However, it should be borne in mind that this practice may be dangerous. The agglutination caused by the agglutinogen and agglutinins of the ABO system is tough and not easily broken down by the above treatment, but that caused by most other blood group systems is fragile, and, if present together with rouleaux, will also be dispersed and a false negative obtained.

Techniques

As has been mentioned, it is possible to determine the group of a specimen of blood either by testing the red cells with standard anti-A and anti-B sera (chosen for their good agglutinating power) or by testing the serum with standard group A and group B red cells (chosen for their sensitivity). It is more difficult to test unknown sera than unknown red cells because the strength of the agglutinins varies greatly in different sera. For reliable grouping both cells and serum should be examined and the tests repeated if there is any discrepancy. When using potent serum and red cells of good sensitivity agglutination takes place very rapidly. As the strength of the agglutinin or agglutinogen decreases, however, the speed of the reaction diminishes. Techniques which do not allow sufficient time for the reaction between the weakest agglutinogen and agglutinin can never be reliable.

The two described here are chosen for their reliability. In a grave emergency it may become necessary to risk a less reliable method; these are described and discussed in Chapter 23.

Technique No. 3.1. ABO grouping by the moist chamber slide technique (Plate 3)

Apparatus

Moist chamber—this can vary from a Petri-dish lined with damp filter paper to a properly constructed cabinet to take many hundreds of tests —a useful one for the moderate sized laboratory is described in Chapter 2.

Cell-suspension tubes—round bottomed, 50 mm. × 11 mm.

Slides—Microscope slides or preferably long glass (or perspex) slides with two rows of 10 divisions.

Microscope with 2/3 objective.

Reagents

Normal saline (0·85 per cent solution of NaCl).

Standard anti-A and anti-B sera.

Standard Group O serum.

Standard A, B and O red cells.

Method. This description is for the testing of seven blood samples with A, B and O controls; it can readily be adapted for any number.

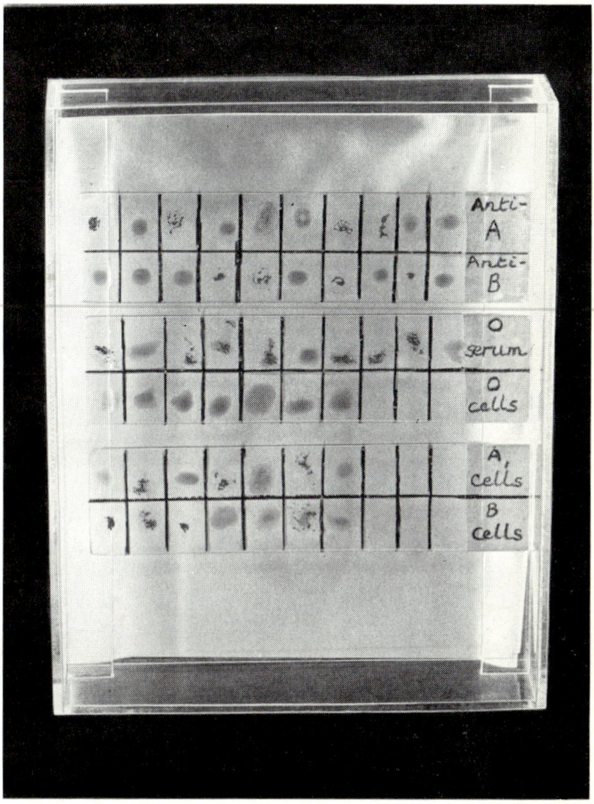

PLATE 3. ABO Grouping by the Moist Chamber technique.

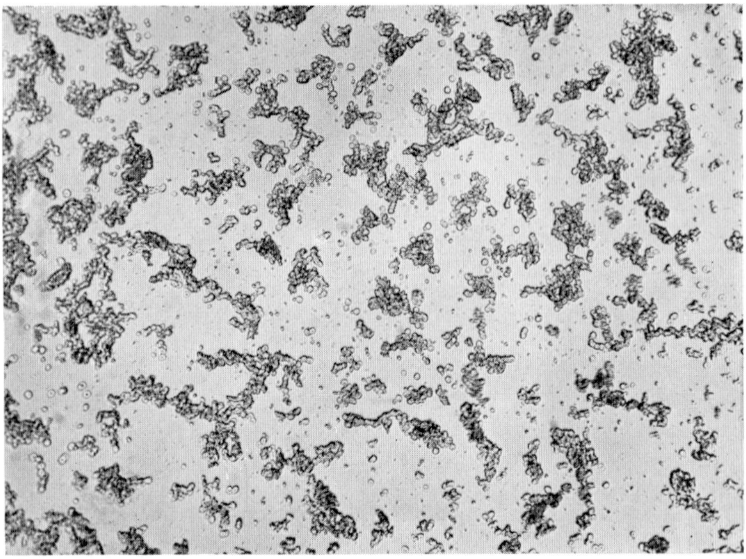

PLATE 4*a*. Typical rouleaux formation (viewed with $\frac{2}{3}''$ objective).

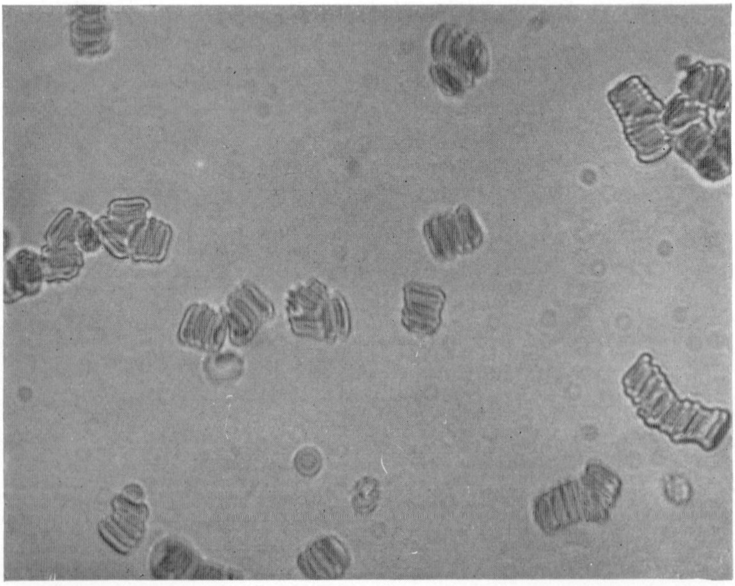

PLATE 4*b*. Typical rouleaux formation (viewed with $\frac{1}{6}''$ objective).

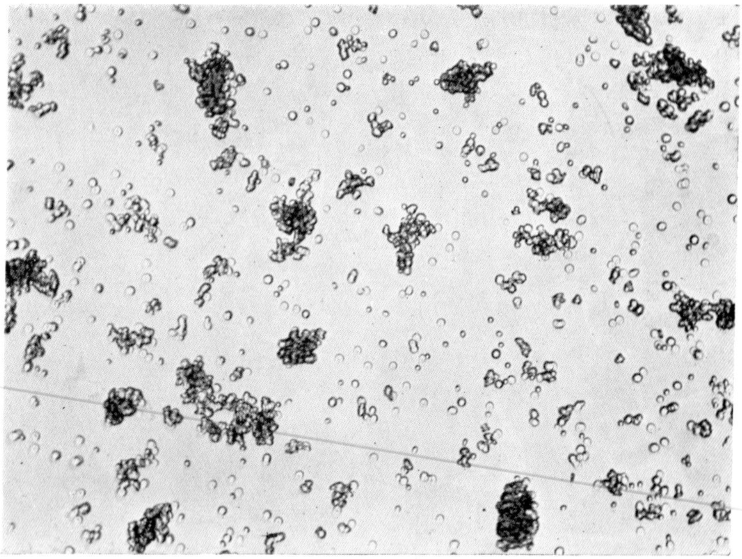

PLATE 5*a*. Typical pseudo-agglutination (from a case of multiple myelomatosis).

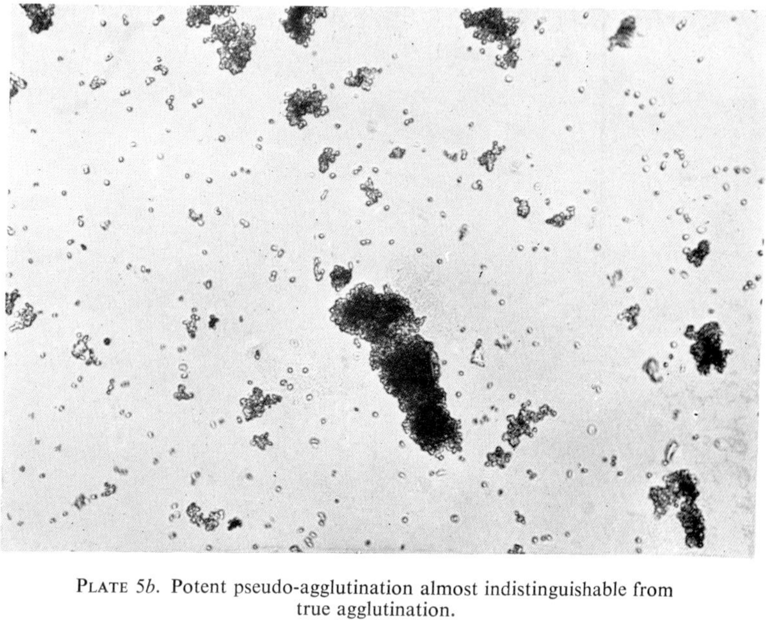

PLATE 5*b*. Potent pseudo-agglutination almost indistinguishable from true agglutination.

Three long slides are placed in the moist chamber giving 6 rows each of 10 divisions (*see* Plate 3).

One drop of anti-A serum is added to each division of row one.

One drop of anti-B serum to each division of row two.

One drop of O serum to each division of row three.

The pipette is carefully rinsed between each row.

The samples to be tested are of clotted blood where the serum has separated (either by standing over-night or by centrifugation) sufficiently for clear serum to be pipetted from the top of the samples while free red cells can be obtained from the bottom of the tube.

Table 3.3

Protocol of ABO Grouping

MOIST CHAMBER SLIDE TECHNIQUE

Tested with	Samples							Controls		
	1	2	3	4	5	6	7	A	B	O
Anti-A	5+	—	5+	—	2+	—	4+	5+	—	—
Anti-B	—	—	—	5+	5+	—	5+	—	5+	—
Group O serum	5+	—	5+	5+	5+	—	5+	5+	5+	—
O red cells	—	—	—	—	—	—	—			
A red cells	—	5+	—	5+	2+	5+	—			
B red cells	5+	5+	5+	—	—	4+	—			
Group	A	O	A	B	for further tests	O	AB			

The first unknown sample is held in the left hand, together with the first suspension tube, one drop of the unknown serum is placed in the first division of rows four, five and six, a 3–5 per cent cell suspension in saline is made in the cell suspension tube and one drop added to the first division of rows one, two and three. The pipette is then rinsed and the tubes exchanged for the second unknown sample and its suspension tube, serum and cells from the second sample being added in the same way to the second division in each row. The process is repeated for each of the seven samples. One drop of a 3–5 per cent suspension of standard Group O cells is run into each division of row four and the last division of rows one, two and three; one drop of group A cells is run into each division of row five and the eighth divisions of rows one, two and three; one drop of group B cells into each division of row six and the ninth division of rows one, two and three. The lid is placed on the moist chamber and the whole gently rocked to ensure mixing of cells and serum in each division.

The tests are allowed to stand at room temperature for 25–30 minutes. The chamber is again gently rocked and the results recorded. The macroscopic readings are checked by removing the slides from the chamber and examining under the lower power (2/3) objective of the microscope. A typical protocol is given in Table 3.3).

Comment

This is the only slide technique which allows adequate time for weak reactions to develop. Agreement should always be found between the results of testing the cells and serum (unless an atypical antibody is present in the serum (*see* section on anomalous results)). If the tests agree, this technique may be regarded as 100 per cent reliable, the main disadvantage being the dimension of the moist chamber required for the performance of a large number of grouping tests at one time.

Technique No. 3.2. ABO grouping by tube technique—standard method (Plate 1)

As this is the technique recommended for use whenever it is possible to leave the tests for at least 1½ hours, both the apparatus used and the technique are described in great detail. Moreover, this is the basic typing technique for all blood group work.

Apparatus

Precipitin tubes, round bottomed glass tubes size 50 mm. × 5·5 mm. internal diameter.
Cell-suspension tubes, round bottomed glass tubes size 50 mm. × 11 mm. internal diameter.
Blocks having 50 holes arranged in 5 rows of 10.
Capillary or Pasteur pipettes graduated to deliver one and two standard volumes. (The standard volume should be of the order of 0·03 ml.)
Microscope slides.
Microscope with 2/3 objective.

Reagents

Normal saline (0·85 per cent solution of NaCl).
Standard anti-A and anti-B sera and standard group O serum (*i.e.* anti-A + anti-B).
Standard group A, group B, and group O red cells.

Testing of Unknown Cells. The method now described allows for the grouping of ten blood specimens, including controls of groups A, B, and O. Small precipitin tubes are placed in the first and second rows of a 50-holed block, and the larger cell suspension tubes in the back row, as in Plate 1. In each tube of the front row are placed 1 volume of anti-A serum and 1 volume of saline, and in each tube of the second row 1 volume of anti-B serum and 1 volume of saline, using the graduated capillary pipette. The addition of saline minimises rouleaux formation. When large numbers of tests are being done the grouping serum may be diluted in bulk with an equal volume of saline and a double volume of this diluted serum placed in each tube. At the end of this stage the tubes are scrutinised carefully to make certain that each contains its allotted quantity of serum. Approximately 0·5 ml. of saline is run into each of the cell suspension tubes in the back row. A 2–5 per cent cell suspension (judged by eye) of the first specimen of red cells to be tested is made with a Pasteur pipette in the corresponding cell suspension tube. Then, using the same Pasteur pipette and without rinsing, 1 volume of cell suspension is measured into the first tubes of both the first and second rows. The pipette is then rinsed three times in normal saline, discarding each rinsing, and the process repeated along the row for each of the specimens to be grouped. Cell suspension tubes in positions 8, 9, and 10 on the block will contain the standard red cells of groups A, B, and O, respectively, as controls. If several blocks of grouping tests are set up at the same time, controls need only be placed in the final block.

The tubes are then tapped to ensure good mixing of the cells and serum and the tests are allowed to stand at room temperature for at least 1½, preferably 2, hours. Each tube is then agitated by tapping with the finger. If the contents show agglutination which is obvious to the naked eye (*see* Plate 6*a* and *b*) a positive result is recorded. The content of each tube not showing obvious agglutination is removed, spread evenly on a microscope slide and examined under the low power of the microscope. Control tubes should be read first, and only if these are satisfactory should the other tests be read.

Testing of Unknown Sera. These tests should be carried out independently of the tests for red cells and are therefore set up in a different block. Two rows of precipitin tubes are placed in the front of the block, as in the cell grouping test. One volume of serum from the first sample is placed in the first tube of both first and second rows, the pipette rinsed, and the process repeated along the row. One volume of a 2–5 per cent suspension of standard group A red cells is placed in each tube of the front row and one volume of a similar suspension of standard group B red cells in each tube of the second row. If the standard cells are run into the control tubes belonging to the cell tests at the same time these controls will serve for both tests otherwise controls must be set up for each test separately. The tubes are shaken and allowed to stand for 2 hours. The reading is the same as for the tests on the unknown cells.

Additional Test, Using Group O Serum. Group O serum contains both anti-A and anti-B agglutinins. It can, therefore, be used to agglutinate all A, B, and AB bloods, leaving only group O bloods unagglutinated. The unknown red cells are incubated with standard group O serum (for criteria *see* Chapter 4) in tubes exactly as for the grouping with anti-A and anti-B sera. This test should be read independently of the other two and then the results correlated. The anti-A in group O serum reacts more strongly than the anti-A in group B serum with some of the low sub-groups of A (A_3, A_x, A_m, etc.) and may prevent such bloods being wrongly diagnosed as group O.

Correlation of Results

The best method of reading and recording the results of a large number of tests is for two people to work together, one reading

Table 3.4

Protocol of ABO Grouping by Tube Technique

Sample No.	Tests on red cells			Tests on serum		Group
	with anti-A serum	with anti-B serum	with Group O (anti-A + anti-B) serum	with A cells	with B cells	
1	C	—	C	—	C	A
2	—	—	—	C	C	O
3	C	—	C	—	C	A
4	—	C	C	C	—	B
5	++	C	C	+	—	For further testing
6	—	—	—	C	C	O
7	C	C	C	—	—	AB
Control A	C	—	C			
Control B	—	C	C			
Control O	—	—	—			

the macroscopic agglutination and preparing microscope slides from the tubes not showing obvious agglutination, while the other examines the prepared slides and records the results. Such a team with practice becomes extremely efficient. If only one worker is available, then he must record his results as they are read; it is permissible, however, to memorise consecutive identical results.

The recorded results are then correlated. Table 3.4 is a facsimile of results obtained on seven unknown red cell samples, together with controls. Sometimes (*e.g.* sample No. 5) the results are not typical. There are several reasons why this might be so; for convenience a list is given here. Some of the items will be better understood when the chapters on the sub-groups of A, Rh antibodies, etc., have been studied.

Anomalous Results

(1) **Weak Reactions.** If agglutination is not clearly visible to the naked eye and has to be read microscopically the reaction is recorded according to the following table:

++ = very large clumps—few free cells.
+ = large clumps—more free cells.
(+) = an even distribution of clumps of about 8–16 cells.
w = weak—an even distribution of clumps of about 3–10 cells.
– = no agglutination.

(For a photograph of these degrees of agglutination *see* Plates 6 and 7.)

The reaction ++ may be taken as denoting definite agglutination. Reactions of + or less mean that the tests must be repeated with further reagents.

(2) **Hæmolysis.** The unknown sera may cause hæmolysis of the standard red cells. If there is good agglutination also (*i.e.* C or ++ reaction), the hæmolysis can be disregarded and the agglutination reaction recorded. If, however, the majority of the cells are hæmolysed so that there is little or no agglutination, a further test is necessary. This is because although the hæmolysis is probably due to the specific anti-A or anti-B hæmolysins, it is not safe to assume that this is so. In these cases three or four serial dilutions of the unknown serum in saline (*see* titration technique No. 4.2, Chapter 4) can be made and tested with red cells of the appropriate ABO group. The dilution giving little or no hæmolysis will normally show agglutination. Alternatively, the serum may be inactivated (*i.e.* heated at 56°C for 30 minutes) to destroy complement and the heated serum retested—by this means hæmolysis is prevented while the agglutination reaction is unimpaired.

(3) **The Weak Agglutinogens of the Sub-groups of A.** Some cells may give consistently poor reactions with anti-A sera because they belong to one of the weaker sub-groups of A. Such blood

should be tested with anti-A and group O sera which have been especially chosen for their good reactivity with weak A agglutinogens.

(4) **Reactions Due to the Cold Agglutinins of the Sub-groups of A.** Typical results given by samples which contain these agglutinins are:

	Anti-A	Anti-B	O serum (anti-A+anti-B)	A cells	B cells
Sample I	C	–	C	+	C
Sample II	+	C	C	(+)	–

If such reactions are obtained, the tests are repeated and, in addition, the red cells tested with anti-A_1 sera and the serum with A_2 cells. (For a description of these reagents and the results which would be obtained *see* Chapter 6.)

(5) **Reactions Due to Other Atypical Agglutinins.** Among the most common atypical agglutinins whose presence in an unknown serum may give rise to anomalous results are the Rh antibodies, in particular anti-D. This difficulty may most easily be overcome by using Rh negative Group A and Group B standard cells. If there are still atypical reactions between the unknown sera and the standard cells these may be due to a variety of atypical antibodies. As a general rule, such cases are investigated by a specialist laboratory which has a large panel of standard cells available (*see also* Chapter 21).

(6) **Auto-agglutinins.** These are agglutinins which if present in the serum of an individual will cause agglutination of his own red cells. The phenomenon is usually observed at temperatures lower than 37°C. Thus if there is an auto-agglutinin in the unknown serum active at the temperature of the test, the red cells will be agglutinated before being tested. Washing the red cells at 37°C or, if necessary, 45°C, may disperse this agglutination and the red cells can be grouped in the usual way. If the results are still not clear cut, a fresh sample must be taken, the cells and serum separated, and the cells washed at 37°C without allowing the sample to cool, so that the agglutinin never becomes attached to the red cells (*see also* Chapter 20).

(7) **Grouping of Cord or Infants' Blood.** The ABO grouping of babies presents difficulty for two reasons. Firstly, the cell agglutinogens may not be fully developed at birth—this is particularly true of the sub-groups of A—and very weak reactions may be obtained. It is therefore recommended that the additional test, using group O sera, should always be used when typing infants' blood. Secondly, infants do not possess their own anti-A and

anti-B agglutinins at birth; these usually start developing at about the third to the sixth month of life. Any antibodies found in the infants' sera at birth have been passively acquired from the maternal serum by passage across the placenta. This means that it is not possible to check the group of the child by means of the antibody content of its serum. It is therefore advisable to test the cells by two different techniques.

Chapter 4

ABO GROUPING SERA—SELECTION AND PREPARATION

The standard sera for blood grouping have to be especially selected, for although all group A individuals have anti-B agglutinins, all group B individuals anti-A agglutinins, and all group O individuals both anti-A and anti-B agglutinins, only about 2 per cent have them in sufficient strength for the certain detection of the weakest agglutinogens.

Criteria

To determine the suitability of a given serum both the titre and the avidity of the agglutinins must be estimated. The determination of the titre involves making serial dilutions of serum in saline in a row of tubes and the addition to each tube of a volume of red cells of the appropriate group to cause agglutination. The reciprocal of the highest dilution of serum still causing agglutination (as viewed under the microscope) is the titre (or titration value) of a particular serum. Experience has shown that to be satisfactory for grouping a serum must have a titre of at least 512 against standard red cells of group A, or 256 against standard red cells of group B.

The avidity of a serum is its power to agglutinate red cells quickly and strongly, forming large clumps. It is possible to find a serum which satisfies the criterion for minimum titration value and yet agglutinates poorly at most dilutions. It is necessary, therefore, to select on the basis of a certain strength of agglutination at a given dilution as well as on the end point of the titre; an anti-A serum must show a V to ++ agglutination, and an anti-B serum a ++ to + agglutination at a dilution of 1 in 64. Sera should show "C" or "complete" agglutination in the four lowest dilutions.

The standard both for titre and avidity is higher for anti-A than for anti-B because there are sub-groups of A (*see* Chapter 6) and a more potent serum is needed for the detection of some of these. Anti-A sera should be titrated with A_2B and, if available, A_3B cells, and are only regarded as satisfactory if they give at least three macroscopic readings with A_2B or one macroscopic reading with A_3B cells.

When group O serum is used as an anti-A + anti-B ($\alpha\beta$) grouping serum it must satisfy the criteria for titre and avidity for both anti-A and anti-B. Fortunately, in most group O sera the anti-A titre is slightly higher than the anti-B, and if the serum satisfies the criteria for anti-B the anti-A is usually satisfactory also. The use of group O ($\alpha\beta$) sera is in the detection of cells belonging to the weaker sub-groups of A (A_3 and A_x). Whenever possible, therefore, sera giving titre of 16 or over with A_x cells should be selected. A description of sub-group A_x is given in Chapter 32.

It is also necessary before issuing ABO grouping sera as specific for agglutinogens A and B to test them against the cells of at least 30 group O individuals. This is a precautionary measure, as the sera may contain atypical agglutinins which would render them unsuitable for grouping purposes. Some of these agglutinins (*e.g.* anti-Lutheran) detect antigens of low frequency and could be missed if the panel of group O cells was too small. Alternatively, a much smaller panel of group O cells, especially selected for their ability to detect atypical antibodies belonging to any of the known blood group systems, can be used (*see also* Chapter 21).

Elimination of Unsuitable Sera

Large numbers of serum samples have to be tested in order to select grouping sera, as only about 2 per cent* of all individuals have anti-A or anti-B agglutinins of sufficient titre and avidity. It is convenient, therefore, to devise a screening method which avoids titrating fully the 98 per cent of sera which are unsuitable. The screening method which we recommend involves making a one in four dilution of each serum, adding red cells, and selecting for full and careful titration those sera causing "C" agglutination at the end of 1 hour. This method is a fairly accurate way of choosing good sera since only about one in ten thus selected have to be discarded upon further testing.

Use of Immune Sera

It is possible to prepare high titre grouping sera by the deliberate injection of A or B substances into human volunteers or animals (usually rabbits). Adequate supplies of grouping sera for routine purposes can be maintained without resorting to this procedure. The chief use of such immune sera is for research purposes (*see* particularly Chapter 32). Animal sera have to be absorbed before use to remove species specific or "anti-Man" agglutinins which agglutinate all human red cells.

* This figure applies to random civilian donors in the south of England. A higher percentage of suitable sera is found in the north of the country. There is also an age-sex relationship, and if young males are tested, up to 20 per cent have antibody titres satisfying the grouping sera criteria.

Snail Anti-A

An anti-A reagent can be prepared from snails. This is an extremely powerful reagent and reacts equally well with A_1 and A_2 blood, though not with A_3. The snail originally used was Helix hortensis, but other snails, in particular Helix aspersa, are equally good. A simple way of obtaining the reagent is to add the contents of a snail's egg to 100 ml. of saline—this reagent is often sufficiently potent to be diluted considerably, especially if tests are performed on enzyme treated red cells. It can be used very dilute in the auto-analyser. The reagent does however react with Group O and Group B cells as shown by the fact that active eluates can be prepared from them. This means that the reagent must be suitably diluted so that the reaction is specific for A.

The snail "anti-A" was thought by Prokop *et al.* (1965) to be recognising a "new" blood group receptor, called by them A_{hel}.

Although this reagent seems attractive, we prefer human anti-A antisera of which there is a quite adequate supply.

The antigens with which these snail reagents and other animal agglutinins react will repay further study. Certainly, although they can distinguish between, for instance, A and not −A, they are by no means identical with the human agglutinins of the same apparent specificity.

Principles of Processing Serum

When a serum has been selected for grouping purposes it is then prepared for use. After the serum has separated from the clot it is collected free of red cells either by gravity or centrifugation. The latter method is to be preferred since it is quicker and improves the yield. Speed is an advantage as the longer the serum is kept in an unfrozen state the greater is the risk of a reduction in titre.

In our experience the best way to sterilize a serum is by Seitz filtration, as this does not appreciably reduce the titre, whereas heating may easily do so. Moreover, Seitz filtration also clarifies serum. Whenever possible sera should be stored frozen solid at − 10 to − 20°C, but this is less essential for anti-A and anti-B sera than for anti-Rh sera. Grouping serum can also be "freeze-dried" without deterioration and it can then be stored at room temperature; this is useful when the serum is for transport, especially to places abroad. Grouping serum should never be kept in capillary tubes, in spite of the fact that it is more economical when only undertaking a few grouping tests on any one occasion. Serious mistakes leading to the death of patients have occurred through using sera stored in this way. For some reason, possibly related to the type of glass used for the making of capillaries, coupled with the greater surface area of serum exposed to it, serum stored in capillaries deteriorates very rapidly and also tends to give false positive reactions. It is possible for a pin-point hole in a capillary to remain undetected and thereby allow the serum to become infected. Moreover, as conditions vary from capillary to capillary no real control is possible.

Techniques

Technique No. 4.1. Screening technique for ABO grouping sera

For anti-A and anti-B a one in four dilution of each of the unknown sera is made in saline with a Pasteur pipette graduated to deliver three unit volumes (*see* Chapter 2). This quantity of saline is placed in a row of precipitin tubes equal in number to the sera to be tested. One unit volume of the first serum under test is added to the first tube and the contents thoroughly mixed. Three volumes of the mixture are then discarded, leaving one volume of a one in four dilution in the tube. The Pasteur pipette is carefully rinsed in saline and then once in the next serum to be tested; it is then ready to be used for making the second one in four dilution. When all the dilutions have been made one unit volume of a 2 per cent suspension of the appropriate standard cells is added and after the tests have stood for exactly 1 hour they are examined macroscopically for agglutination. Only those sera showing a "C" reaction are selected for full titration. About one in ten selected by this method prove unsuitable when titrated in full.

Screening for Group O ($\alpha\beta$) sera is best done by testing one volume of serum with one volume of $A_{\times}$ cells at room temperature for 1 hour. Sera giving visual agglutination will usually prove suitable on full titration.

Technique No. 4.2. Titration of agglutinins (anti-A and anti-B)

The method of performing and reading the titrations is a slight modification of that described by Taylor and Ikin (1939). The titrations are carried out in precipitin tubes, the diluent being normal saline. The standard red cells should be less than 24 hours old when used. With a Pasteur pipette graduated to deliver a constant unit volume (approximately 0·03 ml.) twofold dilutions of serum are made in a row of tubes. To each of these serial dilutions 1 volume of the appropriate red cell suspension (4–5 per cent in terms of whole blood) in saline is added and the tubes shaken. The titrations are made in duplicate and are allowed to stand for 2 hours at room temperature. The cell deposit is then agitated by tapping the tube sharply, and the degree of agglutination read. No reaction is scored as negative until it has been examined microscopically, when an even distribution of clumps of three or more cells is accepted as evidence of agglutination. The titre of the serum is expressed as the reciprocal of the greatest dilution causing agglutination (the cell-suspension volume is neglected in calculating the dilution).* Some workers express the titre as the reciprocal of the highest dilution showing at least a (+) reaction, but in our experience this is a much more variable end-point and we do not recommend its adoption. In any case, when a titration value is quoted the method used and the end-point accepted should always be stated. A useful method of scoring reactions is given below.

Comment. The experimental error of this technique in the hands of an experienced worker rarely exceeds one dilution, in spite of the fact that the unit volume employed is small. The titration values are higher than those obtained when the serial dilutions are made with standard graduated pipettes, using a separate pipette for each dilution, because inevitably there is a slight carry-over from tube to tube when the same pipette is used for the whole titration. This does not affect the validity of the results as only comparative values are required, and indeed no absolute standard of antibody strength exists. This means that the same titration method must be used throughout any series of estimations, and in stating any results or standards the method employed must be clearly indicated.

Sometimes a modification of the Pasteur pipette method is used, in which, instead of measured volumes, drops are used. This modification introduces a large source of error as the drops of saline, of serum and of cell suspension are not the same size. This objection is even more valid when, as we shall see later, it is sometimes necessary to perform titrations using a protein diluent. With practice it is almost, if not quite, as quick to use a graduated Pasteur pipette as to use a dropping pipette.

Macroscopic

C = complete agglutination—large agglutinates surrounded by clear fluid (Plate 6*a*).

V = visual agglutination—while the agglutinates are still visible to the naked eye the surrounding fluid is pink (Plate 6*b*).

* Titres above 512 are usually approximated to the nearest thousand.

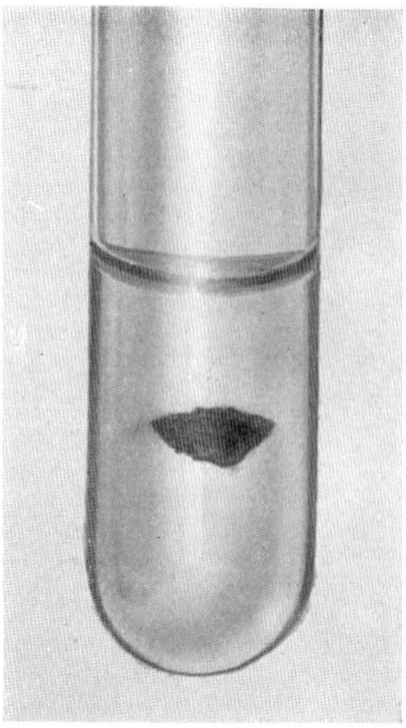

PLATE 6*a*. Complete agglutination.

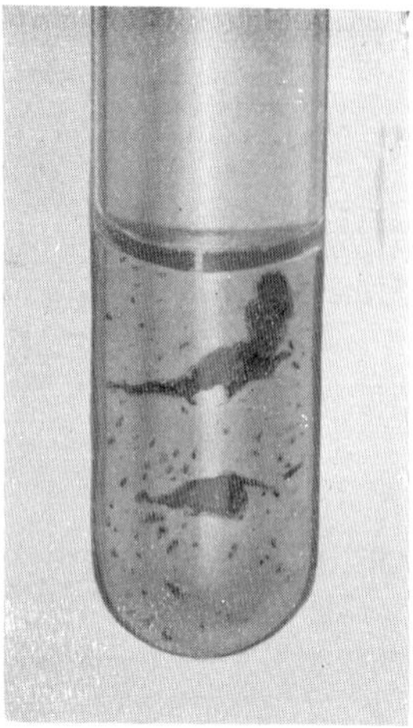

PLATE 6*b*. Visual agglutination.

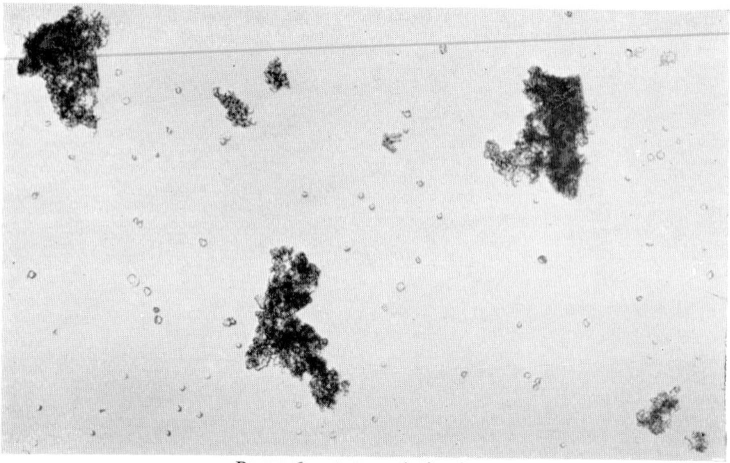

PLATE 6*c*. ++ agglutination.

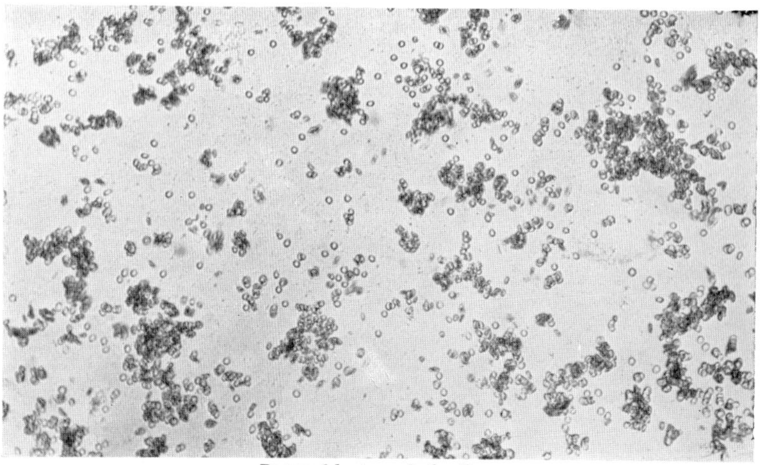

PLATE 6*d*. + agglutination.

p. 44

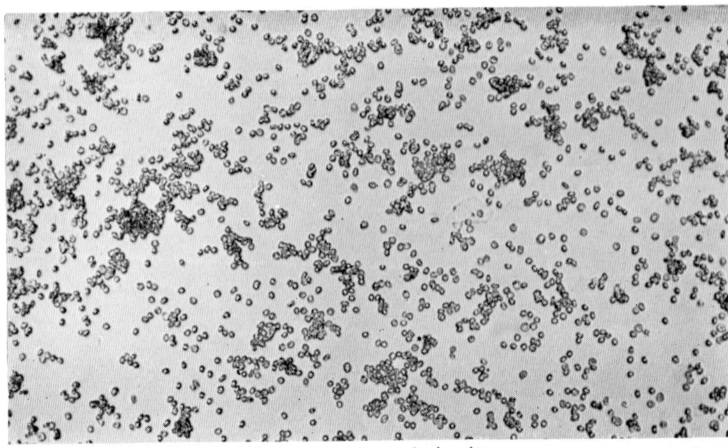
PLATE 7*a*. (+) agglutination.

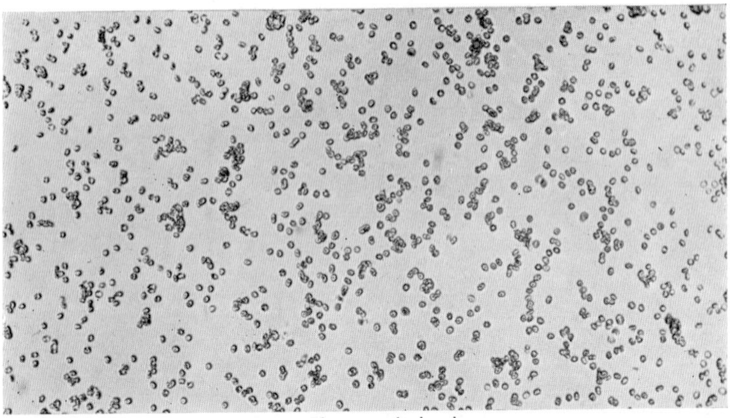
PLATE 7*b*. w agglutination.

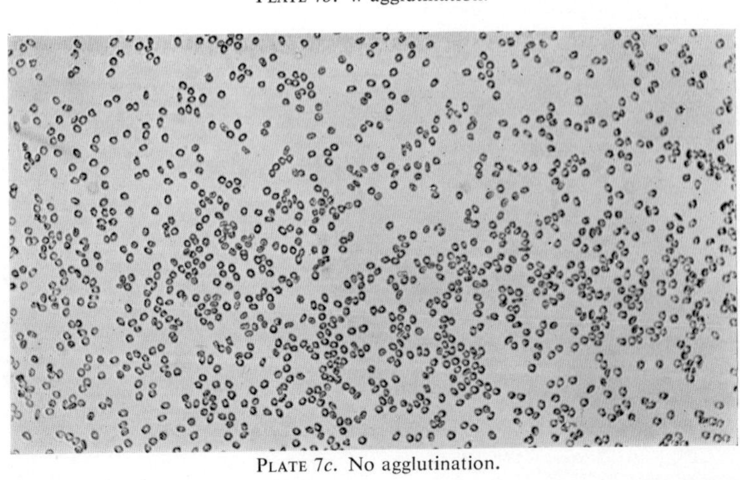
PLATE 7*c*. No agglutination.

Microscopic

++ = very large clumps—few free cells (Plate 6*c*).
+ = large clumps—more free cells (Plate 6*d*).
(+) = an even distribution of clumps of about 8–16 cells (Plate 7*a*).
w = weak—an even distribution of clumps of about 3–10 cells (Plate 7*b*).
— = no agglutination (Plate 7*c*).

Technique No. 4.3. Titration of agglutinins using standard graduated pipettes

Serial dilutions of not less than 0·5 ml. of the serum are made in saline with standard graduated 1 ml. "blow-out" pipettes, using a fresh pipette for each dilution. Then 0·1 ml. of each dilution, beginning with the weakest, is placed (using a standard "run-out" pipette) in each of a row of precipitin tubes, and 0·1 ml. of standard cells added to each. The tests are allowed to stand for 2 hours at room temperature and then read in the same way as for technique No. 4.2.

The disadvantages of this method are that it requires larger volumes of serum and is more time-consuming.

Technique No. 4.4. Master titres

If it is required for any reason to titrate a serum against several different samples of red cells (*e.g.* when comparing the agglutinogen content of different cells of the same group, or when titrating more than one antibody in a serum containing a mixture) a "master" titre is made.

To be comparable with titrations made by technique No. 4.2 the master titre should be made with the master titre pipette shown in Fig. 2.1G. On the other hand, to be comparable with results obtained by technique No. 4.3 the master dilutions are made using a fresh standard graduated pipette for each dilution.

After the dilutions have been made the one volume graduated Pasteur pipette (Fig. 2.1C) can be used to run out (commencing with the weakest dilution) as many rows of dilutions as there are different cells to be added. It is advisable that the "master" dilutions should be made in duplicate, as any error would affect all the titres involved.

Technique No. 4.5. Method of preparation of grouping serum

Serum is rendered sterile by Seitz filtration. For this purpose the serum is separated from the clot and made absolutely cell free. If this is done by centrifugation and the time between the opening of the blood bottle and the filtering of the serum is a matter of a few hours only, then no sterile precautions need be taken until after the serum is Seitz filtered. If the method of pouring off the serum and allowing it to stand for a day or two to settle is adopted, then aseptic precautions should be taken from the beginning of the manipulation. Cloudy or fatty serum should be clarified by passing it through a clarifying (grade 4) Seitz filter pad. For the actual sterilisation the Seitz pad HPEK must be used.

If for any reason the blood instead of being taken into a dry sterile bottle and allowed to clot has been collected into anticoagulant, the plasma can be converted into serum and then processed. The most convenient way is to add 25 gm. of kaolin to each 200 ml. of plasma and shake gently for 5 minutes.

The filtered serum is stored in sterile bottles in suitable quantities, *e.g.* 10 ml. for blood bank use, 1 ml. for routine hospital use. It should be kept frozen solid.

Chapter 5

ISO-IMMUNISATION TO THE BLOOD GROUP ANTIGENS A AND B

Iso-immunisation is the process by which antibodies are formed in an individual in response to the introduction of an antigen from another member of the same species, the individual himself lacking the particular antigen (*see also* Chapter 1). In many antigen-antibody systems the mere presence of an antibody shows that immunisation has taken place but in the ABO blood group system this is not so. In this system individuals who lack either the A or B antigen and so are capable of being stimulated to produce immune antibodies to these antigens, already have naturally occurring agglutinins of the same specificity in their serum. To show that immune anti-A or anti-B agglutinins have been produced, therefore, it is necessary to demonstrate that a change has occurred in the serum after the antigenic stimulus. The easiest way to do this is to show a rise in titre. Immune responses due to blood group antigens are usually, therefore, measured by titrating the serum of an individual both before and after the antigenic stimulus is given.

In the human species there are three ways in which iso-immunisation due to blood group antigens may take place.

(1) By deliberate injection of A or B antigens in the form of red cells or soluble group specific substance.

(2) By transfusion of blood of incompatible group, *e.g.* group A blood to a group B individual.

(3) By pregnancy. In heterospecific blood group pregnancy the mother almost always produces immune antibodies in response to stimulation by the agglutinogen of the fœtus, *e.g.* a mother of group A carrying a group B fœtus will produce immune anti-B antibodies.

A graphical representation of the changes in titre of the anti-A and anti-B agglutinins of a typical group O individual who had been inadvertently transfused with 200 ml. of group A blood is shown in Fig. 5.1. It will be seen that the anti-A titre falls suddenly immediately after the transfusion due to the absorption of the recipient's anti-A agglutinins by the transfused A cells; this is the negative phase. The group A cells are eliminated from the recipient's circulation and immune anti-A agglutinins are produced; these cause the anti-A titre to rise, until 10–15 days after the transfusion when the peak titre is attained. Thereafter the titre returns slowly towards its normal value, becoming stationary slightly above the pre-stimulation level after several weeks. The anti-B titre on the other hand does not show any large changes—there is a slight increase but whereas the anti-A titre has increased from 256 to 8000, a 32-fold increase, the anti-B has risen merely from 128 to 256, a twofold increase; moreover this alteration in the anti-B titre is within the limits of day to day variation and the experimental error of the titration technique, such small variations often being recorded when the titration values of the agglutinins in a normal non-immune control are being estimated over a period of time. It will be realised, therefore, that merely from studying the changes in titre of the anti-A and anti-B iso-agglutinins the group of the transfused blood could have been determined even if the remains in the bottle given had not been available.

Fig. 5.2 shows the changes in titre of the anti-B agglutinin of a group A mother whose infant was group B. During pregnancy the titre rises slightly but the biggest increase takes place after delivery, the peak being attained at the 10–15th day. It will be seen that the immune response curve is very similar in shape whether the stimulus is an injection of incompatible blood or a pregnancy.

Both these figures show titres measuring only agglutinating antibodies (agglutinins). Although most agglutinins are IgM globulins, after an immune response the IgG fraction commonly contains agglutinins too. This fact is not always appreciated as the idea that agglutinins are entirely IgM and incomplete antibodies entirely IgG has been widely proliferated. More recent work has also shown, in immune sera, small amounts of blood group antibody of type IgA and some incomplete antibodies of IgM.

Immune anti-A and/or anti-B sera are characterised by being rich in antibodies of the incomplete type IgG and potent specific anti-A and/or anti-B hæmolysins IgG and IgM. It should not, however, be assumed that anti-A and anti-B incomplete antibodies and hæmolysins are entirely absent from non-immune sera. There is evidence that they are present in these sera, but in such small quantities that they are difficult to detect.* In immune sera the

* If red cells from a patient suffering from paroxysmal nocturnal hæmoglobinuria (called for convenience PNH cells) are used, they are lysed to a titre comparable to the agglutinin titre of the same serum.

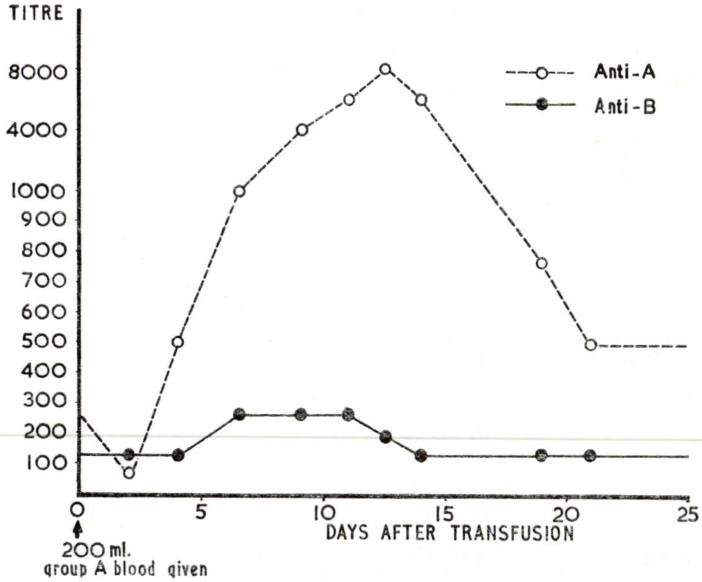

FIG. 5.1. Changes in iso-agglutinin titre following incompatible transfusion of group A blood to group O recipient. Typical immune response.

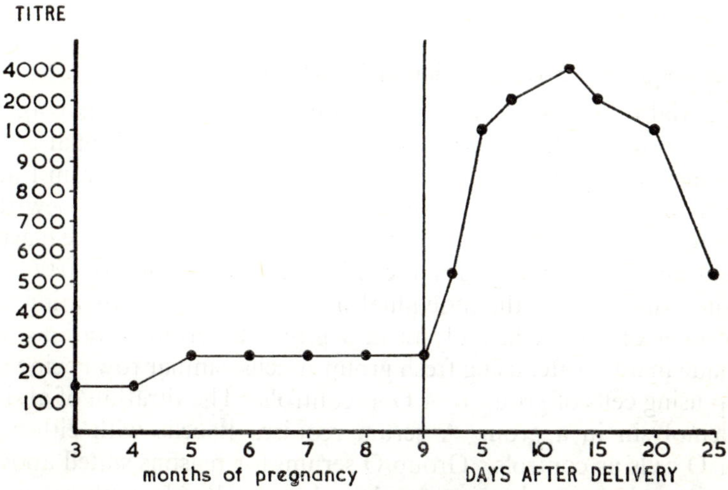

FIG. 5.2. Changes in titre of the anti-B iso-agglutinin of a group A mother; immune response to a group B fœtus *in utero*.

activity of all varieties of antibody present is so much increased that they can more readily be observed. However, incomplete anti-A and anti-B antibodies are difficult to demonstrate even in immune sera since their presence is masked by anti-A and anti-B agglutinins.

If the titre of the incomplete antibody is considerably higher than that of the agglutinins (which is often the case), then the incomplete antibodies may be demonstrated by anti-human globulin (with a specially selected reagent) or papain techniques. Another method takes advantage of the fact that agglutinins are more readily neutralised by A and B group specific substances than are incomplete antibodies (*see* Chapter 25).

There is an almost constant association of hæmolytic properties with immune anti-A and anti-B sera. The titres of the hæmolysins, however, are very much lower than the agglutinin titres of the same sera and usually range between 1 and 16 (except against PNH cells—*see* above). When dealing with immune group O sera it is usual to find hæmolysis of both group A and group B red cells (but never group O) irrespective of whether the immune response has been due to the A or B antigen. Normally the greater titre of hæmolysin is found in association with whichever of the two antibodies (anti-A or anti-B) corresponds in specificity to the stimulating antigen. It is also characteristic of immune anti-A sera to react with A_p cells (pig cells), *see* Chapters 25 and 32.

Technique No. 5.1. Titration of iso-hæmolysins

Serial dilutions of the serum are made by technique No. 4.2 in the serum which is being used as the source of additional complement (*see* below). A convenient range of dilutions is from 1 in 1 to 1 in 32. In order to have adequate fluid in which to view the the colouration caused by hæmolysis it is advisable to make master dilutions large enough for the use of a unit volume of 0·06 ml. when running out the individual titrations. When estimating the content of anti-A hæmolysin in a group B serum, titrations are made in duplicate, using fresh group A cells, similar rows being set up using cells of group B or O as controls. The titration of anti-B hæmolysin in a group A serum requires B cells with either A or O cells as controls. Group O serum, for reasons stated above, is titrated against both group A and group B cells with group O cells as control. After the serial dilutions are made a half volume (0·03 ml.) of packed well-washed cells of the appropriate group is added to each tube. The tests are then incubated at 37°C for

2 hours. Control tubes are set up containing a unit volume of complement serum mixed with each kind of red cell used in the test. At least once during and at the end of the incubation period the tubes are shaken. Then they are centrifuged and the supernatant fluid from each is pipetted into a separate row of clean tubes. Care must be exercised lest red cells are drawn up with the fluid. The degree of hæmolysis is read by holding the tubes in a good light, preferably daylight, against a white background. Each dilution of serum should be read by comparison with the corresponding dilution tested with group O cells; thus, any colouration produced may be matched against a negative control. A convenient method of scoring results is as follows:

++++ = complete hæmolysis.
+++ = deep red serum.
++ = serum red.
+ = serum less red.
± = traces of hæmolysis.
— = colour identical with negative control.

The hæmolysin titre is expressed as the reciprocal of the highest dilution showing hæmolysis.

If the titration is carried out on a serum which has been drawn within 24 hours it is worth while titrating in saline as its own complement may give better results than complement added from another source in spite of the fact that the complement as well as the hæmolysin is being diluted. However, in some cases and indeed in all if the serum is less fresh, complement from another source is necessary so fresh human complement is usually used. When selecting this it must be borne in mind (*see* Chapter 8) that sera of groups A, B or AB will contain, in varying amounts, soluble A or B antigens which may neutralise any anti-A or anti-B hæmolysin present in the serum under test. It is better therefore to select as source of complement a serum which is of the same group as the test serum. Even so there is the problem of the antibody content of the serum; one may be adding hæmolysin to the system as well as complement. The best source of complement is therefore either serum of the same group as the serum under test or group O serum, both of which must be of low agglutinin titre and giving no iso-hæmolysis.

Comment. The subject of iso-hæmolysis and iso-hæmolysin technique has been dealt with here because it is mainly in immune sera that iso-hæmolysins are found in appreciable titre. The mere finding of an iso-hæmolysin, however, cannot be taken to be

3

indicative of an immune serum. The only way to show that iso-immunisation to the A or B antigens has occurred is to demonstrate an increase in the strength of the corresponding antibody. As previously stated this can be most conveniently done by titrating the iso-agglutinin before and at intervals after stimulation by the antigen.

CHAPTER 6

THE ABO SUB-GROUPS

THERE are several sub-groups of A but the main division is into A_1 and A_2 by means of anti-A_1 serum. Anti-A_1 which is specific for A_1 is a normal component of the anti-A found in group B and group O individuals. It can be isolated. This serum is usually prepared by absorbing an anti-A (group B) serum with group A_2 red cells, which remove anti-A and leave anti-A_1. Using anti-A_1 so prepared groups A and AB can be sub-divided into A_1 and A_2, A_1B and A_2B (Table 6.1).

Table 6.1

Reactions of Various Sub-groups of A with Anti-A, Anti-B, and Anti-A_1

Group	Reactions with		
	Anti-A	Anti-B	Anti-A_1 (α_1)
A_1	C	—	C
A_2	C	—	—
A_1B	C	C	C
A_2B	C	C	—

Titration of a group B (*i.e.* an anti-A) serum against red cells of sub-groups A_1 and A_2, A_1B and A_2B shows that the strength of the A agglutinogen in each of the sub-groups is different. The titration values of the anti-A serum against red cells of each sub-group shows that these strengths are in the order $A_1 > A_1B > A_2 > A_2B$. The range of titre can be considerable. For example, in a particular case using an extremely potent anti-A serum, the titre with A_1 was 16,000, with A_1B 4,000, with A_2 1,000 and A_2B 128. In another case in which the anti-A was of average standard for grouping, the titres were A_1 256, A_1B 128, A_2 64, A_2B 16. These figures show how necessary it is, when selecting anti-A grouping serum, to titrate against red cells of the weakly reacting sub-groups, especially A_2B.

If the titration method is used to differentiate between the sub-groups of A it soon becomes apparent that there are occasional examples of red cells encountered in which the A agglutinogen is even weaker than in the sub-group A_2B. Such red cells are called A_3 and A_3B. These give a characteristic appearance with anti-A sera, which consists of some quite large agglutinates with many free cells. It should be noted that typing with anti-A_1 serum will not allow a distinction to be made between A_2 and A_3 since the cells of both these sub-groups are negative with anti-A_1 serum. Further researches have revealed even weaker sub-groups of A which are all negative with anti-A_1 and differ from A_2 in other ways chiefly in the strength of the agglutinogen. In some this is so weak as not to be detectable with ordinary anti-A grouping serum and it is chiefly on account of these that group O serum is included in routine grouping tests.

These sub-groups are still mainly a subject of research. In Chapter 32 we shall endeavour to summarise some of the fascinating serological and genetical complexities which their study is revealing.

Anti-A_1

Anti-A_1 (α_1) occurs as an atypical cold agglutinin* in the sera of individuals who lack the corresponding antigen.

The frequency of occurrence varies with the sub-group. In A_2 it is about 2 per cent, in A_2B about 26 per cent and in the weaker sub-groups even higher to the extent of being almost a constant feature of some of them. The figures refer to the atypical anti-A_1 agglutinins sufficiently potent to be active at room temperature. If tests are done at 4°C many more will be found.

It must be emphasised that the anti-A_1 component of group B and group O sera is always present and is not a cold agglutinin. Its temperature range is similar to anti-A and anti-B, which, although slightly more active in the cold, show little change of titre with temperature and are always active at 37°C.

When active at room temperature the presence of an anti-A_1 agglutinin in the serum of persons of groups A_2 and A_2B often leads to anomalous blood grouping results. This has already been referred to in Chapter 3. The anomalous results, as might be expected from the percentage occurrence of anti-A_1 agglutinins, are most often associated with sub-group A_2B. For example, although the red cells of an individual of sub-group A_2B will give the normal reactions expected of those of AB, the serum if it contains an anti-A_1 will give the reactions characteristic of group B (*see* Table 6.2). Such individuals cannot be said to belong to group AB until further tests have been carried out. These tests comprise

* For definition *see under* "Agglutinin," Glossary.

typing the red cells with anti-A_1 serum to confirm that they do in fact belong to sub-group A_2B, and testing the serum with sub-group A_2 cells in addition to those of A_1 to show that the atypical agglutinin does not react with A_2 cells and is, therefore, anti-A_1. If anti-A_1 typing serum and cells of sub-group A_2 are not available the serum grouping test may be repeated at 37°C in which case the anti-A_1 being a cold agglutinin will be inactive and the results obtained will be those expected of group AB. However, this second test does not give so satisfactory a proof of the presence of anti-A_1 in a group A_2B sample as does the first.

The question naturally arises as to whether anomalous grouping results can be satisfactorily avoided by using sub-group A_2 cells

Table 6.2

Agglutination Reactions of a Sub-group A_2B, the Serum of which Contains an Anti-A_1 Active at Room Temperature

Sub-group A_2B	Anti-A serum	Anti-B serum	Anti-A_1 serum	Red cells		
				A_1	B	A_2
Reaction of red cells	+	C	–			
Reaction of serum				V	–	–

for routine serum grouping tests rather than A_1. This procedure is not recommended for three main reasons. Firstly, A_2 cells do not react as crisply with the wide range of anti-A agglutinin strengths encountered in routine tests as do A_1 cells. Thus for the sake of avoiding a few anomalous results, the serum grouping tests would be rendered less reliable and more laborious to read as macroscopic agglutination would be less frequent. Secondly, the presence of atypical anti-A_1 agglutinins would go undetected which would mean that agglutinins potent enough for use as anti-A_1 typing sera could not be collected. In addition, and of greater importance, the occasional immune anti-A_1 which is active at 37°C and, therefore, may be of clinical significance, would be missed. Thirdly, A_2 cells will themselves be agglutinated by the anti-H and anti-HI types of atypical cold agglutinins (*see* below), and would thus give rise to a further set of anomalous results.

It is of great importance to realise it is just in the circumstance in which the presence of an atypical anti-A_1 may cause anomalous serum grouping results that the cell grouping test also may give an erroneous result. This takes the form of a false negative which may occur if the anti-A grouping serum being used is not of sufficient potency for the detection of the weak A agglutinogen which is characteristic of these low sub-groups of A. Herein lies the necessity for ensuring an adequate titre of anti-A grouping serum with cells of A_2B and for using group O serum as a check. The most usual mistake to occur if these precautions are omitted is the grouping as B of an A_2B with anti-A_1 in the serum. The use of A_2 cells as an extra serum check on all apparent group B samples will prevent such mistakes being made.

Sera Reacting Preferentially with Group O Cells

Atypical cold agglutinins also appear in the sera of individuals of sub-groups A_1 and A_1B (and rarely of group B). These agglutinins are distinguished by their ability to agglutinate all group O and A_2* cells, whereas cells of other groups are agglutinated only weakly or not at all. This preference for cells of groups O and A_2 resulted in these agglutinins being termed "anti-O" or "anti-A_2" (α_2). Certain animal sera, particularly from oxen, occasionally contain an agglutinin which reacts preferentially with human O and A_2 red cells as also do certain plant extracts (*see* below). It was at first thought that all examples of such agglutinins whether of human or animal origin were of the same type and were detecting a product of the O gene, A_2 cells being agglutinated because they contained an O factor in addition to A. This is now known not to be the case and it is thought that the O gene is a 'silent' gene and does not produce a specific antigen.

The animal sera and seed extracts react with a substance called H. It is this substance on which the enzymes produced by the A and B genes act to produce A and B substances while in group O the H substance is unchanged. Apparently the production of A substance in A_2 uses less H than A_1 or B. We can see therefore why anti-H would react more strongly with O cells than with A_2 and least strongly with B and A_1. Some sera of human origin are also anti-H in specificity. H substance is secreted in saliva (*see* Chapter 8) and so anti-H sera are characterised by being inhibited by secretor saliva. There are, however, rare anti-H sera which are not inhibited by human saliva.

We are left with an assortment of human sera which react preferentially with group O cells. Some of these are detecting an antigen produced as a result of the interaction of the H and I genes (*see* Chapter 32) and they are called anti-HI. The majority

* In this connection A_2 denotes all sub-groups except A_1.

of such antisera are not inhibited by human saliva. Recently, it has been suggested that antibodies should have the superscript ^{s} (*e.g.* anti-H^{s}, anti-HI^{s}) when they are inhibitable by human saliva and the superscript ^{c} (*e.g.* anti-H^{c}, anti-HI^{c}) when they are not inhibitable. Eel serum, one of the animal sera thought to be anti-H, has been shown to be anti-HI^{s} or sometimes a mixture of anti-H^{s} and anti-HI^{s}.

Antibodies to the compound antigens IB and IA can also occur, although they are very rare. Their presence is usually masked by the normal anti-B or anti-A of the serum in which they occur. They can be disclosed by absorbing the sera with cord cells of the appropriate ABO group as these cells are I negative and so do not react with anti-IB or anti-IA.

Those concerned mainly with the more practical aspects of these cold agglutinins should realise that these too can cause anomalous grouping results. When anomalous results are encountered the red cells of the individual should be typed with

Table 6.3

The ABO Blood Group System, Showing the Sub-groups of A, with Particular Reference to the Antibody Content of the Serum

Group	Reactions with anti-A_1 (α_1)	Agglutinins always present (typical)*	Agglutinins sometimes present (atypical)†
A_1	+	Anti-B	Anti-H and anti-HI
A_2 (and A_3, A_x, etc.)	–	Anti-B	Anti-A_1 (α_1)
A_1B	+	None	Anti-H and anti-HI
A_2B (and A_3B, A_xB, etc.)	–	None	Anti-A_1 (α_1)
B	–	Anti-A (α) and anti-A_1 (α_1)	Anti-H and anti-HI
O	–	Anti-A (α) and anti-A_1 (α_1) Anti-B	

* React strongly at 4°C, room temperature, and 37°C.

† React strongly at 4°C, less strongly or not at all at room temperature—very rarely active at 37°C.

anti-A_1 and the serum shown to agglutinate O and A_2 cells either preferentially or exclusively.

The fact that the ABO system has both typical and atypical agglutinins is often found to be confusing, particularly as anti-A_1 occurs in both forms. Table 6.3 clearly differentiates between the two types of agglutinins and indicates the groups in which each antibody may be found.

Plant Agglutinins (Lectins)

It has long been known that extracts of certain seeds will agglutinate human red cells. Most of these extracts are of little importance in routine blood group serology as they do not clearly differentiate the blood groups.

Two extracts are, however, useful in testing for the sub-groups of A. Dolichos biflorus seeds are a rich source of an anti-A lectin which reacts very strongly with the sub-group A_1 much less strongly with A_2 and not at all with the other sub-groups of A. By suitable dilution a specific anti-A_1 reagent can be prepared which is more potent and avid than most, if not all, the anti-A_1 reagents prepared from human serum.

Ulex europæus on the other hand is a good source of anti-H, so that Ulex extracts reacts much more strongly with A_2 and the weaker sub-groups of A than with A_1. It is possible to choose a dilution and technique by which these extracts used in parallel will react antithetically and diagnose the sub-groups A_1 and A_2.

Sub-groups of B

In group B there is no variation in antigen strength comparable to that of A nor is group B divisible into two main sub-groups as A is divided by anti-A_1. However, sub-groups of B do occur and may very rarely be the cause of anomalies in ABO grouping. An account of some of the recent work on the sub-groups of B is given in Chapter 32.

Techniques

Technique No. 6.1. Preparation of human anti-A_1 sera

To choose a suitable group B serum, a number of sera are titrated against A_1 and A_2 cells—a suitable serum has a titre of at least 512 with A_1 cells and shows a difference in titre between the A_1 and A_2 cells of several dilutions.

For the absorption the serum is mixed with half its own volume of packed washed group A_2 red cells (the cells are washed by shaking them in an excess of normal saline, centrifuging and removing the supernatant fluid. This process is repeated three times). The serum-cell mixture is allowed to stand in the ice chest at 3–5°C for 2 hours. The mixture is then centrifuged and the supernatant serum collected. If the absorption has been successful the serum will give no reaction with A_2 cells and a titre of 16 or greater with A_1 cells. If there is still a reaction with A_2 cells it may be necessary to reabsorb with half the quantity of cells but if there is only a slight reaction it is often better to dilute the serum to give a negative reaction with the A_2 cells rather than to reabsorb. Over-absorption may result in the removal of some of the anti-A_1 agglutinins.

Ideally the serum should give macroscopic agglutination with all A_1 and A_1B cells and be negative with A_2 and A_2B cells. In practice it will be found that some A_1 cells give much weaker reactions than others. Moreover, a serum that is negative with almost all A_2 and A_2B cells will occasionally give a weak reaction with cells from a few persons of these groups. It is for this reason that it is advisable to use at least two different anti-A_1 reagents for typing purposes.

Anti-A_1 also occurs in A_2 and A_2B as a cold agglutinin and when it is sufficiently strong (*i.e.* giving a titre of 16 or more at room temperature) such a serum can be used as an anti-A_1 typing serum. The main disadvantage is that being a cold agglutinin small changes in temperature may affect the titre and avidity of the serum very considerably. This difficulty is minimised if a cold water bath or incubator at 12–15°C is available.

The selected and absorbed sera are clarified if necessary and then Seitz-filtered. The sterile serum is stored frozen solid in 1 ml. quantities.

Technique No. 6.2. Sub-grouping with human anti-A_1 sera

The technique is essentially the same as for ABO grouping. One unit volume of an anti-A_1 serum is mixed with one unit volume of a 2 per cent suspension of red cells in a precipitin tube. The mixture, after shaking, is allowed to stand at room temperature for 2 hours before reading. No reaction is scored as negative until it has been examined microscopically. It is important to include controls consisting of known A_1 and A_2 cells with each batch of tests. At least two anti-A_1 sera should be used.

Technique No. 6.3. Preparation of anti-A_1 from Dolichos biflorus

The seeds are ground in a mill; for small quantities a small hand-operated pepper mill is quite satisfactory.

To each gram of meal is added 10 ml. of saline. The mixture is thoroughly agitated, one hour in a shaking machine, and then centrifuged at 3,000 r.p.m. for five minutes and the sediment discarded. The supernatant fluid, even though it is sometimes slightly cloudy, can be used immediately. The appearance is improved by filtration through a clarifying Seitz filter (pad grade 4).

The extract can be freeze-dried, stored and reconstituted when required. This procedure is usually unnecessary, however, as it stores very well frozen at −20°C.

It is tested with a panel of known cells of sub-groups A_1 and A_2 as the extract may need dilution so that it gives clear negatives with A_2 cells (*see* technique No. 6.5).

Technique No. 6.4. Preparation of anti-H from Ulex eropæus for the detection of A_2.

The seeds are ground and the extract made exactly as for Dolichos biflorus (technique No. 6.3).

The resulting extract reacts with almost all human red cells, the reaction declining in strength in the direction $O \rightarrow A_2 \rightarrow B \rightarrow A_2B \rightarrow A_1 \rightarrow A_1B$. For use to detect A_2 it is essential that the extract is used at a suitable dilution and technique so that the A_1 and A_1B groups are negative and the A_2 and A_2B groups positive (*see* technique No. 6.5).

Technique 6.5. Sub-typing using Dolichos and Ulex extracts

This is most conveniently done by a slide technique as in tubes the Dolichos extract may cross react with A_2 and O cells and the Ulex with A_1. A suitable dilution of extract is chosen so that in 30–60 seconds the positive reactions are strong and there is no reaction in the negative controls.

One drop of a 5 per cent saline suspension of the unknown cells is mixed with one drop of Dolichos extract on a long slide, the controls being known A_1 and A_2 cells. At the same time one drop of the 5 per cent suspension is mixed with Ulex extract, the controls being O, A_2 and A_1 cells. A_1 cells are strongly agglutinated by the Dolichos and are negative with the Ulex. A_2 cells are positive with Ulex and negative with Dolichos. Occasionally a sample is encountered which gives weak positive reactions with both extracts; this belongs to a rare type known as A_{int}. It is important that the tests are read as soon as the positive control is well developed and while the negative control is still completely unagglutinated. If the tests are read later, false positive results will certainly be obtained.

Practical Importance

Although of considerable academic interest the sub-groups of A are of limited practical importance. Anomalous grouping results due primarily to the occurrence of atypical anti-A_1 agglutinins will be encountered sooner or later and must be dealt with according to the methods described above. As a general rule cold agglutinins such as anti-A_1 and anti-H can be disregarded when selecting blood for transfusion. However, these antibodies are sometimes stimulated by transfusion or pregnancy, in which case, not only do they increase in titre but also become active at higher temperatures. It is only when they reach 37°C that blood of the same sub-group as the recipient must be selected for transfusion.

CHAPTER 7

THE INHERITANCE OF THE ABO BLOOD GROUPS

THE general subject of human inheritance is too wide to be dealt with here. It is assumed that the reader will have an adequate knowledge of the principles underlying the Mendelian theory of inheritance. Its application to blood groups in general has been discussed briefly in Chapter 1. All the genetic terms used in this chapter are defined briefly in the Glossary to which reference should be made by any to whom the sense in which we have used them may not be quite clear.

The characters A, B, and O will be considered first; once the mode of inheritance of these is understood it is comparatively simple to expand the scheme to include the sub-groups of A.

Table 7.1

The ABO Groups and Their Corresponding Genotypes

Blood group or phenotype	Genotypes
A	AA AO
B	BB BO
O	OO
AB	AB

According to the generally accepted theory of Bernstein the characters A, B, and O are inherited by means of three allelomorphic genes, also called A, B, and O. Every individual has two chromosomes each carrying either A, B, or O, one chromosome from each parent. Thus the possible ABO genotypes are AA, AO, BB, BO, AB, and OO. ABO typing is normally only carried out using the two anti-sera, anti-A and anti-B detecting the characters A and B. This divides the population into the four blood groups, group A (phenotype A) comprising two genotypes AA (homozygous) and AO (heterozygous), group B (phenotype B) comprising two genotypes BB (homozygous) and BO (heterozygous), group O (phenotype O) genotype OO (homozygous) and group AB where the phenotype and the genotype are both AB (heterozygous) (Table 7.1).

To illustrate the mode of inheritance a particular type of mating, *e.g.* that in which a group A male mates with a group B female, can be considered. The group A male may be of genotype AA or

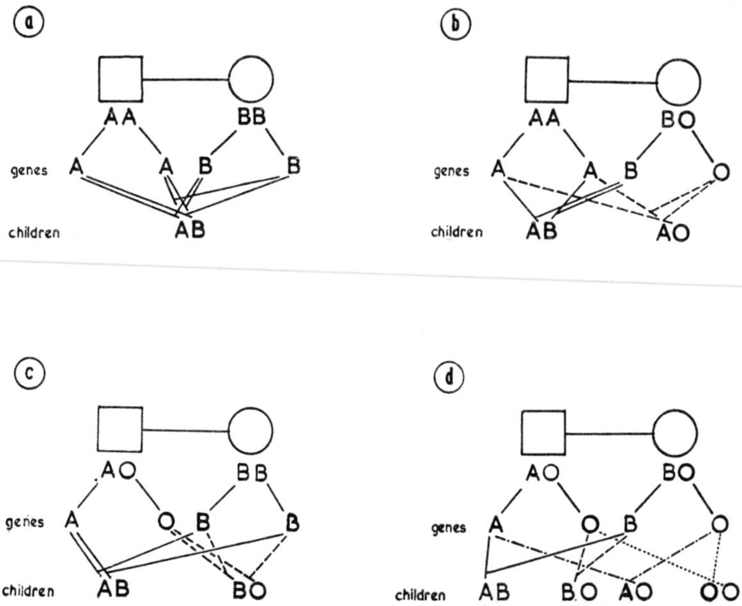

FIG. 7.1. The four genotype matings included in the phenotype mating A × B, and the children arising therefrom.

AO and similarly the group B female may be of the genotype BB or BO, therefore within this one mating four subdivisions exist, namely (*a*) AA with BB, (*b*) AA with BO, (*c*) AO with BB and (*d*) AO with BO. The outcome of the four matings is shown diagrammatically in Fig. 7.1*a–d.*

It will be seen that this mating can result in children of all four blood groups or phenotypes, although it is only in one subdivision, namely subdivision (4) AO with BO, that children of all four blood groups can occur in the same family. From this same subdivision it can be seen that a determination of the groups of relatives will sometimes disclose the genotype of group A or group B individuals, *e.g.* the finding of a group O child in an A × B mating demonstrates the presence of the O gene in both parents, and it follows that any A or B children arising from this particular mating are heterozygous, *i.e.* AO or BO. Table 7.2 shows all the possible ABO matings and the children which can arise from them. Naturally in considering a whole population all the possible genotype combinations will occur for each group of matings, but in

Table 7.2

The Various ABO Matings and the Children which can Arise from Them

Mating		Children	
Phenotypes	Genotypes	Genotypes	Phenotypes
A × A	(1) AA × AA (2) AA × AO (3) AO × AO	(1) AA (2) AA and AO (3) AA, AO, and OO	A and O
A × B	(1) AA × BB (2) AA × BO (3) AO × BB (4) AO × BO	(1) AB (2) AB and AO (3) AB and BO (4) AB, AO, BO, and OO	A, B, AB, and O
A × AB	(1) AA × AB (2) AO × AB	(1) AA and AB (2) AA, AB, AO, and BO	A, B, and AB
A × O	(1) AA × OO (2) AO × OO	(1) AO (2) AO and OO	A and O
B × B	(1) BB × BB (2) BB × BO (3) BO × BO	(1) BB (2) BB and BO (3) BB, BO, and OO	B and O
B × AB	(1) BB × AB (2) BO × AB	(1) AB and BB (2) AB, BB, AO, and BO	A, B, and AB
B × O	(1) BB × OO (2) BO × OO	(1) BO (2) BO and OO	B and O
AB × AB	(1) AB × AB	(1) AA, AB, and BB	A, B, and AB
AB × O	(1) AB × OO	(1) AO and BO	A and B
O × O	(1) OO × OO	(1) OO	O

considering a particular family only one genotype combination will represent the truth. For example, as we have seen there are four possible subdivisions of the A × B mating and in the whole population each one of these four subdivisions will be found; any particular family, however, can only belong to subdivision a, b, c, or d. Sometimes the particular genotype combination will be evident from the phenotypes found but often it will not be possible to determine the genotypes involved.

This means that in Table 7.2, while the two genotype columns are important in enabling us to predict which phenotypes can occur among the offspring of any given mating, they can be omitted for most practical purposes. Table 7.3 is this simplified form of Table 7.2 with the addition of a column which gives the phenotypes which cannot occur among the children of each given mating. It is this column, of course, which is useful in the interpretation of paternity tests. It is obviously never possible to tell whether a man is the father of a given child as there will be many men of the same phenotype, but it is sometimes possible to say that he cannot be the father as, for instance, when he is group O and the child is group AB.

Table 7.3

ABO Matings Showing Possible and Impossible Phenotypes of Children

Mating	Possible phenotypes of children	Impossible phenotypes of children
A × A	A and O	B and AB
A × B	A, B, O, and AB	None
A × AB	A, B, and AB	O
A × O	A and O	B and AB
B × B	B and O	A and AB
B × AB	A, B, and AB	O
B × O	B and O	A and AB
AB × AB	A, B, and AB	O
AB × O	A and B	AB and O
O × O	O	A, B, and AB

Extension to Include Sub-groups of A

The Bernstein theory of inheritance can now be extended to include the sub-groups of A by the simple expedient of replacing A by A_1 and A_2.

Table 7.4 shows the groups or phenotypes with their corresponding genotypes and Table 7.5 the various matings and the groups which can and cannot arise from them. This table applies to the whole population. In considering any particular family, however, it must be remembered that although each parent may belong to any one of the genotypes of which his phenotype is comprised he cannot in fact belong to more than one. The six possible genotype matings included in the one phenotype mating $A_1 \times B$ are shown in Table 7.6 together with the phenotypes which can and cannot be found among the offspring of each mating. Sometimes by studying the phenotypes of the children

Table 7.4

ABO Blood Group Phenotypes and Genotypes, Including Sub-groups of A

Blood group or phenotype	Genotypes
A_1	A_1A_1 A_1O A_1A_2
A_2	A_2A_2 A_2O
B	BB BO
O	OO
A_1B	A_1B
A_2B	A_2B

Table 7.5

ABO Matings, Including the Sub-groups of A

Mating	Possible phenotypes of children	Impossible phenotypes of children
$A_1 \times A_1$	A_1, O, A_2	B, A_1B, A_2B
$A_1 \times A_2$	A_1, A_2, O	B, A_1B, A_2B
$A_1 \times B$	A_1, A_2, B, O, A_1B, A_2B	None
$A_1 \times O$	A_1, A_2, O	B, A_1B, A_2B
$A_1 \times A_1B$	A_1, B, A_1B, A_2B	A_2, O
$A_1 \times A_2B$	A_1, A_2, B, A_1B, A_2B	O
$A_2 \times A_2$	A_2, O	A_1, B, A_1B, A_2B
$A_2 \times B$	A_2, B, O, A_2B	A_1, A_1B
$A_2 \times O$	A_2, O	A_1, B, A_1B, A_2B
$A_2 \times A_1B$	A_1, B, A_2B	A_2, O, A_1B
$A_2 \times A_2B$	A_2, B, A_2B	A_1, O, A_1B
$B \times B$	B, O	A_1, A_2, A_1B, A_2B
$B \times O$	B, O	A_1, A_2, A_1B, A_2B
$B \times A_1B$	A_1, A_1B, B	A_2, O, A_2B
$B \times A_2B$	A_2, B, A_2B	A_1, O, A_1B
$O \times O$	O	A_1, A_2, B, A_1B, A_2B
$O \times A_1B$	A_1, B	A_2, O, A_1B, A_2B
$O \times A_2B$	A_2, B	A_1, O, A_1B, A_2B
$A_1B \times A_1B$	A_1, B, A_1B	A_2, O, A_2B
$A_1B \times A_2B$	A_1, B, A_1B, A_2B	A_2, O
$A_2B \times A_2B$	A_2, B, A_2B	A_1, O, A_1B

it is possible to say to which genotype the parents belong. Moreover, it will be seen that for the mating $A_1 \times B$, A_2 and A_2B children never occur in the same family as B or O children so that

Table 7.6

The Mating $A_1 \times B$

Mating possible genotypes	Possible phenotypes of children	Impossible phenotypes of children
$A_1A_1 \times BB$	A_1B	A_1, B, A_2, A_2B, O
$A_1A_1 \times BO$	A_1B, A_1	B, A_2, A_2B, O
$A_1O \times BB$	A_1B, B	A_1, A_2, A_2B, O
$A_1O \times BO$	A_1, B, A_1B, O	A_2, A_2B
$A_1A_2 \times BB$	A_1B, A_2B	A_1, B, A_2, O
$A_1A_2 \times BO$	A_1, A_2, A_1B, A_2B	B, O

—although, taking all $A_1 \times B$ matings together, all six phenotypes can occur—the finding of, for instance, a group O child in a family where other children are A_2 and A_2B would not be possible if they all had the same parents.

CHAPTER 8

THE GROUP SPECIFIC SUBSTANCES A, B AND H IN TISSUES AND BODY FLUIDS

IT has long been realised that the blood group factors A and B are not confined to the red cells but can be detected in tissue cells and particularly in body fluids. They have a wide distribution and have been found in serum, saliva, gastric juices, ovarian cyst fluid, semen, amniotic fluid, and in smaller quantity in sweat, urine, tears, bile and milk. One of the richest and most readily available sources of group specific substance is saliva, and so it is used extensively in detecting the presence of these substances in any given individual. In about 24 per cent of the population, however, ABO group specific substances are almost absent from the saliva and other body fluids. Those individuals whose saliva contains the appropriate ABO group specific substances are called "secretors" while those whose saliva is devoid of such substances are called "non-secretors". Even in non-secretors a small amount of group specific substance is often detectable using sensitive techniques, *e.g.* mixed agglutination (see Chapter 30).

It has been established that secretion of group specific substances is controlled by a pair of allelomorphic genes, Se and se with Se dominant over se. Thus individuals can be homozygous SeSe, heterozygous Sese or homozygous sese. The first two classes are secretors and the third class, non-secretors. There is evidence that there are two distinct forms of group specific substance, one water soluble present in most body fluids and tissues, and one alcohol soluble present in red cells and almost all other tissues but absent from the secretions. The presence of the water soluble form is controlled by the secretion gene whereas the alcohol soluble form is not so controlled. In other words the tissue cells of every individual, whether secretor or non-secretor, contains a form of group specific substance which can be extracted with alcohol, but the secretor in addition to this possesses the water soluble form which appears in the body fluids. Group O persons are divided into "secretors" and "non-secretors" according to whether their saliva contains H. Secretors of A, B, and AB also have H in their saliva.

The fact that group specific substances are detectable in most tissues and body fluids, has led many workers to attempt their isolation with a view to studying their chemical nature. The richest sources of group specific substances in water soluble form are the body secretions, saliva, gastric juices and the fluid contained in pseudo-mucinous ovarian cysts. A similar non-human material which is rich in a substance showing A specificity is commercial hog pepsin. From these materials a purified form of group specific substance can be extracted. There are several methods but the phenol extraction method is, for practical purposes, the one used today.

When ovarian cyst fluids are used as the source of blood-group substance the crude freeze-dried cyst contents are extracted with cold 95 per cent phenol. The blood-group active material is then usually obtained as phenol-insoluble residue, whereas the contaminating protein goes into solution in phenol. The phenol-insoluble residue is then further purified by fractionation from aqueous solution with ethanol, high-speed centrifugation, etc. Sometimes some of the blood-group active material goes into solution in phenol and this can then be recovered from phenol solution by precipitation with 10 per cent ethanol. Higher concentrations of alcohol are needed to bring down the dissolved protein. If saliva or stomach mucosal linings are used as a source of blood-group substance these are usually digested with pepsin before they are freeze-dried and extracted with phenol. The pepsin treatment does not affect the serological properties of the substances but it alters the solubility in phenol in such a way that most of the material becomes soluble. The blood-group substance can again be recovered from the phenol solution by precipitation with 10 per cent ethanol.

The group specific substance thus prepared shows little or no antigenicity when injected into rabbits unless the substances are first combined with Shiga conjugated protein. In Man the response to the substances is quite marked without prior conjugation with protein. Extremely potent grouping sera can be obtained either in Man or animals by the injection of appropriately prepared substances.

In order to detect group specific substances in solution, advantage is taken of the fact that the soluble substance is capable of neutralising specifically its corresponding antibody. This neutralisation is reflected in a complete or partial inhibition of the agglutinin titre. This is the basis of the inhibition technique, which is of great importance in blood group serology as it can be adapted for many purposes. It can, for instance, be used for the detection of red cell agglutinogens in blood samples in which the red cells are too damaged to agglutinate properly and in forensic medicine it is used for the identification of antigens in blood stains. The tissue cells of the liver, spleen, kidney, etc., can be subjected to the inhibition test in order to find out whether or not they contain A or B substances, but in this case the difficulty of separating the tissue cells from blood cells must be overcome. This is most satisfactorily done by hæmolysing the red cells in the well crushed tissue with distilled water and removing them as stromata after slow centrifugation. Because of the difficulty of ensuring complete removal of stromata, the inhibition technique is not now used for the detection of tissue antigens but the more recent mixed agglutination technique where this problem is overcome. (Coombs, Bedford and Rouillard, 1956.) [*See* technique No. 29.4.]

When detecting the presence of group specific substances it is advisable to test against both anti-A and anti-B agglutinins because except in the case of material from group AB individuals, one or other agglutinin forms a valuable negative control and so confirms the specificity of the group specific substance in question. If the available test material is small in quantity it can be tested against a mixture of anti-A and anti-B agglutinins rather than with each one separately. For this purpose a special mixture of anti-A and anti-B should be made. It is inadvisable to use group O sera as these may contain antibody molecules which cross react with both A and B.

The strength of the anti-A and anti-B agglutinins chosen for inhibition tests should be moderate, a titration value of 32 or 64 being convenient. If more potent sera are used the sensitivity ot the test is decreased. When the group specific substance present in group O individuals is under investigation, anti-H must be used to measure the H content of the saliva. It is also important to include tests with anti-H in the identification of stains from body fluids (*e.g.* saliva, seminal fluid) in forensic work.

The group A cells used, particularly in testing saliva, should be of sub-group A_2 since the A group specific substance more readily neutralises the anti-A (α) component of the serum than the anti-A_1 (α_1). Consequently any inhibition which may occur will be more apparent if group A_2 cells, which only react with the anti-A (α) component, are used for the titration.

A modification of the method can be used in circumstances in which a more precise estimate of the strength of a particular group specific substance is required or when a comparison of the relative strengths of several fluids, *e.g.* salivas, is undertaken. This involves making serial dilutions of the saliva and testing each dilution against the standard anti-serum. By this method it is possible to obtain a titration value for the group specific substance itself.

Techniques

Technique No. 8.1. Preparation of saliva

Some saliva is collected in a suitable container. It is then transferred to a test-tube, diluted with an approximately equal quantity of saline, and placed in a boiling water bath for 10 minutes to destroy enzyme activity. The tube is then centrifuged and the clear supernatant fluid is used in the following tests.

Technique No. 8.2. Inhibition test using undiluted saliva

The crux of the test is the comparison of titration values of anti-A and anti-B sera before and after the addition of saliva from persons of groups A, B, or AB.

The anti-A and anti-B sera chosen should have titres of approximately 64. One unit volume of such an anti-A serum is mixed with one unit volume of saliva and similarly one unit volume of anti-B serum is mixed with one unit volume of saliva. When anti-H is used, equal volumes of ulex europeus extract and saliva are mixed together. It is unlikely that this reagent will require dilution since its titre by saline technique is normally about 64. These mixtures are allowed to stand on the bench for 30 minutes and while waiting for them to absorb the dilutions for the original titres of the anti-A and anti-B sera can be carried out. The red cells of course should not be added at this stage. The procedure for making the dilutions is similar to the method already described for titration of anti-A and anti-B agglutinins (*see* technique No. 4.2) with the exception that a volume of saline is placed in all tubes of the row including the first and one volume only of the serum to be titrated is used and this is placed in the first tube of the row. Thus instead of having undiluted serum in the first tube it is diluted 1 in 2 with saline and is comparable with the serum which is diluted 1 in 2 with saliva. After 30 minutes the serum-saliva mixtures are titrated in exactly the same manner as the original anti-A and anti-B sera. Appropriate red cell suspensions are added to all the tubes and they are allowed to stand on the bench for 2 hours. They are then read and the results scored in the normal manner for titrations.

If the titration value of the anti-A serum is reduced after being mixed with the saliva, then the saliva contains the group specific substance A. Similarly, if the titration value of the anti-B is reduced the saliva contains group specific substance B. Saliva from secretors of all ABO groups will inhibit the anti-H but O and A_2 are most active for H, and A_1 and A_1B least active.

Typical Result

Original titre of anti-A serum	=	64
Titre of anti-A serum + saliva	=	0
Original titre of anti-B serum	=	32
Titre of anti-B serum + saliva	=	32

Conclusion

Reduction in titre of anti-A from 64 to 0 indicates presence of group A substance in the saliva.

No reduction in titre of anti-B indicates absence of group B substance in the saliva.

Therefore saliva is from a secretor individual of group A.

Technique No. 8.3. Inhibition technique using diluted saliva

When saliva from different secretors is being compared the technique given above is too sensitive in that the titre will be neutralised completely using undiluted saliva from all secretors; thus it is necessary to dilute the saliva and then test against a standard quantity of antibody.

The standard serum should be of a titre of 32 or 64 giving two macroscopic reactions with standard cells and the saliva should be tested at dilutions ranging from 1 in 10 to 1 in 500. Suitable intervals obtained by means of standard graduated pipettes are shown in the following table:

Saliva			*Saline*	*Dilution*
0·1 ml.	neat saliva	+	0·9 ml.	$\frac{1}{10}$
0·2 ml.	$\frac{1}{10}$,,	+	0·8 ml.	$\frac{1}{50}$
0·1 ml.	$\frac{1}{10}$,,	+	0·9 ml.	$\frac{1}{100}$
0·1 ml.	$\frac{1}{50}$,,	+	0·2 ml.	$\frac{1}{150}$
0·1 ml.	$\frac{1}{100}$,,	+	0·1 ml.	$\frac{1}{200}$
0·1 ml.	$\frac{1}{50}$,,	+	0·4 ml.	$\frac{1}{250}$
0·1 ml.	$\frac{1}{100}$,,	+	0·2 ml.	$\frac{1}{300}$
0·1 ml.	$\frac{1}{50}$,,	+	0·6 ml.	$\frac{1}{350}$
0·1 ml.	$\frac{1}{100}$,,	+	0·3 ml.	$\frac{1}{400}$
0·1 ml.	$\frac{1}{100}$,,	+	0·4 ml.	$\frac{1}{500}$

Using a Pasteur pipette and starting with the weakest dilution of saliva, one volume of each dilution is pipetted into a row of precipitin tubes, after which an equal volume of test serum is added to each tube, mixed with the saliva dilution and allowed to stand at room temperature for 30 minutes. Then one volume of cells of appropriate group added and the reaction read after a further $1\frac{1}{2}$ to 2 hours at room temperature. In all cases a control of saline + serum is included. Most secretor salivas will give complete inhibition up to a point within the $\frac{1}{100}$ to $\frac{1}{500}$ range. Non-secretors may inhibit slightly at $\frac{1}{10}$ but not at all at $\frac{1}{50}$. If pseudo-mucinous cyst fluids are being tested a much wider range of dilutions should be tested as a screen—for instance $\frac{1}{10}$, $\frac{1}{250}$, $\frac{1}{500}$, $\frac{1}{1000}$, $\frac{1}{5000}$, $\frac{1}{10000}$, and then a further set of dilutions tested, closing in on the highest dilution which is giving complete inhibition.

Typical result											Control
Dilutions of saliva	$\frac{1}{10}$	$\frac{1}{50}$	$\frac{1}{100}$	$\frac{1}{150}$	$\frac{1}{200}$	$\frac{1}{250}$	$\frac{1}{300}$	$\frac{1}{350}$	$\frac{1}{400}$	$\frac{1}{500}$	saline.
Agglutination reaction with standard cells	–	–	–	–	(+)	++	V	V	V	V	V

This shows that up to a dilution of $\frac{1}{150}$ there is enough group specific substance to neutralise completely a titre of 32 of the corresponding antibody and that at $\frac{1}{200}$ and $\frac{1}{250}$ there is partial inhibition. This shows that the saliva is from a secretor but not from one secreting abnormal amounts of group specific substance.

GENERAL BIBLIOGRAPHY FOR ABO SECTION
(*Arranged in chronological order)

LANDSTEINER, K. (1900), "Zur Kenntnis der antifermentativen, lytischen und agglutinierenden Wirkungen des Blutserum und der Lymphe." *Zbl. Bakt.*, **27,** 357.

LANDSTEINER, K. (1901), "Ueber Agglutination-serscheinungen normalen menschlichen Blutes." *Wien, klin. Wschr.*, **14,** 1132.

DECASTELLO, A. V., and STURLI, A. (1902), "Ueber die Isoagglutinine im Serum gesunder und kranker Menschen." *Münch. med. Wschr.*, 1090.

DUNGERN, E. v., and HIRSZFELD, L. (1910), "Ueber Verebung gruppenspezifischer Strukturen des Blutes." *Z. Immun. Forsch*, **6,** 284.

DUNGERN, E. v., and HIRSZFELD, L. (1911), "Ueber gruppenspezifische Strukturen des Blutes III." *Z. Immun. Forsch.*, **8,** 526.

BERNSTEIN, F. (1924), "Ergebnisse einer biostatischen zusammenfassenden Betrachtung über die erblichen Blutstrukturen des Menschen." *Klin. Wschr.*, **3,** 1495.

SCHIFF, F. (1924), "Ueber gruppenspezifische Serumprecipitine." *Klin. Woch.*, **1,** 679.

SCHIFF, F., and ADELSBERGER, L. (1924), "Ueber blutgruppenspezifische Antikörper und Antigene." *Zbl. Bakt., I Orig.*, **93,** 172.

BERNSTEIN, F. (1925), "Zusammenfassende Betrachtungen über die erblichen Blutstrukturen des Menschen." *Z. indukt. Abstamm. U. Vererb. Lehre*, **37,** 237.

LANDSTEINER, K., and VAN DER SCHEER, J. (1925), "On the antigens of red blood corpuscles." *J. exp. Med.*, **41,** 427.

LANDSTEINER, K., and WITT, D. (1926), "Observation on the human blood groups." *J. Immunol.*, **11,** 221.

FRIEDENREICH, V. (1936), "Eine bisher unbekannte Blutgruppeneigenschaft (A_3)." *Z. Immun. Forsch.*, **89,** 409.

TAYLOR, G. L., and IKIN, E. W. (1939), "Observations on the performance of blood-group tests." *Brit. med. J.*, **i,** 1027.

MORGAN, W. T. J., and KING, H. K. (1943), "Studies in immuno-chemistry. The isolation from hog gastric mucin of the polysaccharide-amino acid complex possessing blood group A specificity." *Biochem. J.*, **37,** 640.

WIENER, A. S. (1943), *Blood Groups and Transfusion.* Charles C. Thomas, Springfield, Ill.

BOORMAN, K. E., DODD, B. E., and MOLLISON, P. L. (1945), "Iso-immunisation to the Blood Group Factors A, B and Rh." *J. Path-Bact.*, **57,** 157.

KABAT, E. A., and BESER, A. E. (1945), "Estimation of A and B iso-antibodies in human serum by the quantitative precipitin method." *J. exp. Med.*, **82,** 207.

COOMBS, R. R. A., BEDFORD, D., and ROUILLARD, L. M. (1956), "A and B blood group antigens on human epidermal cells demonstrated by mixed agglutination." *Lancet*, **i,** 461.

KABAT, E. A. (1956), *The Blood Group Substances.* Academic Press Inc., Publishers, New York.

* The full bibliography of the ABO blood groups would fill many pages; here we give a few papers mainly because of their historical interest.

Section 3—The Rh Blood Group System

"And wouldst thou master Rhesus 'Fac',
The E that's 'two', the C that's 'one',
And learn the knack, how not to thwack
The fragile clumps, my son!"

With apologies to E. H., Irish Medical Journal, and to Lewis Carroll

Chapter 9

THE DISCOVERY OF THE Rh BLOOD GROUPS AND Rh TYPING METHODS

Discovery and Importance

In 1940 Landsteiner and Wiener reported the discovery of a human blood factor which they called Rhesus or Rh. They immunised guinea pigs and rabbits with blood from the Macacus rhesus monkey and thereby obtained an anti-serum which after suitable absorption agglutinated not only the red cells of the rhesus monkey but also approximately 85 per cent of a panel of blood samples from the white population of New York. They realised that this serum was detecting a hitherto unknown human blood group antigen and they used it to type as Rh positive those whose red cells were agglutinated by the new antibody and as Rh negative those whose red cells were not so agglutinated. The antibody responsible they called anti-Rh. The distribution of the newly discovered Rh antigen was found to be the same in each ABO blood group, suggesting that the Rh and the ABO blood group systems were unrelated. Later family studies showed that, as expected, the Rh factor was segregating independently of A and B.

The real importance of the Rh factor was only realised when it was shown by Wiener and Peters (1940) that the sera of some people, who had experienced hitherto unexplained incompatible transfusion reactions even when given blood of the correct ABO group, contained antibodies which gave parallel reactions to the animal anti-Rh sera. This meant that the Rh factor was antigenic in man and that the anti-Rh iso-agglutinins which were formed as a result of immunisation could destroy incompatible blood *in vivo*.

Levine and Stetson (1939) had described an atypical antibody which later was shown to be anti-Rh in specificity. This antibody occurred in the serum of a woman delivered of a stillborn fœtus. Shortly after delivery she had required a blood transfusion and was given her husband's blood which caused a hæmolytic transfusion reaction. Levine and Stetson postulated that the antibody had arisen as the result of immunisation of the mother by a fœtal antigen which had been inherited from the father. This became the basis of their work reported in a series of papers in 1941 (Levine *et al.*, 1941*a*, *b*, *c*), which showed that not only could an Rh negative mother become immunised to an Rh positive fœtus *in utero* but also that the antibody could then traverse the placenta and give rise to erythroblastosis fœtalis—or as it is now more generally called "hæmolytic disease of the newborn".

Moreover, they showed that these antibodies were "warm" antibodies reacting more strongly at 37°C, *i.e.* body temperature, than in the cold or at room temperature.

The clinical significance of the Rh factor is, of course, the reason why the Rh system is second only to the ABO system in importance and why methods of Rh testing and antibody detection are so essential a part of the work of any laboratory which deals with blood group serology.

Recent work has shown that the animal anti-serum used by Landsteiner and Wiener was not detecting the antigen which is detected by human anti-Rh serum but another antigen possessed by Rh positive and Rh negative persons but in much greater strength by Rh positives. It has been suggested that this antigen should be re-christened LW after Landsteiner and Wiener who discovered it. Their work stimulated Wiener and Peters and Levine and his co-workers to investigate the human anti-Rh antibodies and was one of the most important discoveries in the history of blood grouping and transfusion. (*See also* Chapter 33.)

Principles of Rh Typing

Since its discovery the Rh system has been found to be composed of a series of antigens each with its corresponding antibody, so that it is much more complicated than was at first realised. However, the original Rh antigen (now called D or Rh_0) and its corresponding antibody, anti-Rh (anti-D or anti-Rh_0) account for over 90 per cent of all haemolytic reactions caused by the Rh blood groups. The techniques of testing are essentially the same for all the various Rh antigens and antibodies. In the interest of simplicity, therefore, tests using anti-D sera and tests for the detection of anti-D antibodies will be dealt with first. When the sub-groups of Rh, the Fisher nomenclature and theory of inheritance of the Rh factor (*see* Chapter 11) have been discussed, the modifications necessary to detect all the various antigens and antibodies will be described (*see* Chapters 12 and 13).

The original anti-Rh typing was done with animal sera but today human sera are almost universally used. Human anti-Rh sera can be obtained from Rh negative women who have recently been delivered of an Rh positive infant suffering from hæmolytic disease of the newborn. Alternatively they can be obtained from human volunteers (usually Rh negative men) who have been deliberately immunised. The selection and preparation of the various types of anti-Rh sera will be dealt with in Chapter 14. For "D-typing" (*i.e.* dividing individuals into the two classes D positive and D negative) the human serum needs to be of the specificity anti-D, of high titre and avidity, and having had any anti-A or anti-B agglutinins removed so that it is suitable for testing blood of all ABO groups.

The standard sera belong to two distinct types called for convenience "saline anti-D" and "albumin anti-D". This is because human anti-D antibodies occur either as agglutinins (or "complete" antibodies), which can agglutinate in a saline medium cells containing the corresponding agglutinogen, or as "incomplete" antibodies, which sensitise the cells in saline but only cause them to agglutinate in a high protein medium. The protein medium usually employed in Rh testing is bovine albumin. This may be obtained from the manufacturers as a 30 per cent solution especially prepared for use in Rh testing. Alternatively it is sometimes supplied in dried form which can be reconstituted to give a 30 per cent solution. Thirty per cent bovine albumin can be diluted to give a 20 per cent solution using AB serum as a diluent. This is preferred by some workers as it makes negative reactions easier to read, there is however a falling off in the strength of the positive reaction using a 20 per cent solution and we do not recommend it.

There are two ways in which the bovine albumin may be introduced into the test if albumin anti-D sera are to be used for Rh typing.

(*a*) The test cells can be suspended in the albumin (making a 2 per cent suspension approximately). This, however, is time-consuming, as red cell suspensions are not so quickly made in albumin as in saline—nor is the rinsing of the pipette so easy! In addition there is considerable wastage of expensive albumin as it is inevitable that more than the requisite amount of cell suspension will be made. This method has now been superseded by (*b*).

(*b*) The serum and saline suspended red cells may be mixed and the test incubated so that the cells have time to become sensitised. The cells are then covered with a layer of bovine albumin without disturbing them. This can be done by removing the supernatant and replacing it with albumin, but it is preferable to run a drop of albumin down the inside of the tube without removing supernatant. Being heavier than the saline-serum mixture the albumin displaces it forming a layer immediately above the red cells. This method involves no undue wastage of albumin.

Controls

Whatever technique is used controls are necessary. For any anti-D testing three controls should be used: (1) known Rh positive cells with the standard anti-D serum, (2) known Rh negative cells with the standard anti-D serum, and (3) the unknown cells with a bland serum (group AB) with the addition of bovine albumin if the technique employed involves its use.

The Positive Control. The cells chosen for this test should be standard Rh positive cells known to be weakly reacting. Anti-D does not normally show "dosage" (*see* Glossary) but as the D antigen in the R_1 phenotype is weaker than in the R_2, ideally cells belonging to group O R_1r should be used (*see* Chapter 12). Where the serum is known to react well with all Rh sub-groups, R_1R_2 red cells may be used. This control should be set up under exactly the same conditions as the Rh(D) typing tests and unless it gives a satisfactory positive reaction all the tests should be repeated.

The Negative Control on the Anti-serum. This consists of known Rh negative cells incubated with the standard serum under exactly the same test conditions as the unknown cells. If the standard serum has had anti-A and/or anti-B agglutinins absorbed out of it, it is as well that the Rh negative cells are of group AB as a negative reaction then shows both that the anti-A and anti-B have been completely removed and that it is not giving false agglutination due to contamination, etc.

Negative Control on the Cells Under Test. In this control the test is repeated replacing the standard serum with an AB serum. It is exceedingly important that it should be included in all slide and enzyme techniques, in tests on cord blood and on blood from patients whose protein balance may be disturbed. It may be omitted when the tube technique is used for testing normal blood samples, *i.e.* from blood donors, from routine ante-natal cases, husbands, etc. provided a saline anti-D is included in the typing.

If this control is positive no positive results obtained with standard antisera can be relied upon and the phenomenon should be fully investigated (*see* Chapter 20). It may be possible to type the cells successfully using suitably diluted saline antisera or alternatively it may be necessary first to elute an antibody from the cells; in the very rare case typing of the cells may be impossible.

Test Sera

It is advisable in all typing to use two different sera of the same specificity. No blood group should be determined on the result of a single reaction. Any discrepancy between the two readings necessitates a further investigation.

Techniques

There are innumerable Rh typing methods, a few are so unreliable as to be best forgotten, most are reasonably accurate in the hands of an experienced worker and one or two are sufficiently proven to be used as the yardstick by which other methods are assessed. It is, perhaps, of interest to note in this connection that almost every worker if asked "What do you do in the event of this method giving you a doubtful result" replies "Oh, then I check it by the tube technique". The methods described in this chapter are those we consider to be the best. In Chapter 22 we describe others which are faster but, we feel, slightly less reliable. There are circumstances which make the adoption of such techniques essential but in our opinion they should be reserved for the case where the condition of the patient warrants the risk being taken. Sometimes the choice of method is dictated by the convenience of the laboratory (less washing-up!) rather than the safety of the patient. If one of the most reliable of the quick methods (*see* Chapter 23, Table 23.2) is selected and used in parallel to the tube technique for part at least of the day to day routine work, experience will be gained which will minimise the risk of errors when the method is used in an emergency.

Technique No. 9.1. Rh typing by the moist chamber slide technique

The apparatus used is the same as for the ABO moist chamber technique (technique No. 3.1). If a saline anti-D is used, one volume of serum is mixed on a slide with one volume of a 5 per cent suspension in saline of washed red cells. If an albumin anti-D is used, equal volumes of albumin, of serum and the red cell suspension are mixed together. The slide is gently rocked and placed in a moist chamber in the 37°C incubator for 30 minutes, controls of known D positive and D negative cells being included. The control on rouleaux formation and pseudo-agglutination must be included also, it will consist of equal volumes of the suspension of unknown cells and group AB serum for the saline anti-D and for the albumin anti-D of equal volumes of cell suspension, of albumin and of group AB serum.

Comment. This method is a good one provided the sera are especially chosen and that all the controls are satisfactory. It is particularly important that the unknown cells under test should be thoroughly washed and that the control suspensions in group AB serum and in bovine albumin are included.

Occasionally weakly reacting D positive blood may appear to be D negative by this technique, but except in cases where the unknown cells are giving pseudo-agglutination with group AB serum alone or with group AB serum and bovine albumin, it is very unlikely that a false positive reaction will be obtained. If the cells are giving pseudo-agglutination, a more detailed investigation will have to be made.

Technique No. 9.2. Standard technique for Rh typing. One-stage method using saline anti-D

Apparatus. The apparatus for this technique is the same as for ABO grouping in tubes, with the addition of a 37°C incubator or water bath.

Reagents

Normal saline.
Two different saline anti-D sera.

Standard group O Rh positive and group O Rh negative red cells.

Precipitin tubes are placed in the first and second rows of a fifty-holed block and the larger cell suspension tubes in the back row.

One unit volume of the first anti-D serum is delivered into each tube of the front row using the standard graduated Pasteur pipette. The second anti-D is run into the second row in the same way. The tubes are then examined to see that each does in fact contain one volume of anti-serum. (This prevents those errors that can arise from serum going outside instead of inside the precipitin tubes, a mistake which can easily happen when dealing with such narrow tubes, or from serum leaking out of the tube through an almost invisible crack.) About 1·5 ml. of saline is run into each of the cell suspension tubes. A 2 per cent cell suspension, judged by eye is then made in the first of these tubes from the first unknown sample—and one volume of this suspension added to the corresponding tubes in rows 1 and 2. The pipette is carefully rinsed at least three times in saline, discarding each rinsing, and the process repeated for each unknown sample to be tested. The known D positive and D negative cells must be included at the end of each batch of tests as controls. The serum-cell mixtures are then tapped to ensure good mixing and the tests incubated at 37°C for 2 hours.

The reading of the reactions is the most difficult part of the test; the clumps are quite easily dispersed by rough handling unless the anti-serum is unusually potent. The cell sediment should, therefore, be removed from the tube with a wider bore Pasteur pipette (*see* Fig. 2E) and very gently spread on to a microscope slide (for details of preparing film *see* Chapter 2). The actual degree of agglutination should be recorded. (*See* Plates 6 and 7 for appropriate symbols.) It is advisable to check every test microscopically even when the agglutination can be seen with the naked eye, because occasionally macroscopic clumping may be observed which is not true agglutination and microscopically a "mixed blood" appearance would be recognised.

Technique No. 9.3. Standard technique for Rh typing. Two-stage method (Albumin addition)

The tests are put up exactly as described above but the reagents used are anti-D sera containing incomplete antibodies, "albumin" sera and an AB serum as the negative control in the cells under test. The tests are incubated for 1 to 1½ hours at 37°C. Then one drop of bovine albumin is allowed to run down the side of each tube, taking care not to disturb the cell sediment. The albumin displaces the serum-saline mixture forming a layer immediately above the cell button. The tests are incubated for a further 30 minutes. It will be found that the agglutinates formed using this method are not easily broken down so that the tubes can be gently shaken, the positive reaction will almost invariably be macroscopic but all negatives are checked microscopically as weak positive reactions are occasionally encountered usually denoting the presence of the D^u antigen (*see* below).

Comment. This is a very convenient and reliable technique. The time factor is not critical, the first stage must be long enough to allow the cells to sediment, the second can be reduced to 15–20 minutes when the serum used is potent, on the other hand either stage can be left for 2–3 hours without detriment. This flexibility can be of considerable advantage in a busy laboratory. A certain amount of experience is needed in reading the negative reactions as there is sometimes a tendency for the cells to agglomerate; gentle rolling of the microscope slide will however disperse such clumps while having no such effect on the true agglutinates.

Interpretation of Results

D-typing is always performed with two anti-D sera. A negative result with both sera will mean that the blood sample under test is probably D-negative—it should not, however, be regarded as completely Rh negative without further testing for the other Rh antigens (*see* Chapter 12). This further testing can be omitted in an emergency since a patient who is negative with two anti-D sera must always receive Rh negative blood. A positive result (V or ++) with both anti-D sera will mean that the sample is almost certainly Rh positive and for all practical purposes can be so considered. High grade D^u red cells (*see* Chapter 12) may also be positive with both anti-D sera, but such cells are treated as Rh positive for all practical purposes. Samples which give doubtful reactions [+, (+) or w] with one or both anti-sera should be re-tested, if possible, with a larger range of anti-D sera. If the blood sample is more than 48 hours old it is as well in these doubtful cases to wash the red cells with saline at 37°C as this will appreciably restore their diminished agglutinability. A negative result with one serum and a positive with the other is also an indication for testing against a number of anti-D sera. The reasons for these anomalous results (other than technical faults) are dealt with fully when the subject of D^u is considered in Chapters 11, 12 and 33.

CHAPTER 10

METHODS OF DETECTION OF ANTI-D ANTIBODIES

Rh antibodies are with only one or two exceptions immune antibodies. Therefore the vast majority of D negative individuals will not have anti-D antibodies in their serum. When such antibodies have been formed as the result of immunisation they are of such clinical importance, especially in the ætiology of hæmolytic disease of the newborn, that it is essential that their presence should be detected.

The tests for their detection fall into five main divisions.

(1) Saline agglutination tests.
(2) Tests in a high protein medium—especially bovine albumin.
(3) Tests using anti-human globulin ("Coombs tests").
(4) Tests using red cells partially digested with proteolytic enzymes.
(5) Blocking tests.

The general principles of the tests will be dealt with quite shortly, then will follow a full description of at least one method of each type. These methods while not exhaustive include sufficient techniques for the full investigation of any serum for the presence of Rh antibodies. Finally the correlation between the tests and the antibodies which they demonstrate will be considered.

(1) **Saline Agglutination Tests**

When anti-D is present in a serum as an agglutinin, mixture with a saline suspension of cells having the D antigen results in agglutination. As mentioned in the previous chapter, the agglutination is often readily dispersed by rough handling of the agglutinates. This is particularly true when the anti-D is present in low titre as often will be the case when unknown sera are being tested for antibodies.

(2) **Tests in High Protein Media**

It has been found that there are antibodies which fail to agglutinate red cells in saline but do so in a "high protein" medium. One of the first used was the natural one, human serum—the resulting agglomeration of cells being called "conglutination".

Various other media were tried; the most effective was found to be bovine albumin, fraction 5 of the Cohn separation. Incomplete anti-D antibodies will cause firm agglutination of D-positive red cells suspended in 20–30 per cent bovine albumin. No other protein medium has been found to be as effective as bovine albumin while giving negative reactions free from pseudo-agglutination.

(3) Tests Using Anti-human Globulin

Human globulin if injected into an animal of another species will act as an antigen and cause the animal to produce specific anti-human globulin antibodies. These antibodies are capable of reacting with all human globulin molecules including those which are antibodies. The reaction will still take place even if the antibodies (*e.g.* anti-D) are already specifically attached to red cells. In these circumstances the red cells will be clumped. Anti-human globulin (AHG or Coombs' reagent) is serum from animals, usually rabbits, immunised with either whole human serum or the precipitated globulin fraction. Unwanted antibodies are removed leaving a serum specific for human globulin. (For details of the preparation and standardisation of anti-human globulin *see* Appendix I.) In the present chapter the method of using the anti-human globulin reaction to detect incomplete anti-D antibodies in human serum is described in great detail, for once the basic technique has been mastered it will be found easy to adapt it for other purposes.

(4) Tests Involving the Use of Proteolytic Enzymes

It has been stated that incomplete antibodies will not cause agglutination of red cells in a saline medium. This is true of untreated red cells but Pickles discovered in 1946 that cholera filtrate would modify red cells to make them agglutinable in saline by incomplete antibodies. It was felt that this was due to a proteolytic action on the red cell surface and other enzymes known to have proteolytic activity were tested. Many of them were found to have the same effect and today four are in general use, namely papain, trypsin, ficin and bromelin. We shall describe techniques using all these enzymes although our personal preference is for papain. The mechanism by which these enzymes render cells capable of being agglutinated by incomplete antibodies is by no means fully understood. It is probably partly a direct result of proteolytic action which may expose receptors which were originally below the red cell surface making it easier for the small incomplete antibodies not only to combine with the cells but to link them together to form agglutinates. It is also probably due to changes in electrical charge upon the cells which enables them to approach each other more easily. Most enzyme techniques are two-stage with the cells being first modified by the enzyme and then exposed to the antibody containing serum. It is however also possible to adjust the potency of enzyme preparation, usually by means of an activator, so that the cells are adequately digested even in the presence of serum, making a one-stage test possible. The advantages of the enzyme techniques are sensitivity, avidity and speed of reaction. The main disadvantage is that some sera contain auto-antibodies against enzyme-treated cells which normally react with all of the test cells used. These have to be removed before the serum can be tested for iso-antibodies.

(5) **Blocking Test**

The blocking test is the test which was used originally to demonstrate the presence of "incomplete" antibodies. It cannot, however, be used to detect the presence of incomplete antibodies in a mixture of complete and incomplete unless the serum is first treated to remove the complete antibody. Moreover, not all types of incomplete antibody are capable of blocking red cell receptors.

The blocking antibodies will sensitise red cells in a saline diluent but will not cause them to agglutinate. In the presence of excess of anti-D incomplete antibody all the D receptors of the red cells will have this antibody attached to them and are said to be "blocked", that is incapable of taking up more antibody. When such blocked cells are mixed with serum containing saline anti-D agglutinins there are no free D receptors with which the agglutinins can react, therefore no agglutination takes place. The absence of agglutination between cells containing the D antigen and serum containing anti-D agglutinins clearly demonstrates the presence of anti-D blocking incomplete antibodies attached to the D receptors.

Techniques

In the following techniques standard cells from one D-positive and one D-negative individual are used; these will detect the presence of an antibody. For the complete establishment of the identity of the antibody further tests are necessary; these are discussed after the various Rh antibodies are described (Chapter 13).

Technique No. 10.1. Detection of Rh antibodies—saline

One unit volume of the serum under test is placed in each of two precipitin tubes by means of the graduated Pasteur pipette. To one is added one unit volume of D positive and to the other one unit volume of D negative red cells (2 per cent suspensions in normal saline). The tests are incubated at 37°C for at least 2 hours. Whenever possible the tests are left for 3–4 hours as the agglutination becomes "tighter" and thus more easily read. The cell sediment is examined for agglutination under the low power (2/3) of the microscope (for preparation of film *see* Chapter 2). It must be emphasised that the gentle handling of the sedimented cells in making the smear is even more important in all antibody detection tests than it is in the Rh typing of red cells. For typing red cells potent known sera are used and the degree of agglutination will be much greater than will often be the case when a search for antibodies is being made in entirely unknown sera. Results are recorded as for Rh typing.

Comment. The saline technique is the best for the detection of agglutinins and, therefore, should always be included in any antibody detection routine.

Technique No. 10.2. Detection of Rh antibodies—albumin

One volume of a 2 per cent suspension in saline of standard cells is mixed with one volume of unknown serum, each serum being tested with D positive and D negative cells. The mixtures are then incubated for 1½ hours at 37°C. Then one volume of 30 per cent bovine albumin is allowed to run down the side of each tube to form a layer over the red cell button, care being taken that the red cells are not disturbed. The tests are re-incubated for a further 30 minutes at 37°C, then read.

Comment. This test should only be used in conjunction with anti-globulin and/or enzyme techniques.

Technique No. 10.3a. Indirect anti-human globulin (Coombs) test*

This test has three stages: (1) sensitisation of the red cells; (2) washing the cells free of all traces of serum; (3) mixing the washed red cells with the anti-human globulin serum (Coombs reagent).

There are an almost bewildering number of modifications of

* When the indirect anti-human globulin is used as a typing technique (*e.g.* techniques Nos. 10.10 and 17.1 it is essential to include the direct anti-human globulin (10.3b) on the unknown cells as a negative control. If this control is positive *see* Chapters 20 and 26.

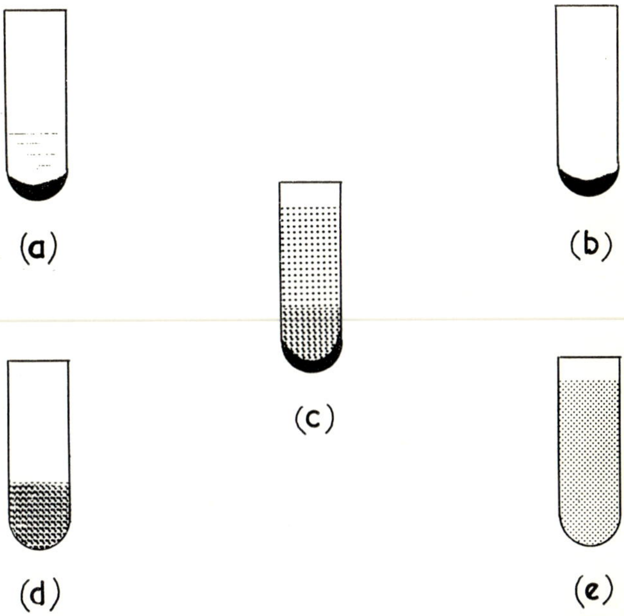

FIG. 10.1. Washing of red cells for Coombs tests.

(*a*) Red cell button and clear supernatant.
(*b*) Supernatant removed.
(*c*) Incorrect washing. Uneven suspension of cells can be corrected by mixing with a Pasteur pipette or tapping with the finger, inversion and vigorous shaking.
(*d*) Correct washing—Stage I. Re-suspension of cells in a small quantity of saline (shake rack or tap tubes individually to ensure even suspension).
(*e*) Correct washing—Stage II. Tube filled with saline to give an even suspension throughout.

p. 86

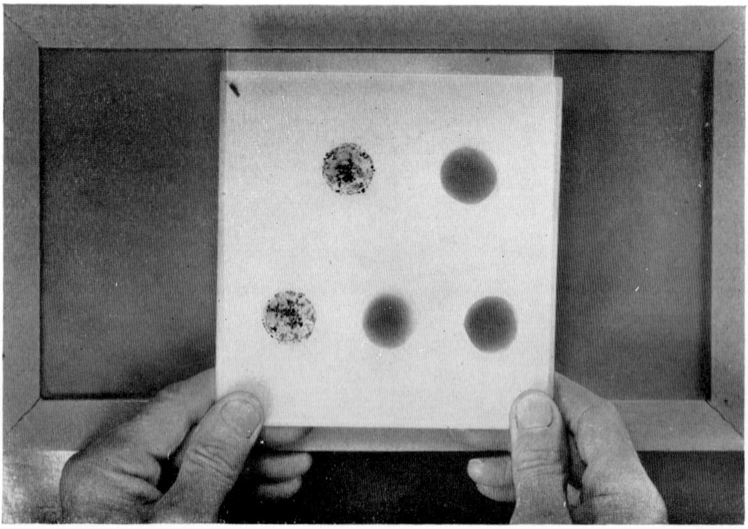

PLATE 8. Reading of the Coombs test (from above).

To face p. 87]

this technique but the following method has been selected as one giving very satisfactory results.

(1) *Sensitisation.* Two unit volumes (0·03 ml. each) of the serum to be tested are mixed with 4 volumes of approximately 5 per cent D positive red cells and a further two volumes are mixed with 4 volumes of 5 per cent D negative red cells in the 50 mm. × 11 mm. cell suspension tubes. The cells used should have been washed three times as traces of plasma may result in small clots which interfere with the reading of the results.

The same D positive and D negative red cells are mixed with a serum containing weak, incomplete anti-D antibodies to act as positive and negative controls. The tests are incubated at 37° for 1 hour.

(2) *Washing.* The supernatant fluid is discarded and the cell sediment washed three times in saline. The thorough washing of the red cells at this stage is most important as any free globulin (even as little as one part in several thousand parts of saline) left in solution will react with and so diminish the activity of the anti-human globulin serum. For each wash therefore the cells are completely re-suspended in at least 100 times their own volume of clean saline.

It is the complete suspension of the cells, especially after centrifugation, which often presents difficulty. Fig. 10.1 shows both correct and incorrect washing of tests. An adequate method for washing is achieved by the addition of a small quantity of saline 10.1(*d*) in which the cells are evenly suspended either by a vigorous jarring of the rack or by lifting each tube and tapping with the finger. The tube is then filled to the top with saline and the result is an even suspension of cells in sufficient saline for adequate washing 10.1(*e*). Of course if a jet of saline of sufficient force to cause even suspension of cells can be directed into each tube, then no further handling of the tubes is necessary, but in our experience this is difficult to achieve.

(3) *Mixture with Anti-human Globulin.* Directions for the dilution of the anti-human globulin with saline will be supplied with the reagent. The recommended dilution will probably be between 1 in 50 and 1 in 100. Great care must be exercised to ensure that all glassware used in making up and putting out anti-human globulin reagent is absolutely clean and free from traces of human serum which would inevitably react with some of the anti-human globulin in the reagent. If contamination of the diluted reagent is suspected, it should be centrifuged: the appearance of a white film on the bottom of the tube will confirm the suspicion of

contamination with serum and the reagent should be discarded. Unused diluted reagent can be kept frozen at −20°C for about a week provided it is not thawed and re-frozen more than once a day and is always carefully checked by controls. The mixture of cells with human globulin is best performed on an opalescent tile but microscope slides can be used if preferred. The tile must be scrupulously cleaned with soap and water and rinsed thoroughly under running water and polished with a clean dry cloth. One drop of diluted reagent is then mixed with one drop of weakly sensitised D positive control cells to ensure that the reagent is active. Mixture can be conveniently effected with a small plastic rod. Glass slides or glass mixing rods are not recommended since the presence of colloidal silica in the test fluid may cause false agglutination to occur.

The tile or slide is gently rocked (it must not be shaken or jarred), left to stand for a few minutes, rocked once more and the result read macroscopically over a light. The D negative control cells are set out at the same time. It is also recommended that washed group AB cells should be included as a further negative control to ensure that the reagent is not giving "non-specific" agglutination due to insufficient absorption from the serum of "anti-man" antibodies. If these controls are satisfactory, the tests are then set out in a similar manner, positive and negative controls being included in each batch of tests—these act as "time controls" the tests being read after the positive control shows definite agglutination and before the appearance of any "non-specific" agglutination in the negative controls (Plate 8).

Comment. This is a very delicate test, involving great care at every stage for reliable results. False positives are most likely to be obtained through dust particles in saline, colloidal silica or small plasma clots, false negatives through the reagent becoming inactive due to contamination with serum proteins. It cannot be recommended for large-scale routine work where time is not available for the unhurried performance of a complicated test. It is the best single test for incomplete antibodies of all types and should always be used in direct matching and special investigations.

Technique No. 10.3b. Direct anti-human globulin (Coombs) test

The object of this test is to determine whether the red cells of certain patients (notably hæmolytic anæmias and infants thought to be suffering from hæmolytic disease of the newborn) have become sensitised by antibodies *in vivo*. The test is distinguished from that described above (10.3a) in that the first stage, *viz.* incubation of test serum with red cells in order to sensitise them, is omitted.

The red cells suspected to be sensitised *in vivo* are carefully washed at least three times in a large volume of saline. They are then mixed with anti-human globulin serum (Coombs reagent) on a tile and read exactly in the manner described above. An extra control of the patient's washed red cells with a drop of saline to replace the anti-human globulin reagent is included. The development of agglutination in the anti-human globulin-red cell mixture shows that the red cells are sensitised by antibody. It should be noted that while this test reveals the presence of incomplete antibodies on the red cells it does not identify their specificity. This must be determined in other ways, one of which is to elute the antibody by technique No. 21.3, 26.4, 26.10, or 26.11 and to test the eluate with a panel of standard cells by technique No. 21.1.

Technique No. 10.4. Trypsin technique

There are several preparations of trypsin which can be used partially to digest the test red cells. (*See* Appendix I.)

Preparation of Trypsin treated Cells. The standard D positive and D negative red cells are freshly bled into 3·8 per cent tri-sodium citrate, separated by centrifugation and washed twice with 0·85 per cent saline.

The washed packed cells then have the buffered trypsin solution added to them in the proportion of four parts of solution to each part of packed cells—both solution and cells should be at 37°C for at least 5 minutes before being mixed.

The red cell/enzyme mixture is incubated at 37°C for $\frac{1}{2}$ to $\frac{3}{4}$ hour, *i.e.* sufficient time to render the D positive cells agglutinable by an incomplete anti-D but not so long that they become pan-agglutinable or even completely hæmolysed.

The red cells are then washed twice with an excess of warm (37°C) saline and stored in bulk in the hot room or water bath until needed. Before adding the trypsin-treated cells to the test sera, a 4 per cent suspension of the cells is made in warm saline.

Antibody Detection. One unit volume of each of the unknown sera is measured into each of two precipitin tubes and left at 37°C for 10 minutes before the addition of an equal volume of trypsin-treated red cells, D positive to one set of tubes and D negative to the other. They are then incubated for 1 hour. The tests are read by gently tapping the tubes and examining them macroscopically for agglutination, negatives are confirmed microscopically. A control serum known to contain a weak anti-D antibody is included in each batch of tests; only if this gives a macroscopic positive with the D positive and a clear negative with the D negative cells should the rest of the tests be read.

Comment. This is a very sensitive and useful technique. Occasionally sera are encountered which give pan-agglutination with trypsin treated red cells. The antibody responsible for the pan-agglutination can usually be quite easily removed by incubating the serum with an equal volume of the patient's own trypsin treated red cells. The absorbed serum can then be re-examined for the presence of specific antibodies with the standard trypsin treated cells.

Technique No. 10.5a. Löw's papain technique for antibody detection—one stage

Equal volumes of the serum to be tested, papain (for preparation *see* Appendix I) and a 2 per cent suspension of red cells are placed in a precipitin tube, taking care to adhere strictly to the order: (*a*) serum, (*b*) papain, (*c*) red cells. It is also important that the serum/papain mixture should not be allowed to stand on the bench for more than about five minutes before the red cells are added. It has been noted that the best results are obtained if the red cells are allowed to sink through the fluid during the incubation period. Therefore the contents of the tubes are not mixed up at the initial stage. This is known as a layering technique. The test is read after precisely one hour's incubation, controls of known D positive and D negative cells with a weak incomplete anti-D being included with each batch of tests.

Comment. This is a good and efficient technique and is excellent for the detection of Rh antibodies. In fact anti-D antibodies may be detectable by this technique when they are not apparent by any non-enzyme technique, even the anti-human globulin. It does, however, give positives when certain other antibodies are present such as anti-P_1 anti-Lewis, anti-H, etc., so that care must be taken in the establishment of the specificity of any antibody detected by this method. Auto-antibodies are also encountered and can be removed by absorption of the serum with an equal volume of the patient's own papain treated cells, after which the absorbed serum is retested.

The technique is also useful as a typing technique if the typing serum being used works best in papain or is a "papain type" antibody. Anti-e is often such an antibody.

Technique No. 10.5b. Papain technique—two stage

To treat cells with papain either a saturated solution of papain or the Löw's papain which contains cystine as an activator (*see* Appendix I) can be used.

The use of Löw's papain is preferable because it is a standard solution and the digestion time can be cut to 15 minutes.

For the preparation of papain treated cells, washed, packed cells are used as for the trypsin technique. One part of the Löw's papain is added to one part of 50 per cent of suspension of cells and incubated for 15–20 minutes. The red cells are then washed twice with an excess of warm (37°C) saline and stored at 37°C until needed.

Antibody Detection. One unit volume of each of the unknown sera is measured into a precipitin tube and left at 37°C for 10 minutes after which one volume of a 2 per cent suspension of papain treated cells is added. The test is incubated at 37°C for 1 hour—the sediment re-suspended by gentle tapping and the degree of agglutination read macroscopically and if necessary microscopically. The sensitivity can be increased by slow centrifugation before reading.

Comment. This technique is slightly more sensitive than even the one stage papain test. It has the same disadvantages as the one stage technique, in that it detects some cold antibodies and auto-antibodies. The latter can be removed by absorbtion of the serum with the patient's own papain treated cells and the absorbed serum retested.

Technique No. 10.6. Detection of Rh antibodies using bromelin

A solution of bromelin is prepared as described in Appendix I. The original technique using bromelin was one where cells, serum and bromelin solution were centrifuged at 1,500 r.p.m. for 1–2 minutes, without prior incubation. This has been found to be very unreliable. The following technique is standard in a number of laboratories in England.

The stock solution of bromelin is diluted 1 in 2 in saline, buffered with Sorensen's buffer ph 7·3 on the day of use. If kept, the diluted bromelin deteriorates rapidly.

Equal volumes of diluted bromelin solution, serum and red cells are placed in a precipitin tube and incubated at 37°C for 1 hour. The sediment is gently agitated and the tests read macroscopically for agglutination.

Comment. This technique is by no means as sensitive as papain for the detection of anti-D. The fact that fewer cold antibodies and auto-antibodies are detected by it does not compensate for its failure to detect some weak Rh antibodies. A further disadvantage is that batches of bromelin vary so that the sensitivity of the test varies also. Moreover the enzyme is less stable than papain or trypsin.

Technique No. 10.7. Detection of Rh antibodies using ficin

For the preparation of stock solution and Hendry's buffer *see* Appendix I.

Ficin Treatment of Cells. Ficin for use is made by adding 1 volume of stock solution to 39 volumes of Hendry's buffer. These 40 volumes are warmed to 37°C when one volume of packed washed cells is added and the mixture incubated for exactly 15 minutes at 37°C. The cells are then washed three times in saline and stored at 37°C until needed.

Antibody Detection. One volume of test serum is measured into each of two precipitin tubes and left at 37°C for 10 minutes, after which one volume of ficin treated cells is added, D-positive cells to the first tube and D-negative to the second. They are incubated for 1 hour and then read macroscopically for agglutination.

Comment. This is a very sensitive technique. Its main disadvantages are firstly the care that must be taken with powdered ficin and secondly that the digestion time is very critical, a few moments over or under can result respectively in a false positive or a false negative reaction being obtained. Like the other enzyme techniques auto-antibodies are often detected which have to be removed by absorption with the patient's own treated cells before the test with standard cells can be performed.

Technique No. 10.8. Blocking test

This is not so sensitive a test for the presence of incomplete antibodies as either the albumin or the Coombs test but it is the only test that demonstrates their "blocking" nature and thus shows that complete and incomplete antibodies even when of the same specificity are not identical.

One unit volume of unknown serum is mixed with one unit volume of a 2 per cent red cell suspension in saline of D-positive cells. The tests are incubated at 37°C for 1 hour.

The controls on this test consist of (1) one unit volume of group AB serum, and (2) one unit volume of a serum known to contain incomplete anti-D, to each of which are added one volume of the 2 per cent suspension of D-positive cells. These are incubated for 1 hour at 37°C with the tests on the unknown sera. Then a unit volume of a saline agglutinating anti-D which has been diluted to give a ++ reaction is added to each tube. The tubes are well shaken and allowed to stand for a further 1½ hours after which

Table 10.1

Specimen Results Obtained by the Blocking Test

Serial No. of serum tested	Reaction after first stage	Reaction after second stage	Conclusion
1213	–	++	No antibody demonstrated
1306	–	(+)	Incomplete anti-D present
1175	–	–	Incomplete anti-D present
Control (1), AB serum	–	++	No antibody present
Control (2), incomplete anti-D	–	–	Incomplete anti-D present

they are examined for agglutination. Absence of agglutination or definitely diminished agglutination in the test as compared with control tube (1) together with no agglutination in control tube (2) indicates the presence of blocking antibody in the unknown serum. (*See* Table 10.1 for specimen results.)

It will be realised that this test for incomplete antibodies cannot be performed in the presence of saline agglutinins as the test cells would be agglutinated during the first stage. If for any reason it is important to show whether a serum does in fact contain incomplete as well as complete antibodies, it is necessary first to inactivate the latter. This may be done in several ways; probably the easiest is to dilute the serum with an equal part of saline (to minimise the risk of coagulation) and then heat at 70°C for approximately 10 minutes. The exact time needed to destroy all the agglutinins without appreciably increasing the viscosity of the serum varies and must be determined by trial and error.

Comment. This is not a sensitive technique and is only used when it is required to prove that a given antibody can specifically block red cell receptors.

Titration of Rh Antibodies

Technique No. 10.9. Saline. Serial dilutions of the serum are made in saline as in technique No. 4.2 (or if desired techniques

Nos. 4.3 or 4.4) and incubated at 37°C for 2 hours with standard D-positive red cells (2 per cent suspension) in saline. The tests are read taking the usual precautions against breaking down the agglutinates. The results are recorded as for ABO titres. *See* Plates 6 and 7.

Technique No. 10.10. Albumin two-stage method. Tests are set up as for technique No. 10.9 but using AB serum as diluent. After 1½ hours' incubation bovine albumin is added without disturbing the cells. After a further 30 minutes' incubation the tests are read in the usual manner.

Technique No. 10.11. Indirect anti-human globulin (Coombs) technique. Serial dilutions of the serum are made in saline using double unit volumes (0·06 ml.) in the cell-suspension tubes. A half unit volume (0·015 ml.) of packed washed D-positive red cells is added to each tube. From this point the procedure is exactly as in technique No. 10.3a.

Technique No. 10.12a. Two-stage Papain or Trypsin. The serial dilutions of serum are made in saline and warmed to 37°C before the addition to each tube of an equal volume of papain treated or trypsin treated D-positive red cells. The tests are incubated for 1 hour, centrifuged and read by tapping the tubes and examining the contents macroscopically and if necessary microscopically for agglutination.

Technique No. 10.12b. One-stage Papain. The serial dilutions are made as for technique No. 10.10 (it is important to use AB serum as diluent as if saline is used the enzyme will over papainise the cells and give false positive reactions), after which one volume of Löw's papain is added to each tube. This is followed immediately by an equal volume of a 2 per cent suspension in saline of D-positive red cells. Care is taken to layer the serum, papain and red cells, if they are mixed the titre will be substantially reduced. The tubes are incubated for exactly 1 hour and then read, first tapping the tube twice gently before examining the contents macroscopically and, if negative, microscopically.

Technique No. 10.13. Blocking Titre. Serial dilutions of the serum containing blocking antibody are made and one volume of a 2 per cent suspension of D-positive red cells added to each tube. A control consisting of equal volumes of AB serum and the D-positive cells is set up at the same time. After 1 hour's incubation at 37°C a unit volume of a saline anti-D diluted to give a ++ reaction is added to each tube. The tubes are well shaken and incubated for a further 1½ hours. The tests are read with the usual Rh precautions (for a specimen protocol *see* Table 10.2).

Table 10.2

Protocol of Blocking Titre

	Dilutions of serum containing incomplete antibody								Control of AB serum
	Neat	$\frac{1}{2}$	$\frac{1}{4}$	$\frac{1}{8}$	$\frac{1}{16}$	$\frac{1}{32}$	$\frac{1}{64}$	$\frac{1}{128}$	
Reaction of added saline anti-D with D-positive red cells	−	−	−	w	(+)	+	++	++	++

Interpretation of Results

Sera are usually tested by at least two of the techniques, Nos. 10.1–5b in parallel; *e.g.* in the testing of Rh negative women ante-natally it is recommended that the saline (No. 10.1) albumin addition (No. 10.2) and the papain (10.5a or b) or trypsin (10.4) are used. Various patterns of reaction that may be obtained are shown in Table 10.3.

Table 10.3

Results that may be obtained in Antibody Tests

	Sal.		Albumin		Papain		Conclusion and further investigation	
	D+	D−	D+	D−	D+	D−		
1.	+	−	+	−	+	−	Anti-D	Check with further D+ and D− cells and titrate (1–3)
2.	−	−	+	−	+	−	Anti-D incomplete type	
3.	−	−	−	−	+	−	Anti-D incomplete type found either at beginning or end of immune process	
4.	+	+	+	+	+	+	Not anti-D	Needs full antibody investigation
5.	−	−	+	+	+	+	Not anti-D	,,

The finding of a positive reaction with D positive cells and a negative reaction with D negative cells with serum from an individual whose own cells are D negative means that there is a high probability that the antibody is in fact anti-D. Nevertheless, a confirmatory test with a slightly larger panel of known cells should be done. Three examples of D positive and two of D negative cells are adequate and should be used by the techniques by which the antibody is reacting best and it should only be reported as anti-D if clear-cut positives (ranging + to C) or negatives are obtained. If the positive reactions are inconclusive ((+) or w) the tests should be repeated and if still weak the presence of anti-D antibody should not be considered conclusive until confirmed in a later sample. It must be realised that a serum behaving like anti-D in the above tests may, in fact, be a mixture of Rh antibodies (*see* Chapter 13). Occasionally, as in examples 4 and 5, Table 10.3, the antibody belongs to one of the other blood group systems (*see* Section 4 in Chapter 21).

Classes of Rh Antibody

The results of saline, albumin, anti-human globulin, blocking and enzyme techniques in parallel in tests for Rh antibodies have revealed differences which have enabled four classes of Rh antibody to be clearly distinguished and there may be others.

The four classes are as follows:

(*a*) Agglutinin which is characterised by its ability to agglutinate red cells in saline suspension.
(*b*) Cryptagglutinoid which is an incomplete antibody detectable by albumin, anti-human globulin and enzyme techniques but which does not block nor agglutinate red cells in saline.
(*c*) Agglutinoid which is not reactive by saline or albumin methods, but is detectable with anti-human globulin, blocking and possibly by enzyme tests.
(*d*) "Papain type" antibody which is negative or at most weak with anti-human globulin and albumin and is best detected by papain technique, although it is sometimes reactive by ficin or trypsin.

The reactions of these antibodies are to be found in Table 10.4. In any given serum these are unlikely to be so clear cut, as the serum probably will contain at least two and possibly all four types of antibody in varying proportions and the different kinds may mask each other. These points are particularly relevant in the interpretation of titres.

The four classes of Rh antibody described above are, as mentioned, based on differences of behaviour of the antibodies in certain techniques. These are related to the classes of immunoglobulins, as follows:

(*a*) mostly IgM with some IgG,
(*b*) and (*c*) IgG and may also be active in the IgA class;
(*d*) is IgM.

Interpretation of Titres

In routine work titres are carried out by saline or albumin techniques in parallel and in special cases by anti-human globulin and/or enzyme techniques in addition. The finding of a negative or low titre in saline in association with a moderate or high titre in albumin only establishes the presence of cryptagglutinoids (*see* Table 10.4). It cannot even be assumed that agglutinins are absent since in the presence of agglutinoids (blocking antibodies) the agglutinins may be prevented from reacting with the red cells. Evidence that this is sometimes the state of affairs is obtained when sera are analysed by salting out and electrophoresis or fractionated by column chromatography. It should be noted that a titre of 1 or 2 with red cells suspended in saline is not good evidence for saline/agglutinins since, at these low dilutions, there may be sufficient concentration of protein for agglutination of the cells to be caused by incomplete antibody.

A moderate or high titre by saline technique establishes unequivocably the presence of agglutinins, but unless the titre in albumin is at least two dilutions higher, the assumption that incomplete antibodies are present also cannot be made without further tests, *e.g.* after heating the serum, etc.

Table 10.4

Classes of Rh Antibodies and Techniques for their Detection and Differentiation

Classes of Rh antibody	Reactions by various techniques					
	Saline	Albumin	A.H.G.	Trypsin	Papain	Blocking
Agglutinin	+	+	+	+	+	–
Cryptagglutinoid	–	+	+	+	+	weak or –
Agglutinoid	–	–	+	?	?	+
Papain type antibody	–	–	weak or –	weak or –	+	–

CHAPTER 11

THE VARIOUS Rh ANTIGENS WITH SPECIAL REFERENCE TO THE FISHER NOMENCLATURE AND THEORY OF INHERITANCE

IT was not long before it was realised that important though the first described Rh antigen (now called D) and its corresponding antibody (anti-D) were, they were not by any means the whole of the Rh system.

In 1941 American workers noted that not all so called anti-Rh sera gave parallel results and it seemed, therefore, that more than one Rh antigen and its corresponding antibody might exist. Moreover the reactions obtained with some of the anti-sera suggested that they were in fact a mixture of two Rh antibodies. In addition another antibody was found which agglutinated all Rh negative red cells as well as many which were Rh positive. This antibody was called anti-Hr to show that its reactions were in some measure antithetical to those of anti-Rh. With these new antibodies it was found possible to subdivide the original Rh positive and Rh negative groups.

Concurrently with the American work three antibodies, which were obviously related to the Rh system, were being investigated in England.

One of these, which agglutinated the red cells of about 70 per cent of all individuals, was obviously related to anti-Rh in that almost all the red cells which were positive with this serum were also Rh positive. This antibody was called anti-Rh_1.

The second antibody was also related to anti-Rh in that almost all the cells with which it gave a positive reaction were Rh positive but differed strikingly in that it only agglutinated some 30 per cent of the samples with which it was tested. This antibody was called anti-Rh_2.

The third antibody agglutinated the cells of all Rh negative individuals and some Rh positives (including all those positive with anti-Rh_2) giving an overall frequency for the antigen it was detecting of approximately 80 per cent. This antibody was called "St" after the woman in whom it was found, pending a nomenclature which would describe its place in the Rh system.

This antibody was later found to be identical with the anti-Hr mentioned above.

These three sera enabled the English workers also to subdivide the Rh positive and Rh negative groups and it was very satisfying that the subdivisions made quite independently on both sides of the Atlantic were in all essentials the same.

This pattern of discovery, *i.e.* the finding of antibodies which are obviously reacting with antigens related to but not identical with the original antigen, is one which recurs in almost all blood group systems. A theory then has to be formulated to explain how the various sub-groups arise and are inherited. There are two main theories about the origin and inheritance of the Rh subtypes. We shall here describe in most detail that of Fisher because, in our opinion, it is the clearest way to approach the subject and to gain a working knowledge of the main Rh subgroups and the antibodies with which they react. In Tables 11.1 and 11.2 the Wiener nomenclature is given in parallel to that of Fisher for the benefit of those readers who may wish to convert one to the other. A short paragraph explaining Wiener's theory appears below.

From a study of the results obtained Fisher noticed that the reactions of anti-Rh_1 and the serum St were antithetical and so he postulated that the genes responsible for the production of the antigens recognised by those two antibodies were allelomorphic. He chose to call them C and c. The two remaining antibodies, anti-Rh and anti-Rh_2 were not showing antithetical reactions. The antigen picked out by anti-Rh was called D and the antibody anti-D. Similarly the antigen picked out by anti-Rh_2 was called E and so anti-Rh_2 was called anti-E. It seemed likely that the genes for these antigens also would have allelomorphs which would fit into the system and be called d and e. Thus an Rh system controlled by three pairs of allelomorphic genes Cc, Dd and Ee had been formulated. Since many family studies with the four anti-sera had been made without a single example of a cross-over being found it was assumed that the genes must be very closely linked.

Support for the theory was obtained through the discovery of an antibody which gave the exact reactions predicted for anti-e. Later the eighth gene combination R_y (CdE) was found.

However, an antibody with the predicted reactions for 'd' has not been discovered, despite several false alarms, and 'd' is now regarded as being 'silent'.

Table 11.2 shows the reactions between the antigens formed by the eight gene complexes and the four most commonly used

Table 11.1

The Eight Rh Gene Complexes

Fisher notation	Common notation	Wiener notation	Frequency
CDe	R_1	R^1	0·421
cDE	R_2	R^2	0·141
cDe	R_0	R^0	0·026
CDE	R_z	R^z	0·002
Cde	R′	r'	0·010
cdE	R″	r''	0·012
CdE	R_y	r^y	very low
cde	r	r	0·389

Note. All figures quoted in this table apply to the English population, being based on the figures quoted in *Blood Groups in Man*, Race & Sanger, 1954.

Table 11.2

The Eight Rh Blood Types and their Reactions with the Four most commonly used Anti-sera

Wiener		Fisher	Reactions with Serum			
Agglutinogen	Blood Factors	Antigen Complex	**Anti-rh′** Anti-C	**Anti-rh″** Anti-E	**Anti-Rh_0** Anti-D	**Anti-hr′** Anti-c
Rh_0	**Rh_0, hr′, hr″ and hr**	cDe	−	−	+	+
Rh_1	**Rh_0, rh′ and hr″**	CDe	+	−	+	−
Rh_2	**Rh_0, rh″ and hr′**	cDE	−	+	+	−
Rh_z	**Rh_0, rh′ and rh″**	CDE	+	+	+	−
rh	**hr′, hr″ and hr**	cde	−	−	−	+
rh′	**rh′ and hr″**	Cde	+	−	−	−
rh″	**rh″ and hr′**	cdE	−	+	−	+
rhy	**rh′ and rh″**	CdE	+	+	−	−

antibodies. It is of course an over-simplification as it is not possible to test single antigen complexes with the anti-sera because every individual will have two of these gene combinations making up his genotype, one inherited from each parent.

In Table 11.3 the 36 Rh genotypes are arranged in groups according to their reactions with the four generally available anti-sera.

and with anti-e for the C negative E positives. (The only place where the use of such a rare serum is justified by the additional information obtained.) These groups are the Rh phenotypes into which individuals can be classified according to the pattern of reactions their blood gives with the various anti-sera. The number of phenotypes that can be distinguished depends of course on the number of different anti-sera with which red cells are tested; *e.g.* if anti-D alone is used only two phenotypes D-positive and D-negative can be distinguished. Table 11.4 presents the same information in terms of Wiener nomenclature.

It can be seen from Table 11.3 that on the reactions with the four anti-sera and anti-e, where indicated, there are fourteen Rh sub-types or phenotypes. In a few cases, *e.g.* rr (cde.cde) and R′R′ (Cde.Cde) the phenotype discloses the only possible genotype but some of the other phenotype groups include many genotypes, *e.g.* the phenotype R_1R_2 giving the pattern ++++.

It will be appreciated by now that in only a few cases will tests, even with all the available anti-sera, disclose the actual genotype of an individual. At best a probable genotype may be deduced from the frequency with which each occurs within a particular phenotype, *e.g.* within the phenotype whose pattern of reaction is ++++ the genotype R_1R_2 (CDe.cDE) is 88·4 per cent of the phenotype. This means that the probable genotype, therefore, of an individual in this phenotype is R_1R_2 (CDe.cDE). This subject will be referred to again when discussing the interpretation of "genotyping" tests on husbands of women who have formed Rh antibodies. (*See* Chapter 25.)

A more accurate assessment of genotype can sometimes be made with the aid of family studies.

The mode of inheritance of the Rh gene combinations is illustrated in the particular mating R_1R_2 (CDe.cDE) × R_1r (CDe.cde) (Fig. 11.1). The Rh gene combinations being composed of closely linked genes on adjacent loci on a single chromosome are inherited as a unit and behave in this connexion like simple Mendelian dominants. This means that for any given antigen combination (*e.g.* CDe) to appear in the blood of a child it must be present in the blood of one or both parents.

Full tables giving all the possible matings to include every Rh sub-type and the sub-types of the children arising from such matings are too unwieldy to be given. Any required portion of such a table can readily be compiled when needed. For an example the mating R_1R_2 and R_1r can be taken. The phenotype R_1R_2 includes nine genotypes, namely, R_1R_2, $R'R_2$, R_1R'', R_0R_Z, R_Zr,

Table 11.3

The Rh Genotypes Arranged in Phenotypes

Reactions					Phenotypes			Genotypes			
					Name		Occurrence in total population	Name		Occurrence in total population	Occurrence in phenotype
C	D	E	c	e	Common English usage	Fisher	%	Common English usage	Fisher	%	%
–	–	–	+		rr	ccddee	15·102	rr	cdecde	15·102	100
–	–	+	+	+	R″r	ccddEe	0·924	R″r	cdEcde	0·924	100
+	–	–	+		R′r	Ccddee	0·764	R′r	Cdecde	0·764	100
+	–	+	+		R′R″	CcddEe	0·023	R′R″ R_yr R″R_y	CdecdE CdEcde cdECdE	0·023 0·000 0·000	100·0 0·0 0·0
–	–	+	+	–	R″R″	ccddEE	0·014	R″R″	cdEcdE	0·014	100
+	–	–	–		R′R′	CCddee	0·010	R′R′	CdeCde	0·010	100
+	–	+	–	+	R′R_y	CCddEe	0·000	R′R_y	CdeCdE	0·000	100
+	–	+	–	–	Ry Ry	CCddEE	0·000	R_yR_y	CdECdE	0·000	100
+	+	–	+		R_1r	CcDee	34·890	R_1r R_1R_0 R′R_0	CDecde CDecDe CdecDe	32·681 2·159 0·050	93·7 6·2 0·1

+	+	−	−		R_1R_1	CCDee	18·508	R_1R_1 R_1R'	CDeCDe CDeCde	17·680 0·828	95·5 4·5
+	+	+	+		R_1R_2	CcDEe	13·417	R_1R_2 R_1R'' $R'R_2$ R_zr R_2R_z R_0R_z $R''R_z$ R_2R_y R_0R_y	CDecDE CDecdE CdecDE CDEcde cDECDE cDeCDE cdECDE cDECdE cDeCdE	11·865 0·999 0·277 0·189 0·069 0·012 0·006 0·000 0·000	88·4 7·5 2·1 1·4 0·5 0·1 0·0 0·0 0·0
−	+	+	+	+	R_2r	ccDEe	11·751	R_2r R_2R_0 R_0R''	cDEcde cDEcDe cDecdE	10·966 0·724 0·061	93·3 6·2 0·5
−	+	+	+	−	R_2R_2	ccDEE	2·326	R_2R_2 R_2R''	cDEcDE cDEcdE	1·991 0·335	85·6 14·4
−	+	−	+		R_0r	ccDee	2·061	R_0r R_0R_0	cDecde cDecDe	1·995 0·066	96·8 3·2
+	+	+	−		R_1R_z	CCDEe	0·211	R_1R_z $R'R_z$ R_zR_z R_1R_y R_yR_z	CDeCDE CdeCDE CDECDE CDeCdE CdECDE	0·205 0·005 0·001 0·000 0·000	97·1 2·4 0·5 0·0 0·0

Table 11.4

The Rh–Hr Phenotypes and Genotypes

Reactions with Anti-sera					Phenotypes		Genotypes
Anti-Rh$_0$	**Anti-rh′**	**Anti-rh″**	**Anti-hr′**	**Anti-hr″**	Name	Frequencies N.Y.C. whites %	
−	−	−	+	+	rh	14·4	rr
−	+	−	+	+	rh′rh	0·46	$r'r$
−	+	−	−	+	rh′rh′	0·0036	$r'r'$
−	−	+	+	+	rh″rh	0·38	$r''r$
−	−	+	+	−	rh″rh″	0·0025	$r''r''$
−	+	+	+	+	rh′rh″	0·006	$r'r''r^yr$
−	+	+	−	+	rhyrh′	0·0001	r^yr'
−	+	+	+	−	rhyrh″	0·0001	r^yr''
−	+	+	−	−	rhyrhy	0·000001	r^yr^y
+	−	−	+	+	Rh$_0$	2·1	R^0R^0 *or* R^0r
+	+	−	+	+	Rh$_1$rh	33·4	$R'r$, $R'R^0$ *or* R^0r'
+	+	−	−	+	Rh$_1$Rh$_1$	17·3	$R'R'$ *or* $R'r'$
+	−	+	+	+	Rh$_2$rh	12·2	R^2r, R^2R^0 *or* R^0r''
+	−	+	+	−	Rh$_2$Rh$_2$	2·4	R^2R^2 *or* R^2r''
+	+	+	+	+	Rh$_1$Rh$_2$	12·9	$R'R^2$, $R'r''$, *or* R^2r', R^zr, R^zR^0, R^0r^y
+	+	+	−	+	Rh$_Z$Rh′	0·2	R^zR', R^zr' *or* $R'r^y$
+	+	+	+	−	Rh$_Z$Rh$_2$	0·07	R^zR^2, R^zr'' *or* R^2r^y
+	+	+	−	−	Rh$_Z$Rh$_Z$	0·0004	R^zR^z *or* R^zr^y

R_yR_0, R_2R_z, $R''R_z$, R_yR_2, and the phenotype group R_1r includes the three genotypes R_1r, R_1R_0, and $R'R_0$. Within this one phenotype mating we have, therefore, twenty-seven possibilities for the genotype mating, each giving rise to different Rh sub-types among

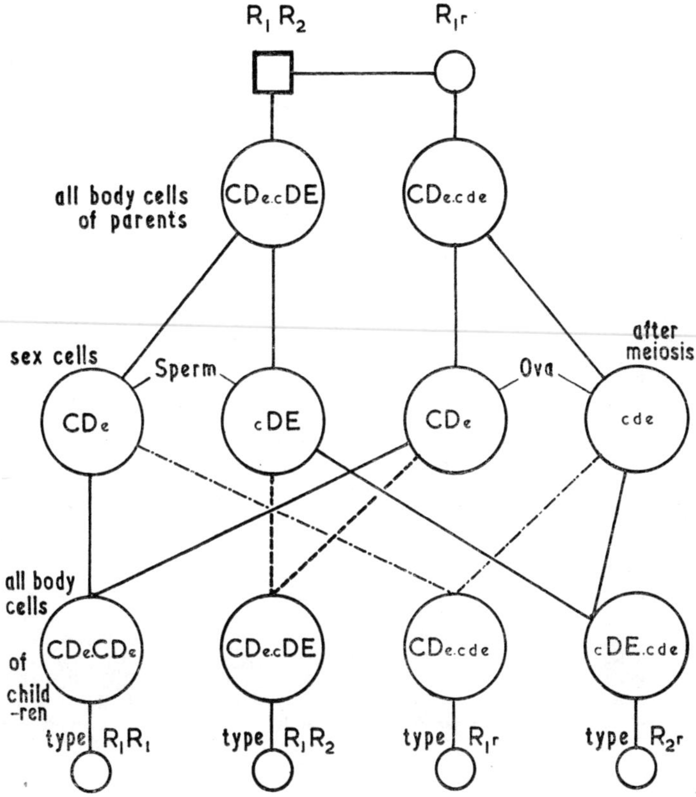

FIG. 11.1. The segregation of the Rh genes—illustrated by the mating $R_1R_2 \times R_1r$

the offspring (Table 11.5). It can be seen that occasionally the phenotype of one or more children of a mating will throw light on the actual genotype of one or the other, or both, parents; in other cases, of course, the phenotype of the children is no help and may even be misleading, *e.g.* when a child whose genotype is really R_zr is thought of as R_1R_2 which is the phenotype to which R_zr belongs.

Some phenotype matings are much less complicated than the example chosen because there are fewer alternative genotypes in each phenotype and in a few cases, *e.g.* rr and $R'r$ the genotype of

Table 11.5

The Phenotype Mating $R_1R_2 \times R_1r$

R_1R_2 phenotype	R_1r phenotype	Percentage occurrence of each genotype mating		Genotype of offspring (with phenotype name given in brackets where it differs from the genotype name)
Possible genotypes	Possible genotypes	Within the total population	Within the phenotype	
R_1R_2	R_1r	7·75	82·83	R_1R_1 R_1r R_1R_2 R_2r
$R'R_2$	R_1r	0·18	1·93	$R_1R'(R_1R_1)$ $R'r$ R_1R_2 R_2r
R_1R''	R_1r	0·65	6·97	R_1R_1 R_1r $R_1R''(R_1R_2)$ $R''r$
R_0R_z	R_1r	0·01	0·09	$R_1R_0(R_1r)$ R_0r R_1R_z $R_zr(R_1R_2)$
R_zr	R_1r	0·12	1·32	R_1R_z $R_zr(R_1R_2)$ R_1r rr
R_yR_0	R_1r	0·00	0·00	$R_1R_y(R_1R_z)$ $R_yr(R'R'')$ $R_1R_0(R_1r)$ R_0r
R_2R_z	R_1r	0·04	0·48	R_1R_2 R_2r R_1R_z $R_zr(R_1R_2)$
$R''R_z$	R_1r	0·00	0·04	$R_1R''(R_1R_2)$ $R''r$ R_1R_z $R_zr(R_1R_2)$
R_yR_2	R_1r	0·00	0·00	$R_1R_y(R_1R_z)$ $R_yr(R'R'')$ R_1R_2 R_2r
R_1R_2	R_1R_0	0·51	5·47	R_1R_1 $R_1R_0(R_1r)$ R_1R_2 $R_2R_0(R_2r)$
$R'R_2$	R_1R_0	0·01	0·13	$R_1R'(R_1R_1)$ $R'R_0(R_1r)$ R_1R_2 $R_2R_0(R_2r)$
R_1R''	R_1R_0	0·04	0·46	R_1R_1 $R_1R_0(R_1r)$ $R_1R''(R_1R_2)$ $R''R_0(R_2r)$
R_0R_z	R_1R_0	0·00	0·01	$R_1R_0(R_1r)$ $R_0R_0(R_0r)$ R_1R_z $R_0R_z(R_1R_2)$
R_zr	R_1R_0	0·01	0·09	R_1R_z $R_zR_0(R_1R_2)$ R_1r R_0r
R_yR_0	R_1R_0	0·00	0·00	$R_1R_y(R_1R_z)$ $R_yR_0(R_1R_2)$ $R_1R_0(R_1r)$ $R_0R_0(R_0r)$
R_2R_z	R_1R_0	0·00	0·03	R_1R_2 $R_2R_0(R_2r)$ R_1R_z $R_0R_z(R_1R_2)$
$R''R_z$	R_1R_0	0·00	0·00	$R_1R''(R_1R_2)$ $R''R_0(R_2r)$ R_1R_z $R_zR_0(R_1R_2)$
R_yR_2	R_1R_0	0·00	0·00	$R_1R_y(R_1R_z)$ $R_yR_0(R_1R_z)$ R_1R_2 $R_2R_0(R_2r)$
R_1R_2	$R'R_0$	0·01	0·13	$R_1R'(R_1R_1)$ $R_1R_0(R_1r)$ $R_2R'(R_1R_2)$ $R_2R_0(R_2r)$
$R'R_2$	$R'R_0$	0·00	0·00	$R'R'$ $R'R_0(R_1r)$ $R_2R'(R_1R_2)$ $R_2R_0(R_2r)$
R_1R''	$R'R_0$	0·00	0·01	$R_1R'(R_1R_1)$ $R_1R_0(R_1r)$ $R'R''$ $R''R_0(R_2r)$
R_0R_z	$R'R_0$	0·00	0·00	$R'R_0(R_1r)$ $R_0R_0(R_0r)$ $R'R_z(R_1R_z)$ $R_0R_z(R_1R_2)$
R_zr	$R'R_0$	0·00	0·00	$R'R_z(R_1R_z)$ $R_0R_z(R_1R_2)$ $R'r$ R_0r
R_yR_0	$R'R_0$	0·00	0·00	$R'R_y$ $R_0R_y(R_1R_2)$ $R'R_0(R_1r)$ $R_0R_0(R_0r)$
R_2R_z	$R'R_0$	0·00	0·00	$R'R_2(R_1R_2)$ $R_2R_0(R_2r)$ $R'R_z(R_1R_z)$ $R_0R_z(R_1R_2)$
$R''R_z$	$R'R_0$	0·00	0·00	$R'R''$ $R''R_0(R_2r)$ $R'R_z(R_1R_z)$ $R_0R_z(R_1R_2)$
R_yR_2	$R'R_0$	0·00	0·00	$R'R_y$ $R_0R_y(R_1R_2)$ $R_2R'(R_1R_2)$ $R_2R_0(R_2r)$

the whole phenotype group is the same. Thus the mating $R'r \times rr$ can be fully considered in the one line table:

Phenotype mating	*Genotypes of children*	*Phenotypes of children*
Genotype $R'r \times rr$	$R'r$ and rr	$R'r$ and rr

In this case of course it is possible to determine the actual genotype with the four anti-sera anti-C, anti-D, anti-E, and anti-c and family studies will merely confirm the findings.

The Theory of Wiener

Wiener favours the concept of one gene instead of three closely linked ones. However, to understand his theory fully, it is necessary to grasp his conception of agglutinogens and blood factors.

He postulates that a gene gives rise to an agglutinogen on the red cell surface and that this in turn possesses a number of blood factors. For example, the gene R^1 (*see* Table 11.1) gives rise to the agglutinogen Rh_1 which possesses the three blood factors $\mathbf{Rh_0}$, ***rh'*** and ***hr''*** (*see* Table 11.2).

It will be a relief to realise that the concept of one gene versus the concept of three closely linked genes has no significance in practical laboratory work beyond the unfortunate existence of a double nomenclature. Although we have found that the subgroups of Rh are more comprehensible to students using the Fisher nomenclature that of Wiener has in its favour an appreciation that the terms "gene" and "antigen" refer to different entities and therefore require distinguishing symbols. The Fisher nomenclature makes no such distinction between genes and antigens. Wiener adopts the convention of italics for genes or genotypes, regular face type for agglutinogens and phenotypes and bold-face type for blood factors and corresponding antibodies. The blood factor **hr** appearing in Table 11.2 refers to the Fisher compound antigen ce (*see* Chapter 33).

Rare Rh Genes

The Rh system is further complicated by such genes as C^w, C^x, c^v, C^u, G, V, etc., but it is not proposed to deal with these until Chapter 33. The antigen D^u however is discussed here because it is a common cause of anomalies in "D" typing.

D^u

Red cells of the type D^u (Table 11.6) are recognised by the fact that they are agglutinated by some anti-D sera but not others. Specific anti-sera have not been found for them. With the same range of anti-D sera different examples of D^u cells behave differently and for convenience may be classified as high grade or low grade. A high grade D^u red cell is one that is agglutinated by the majority of anti-D sera. A type of high grade D^u is sometimes encountered which is agglutinated by all sera but only weakly. A low grade D^u red cell is one which is only agglutinated by one or two of a range of sera with which it is tested, although it is sensitised by most of them, as can be proved by testing with anti-human globulin (Coombs test). Sometimes the D^u is of such a low grade that the fact that it has reacted at all with anti-D can only be detected by the indirect anti-human globulin test, or by pretreating the D^u cells with papain before testing with a powerful incomplete anti-D. In practice it is recommended that both these methods are used (*see* Chapter 12).

It is important to realise that pretreatment of a D^u cell with papain almost invariably renders it agglutinable by almost all anti-D sera.

It has been well established that D^u is inherited, *i.e.* a parent who is D^u can pass on to his child a D^u antigen which behaves towards anti-D sera as does the D^u antigen of the parent. The

Table 11.6

Examples of the Reactions Given by D^u Red Cells

D^u red cells	Reactions with anti-D sera											
	Saline agglutinating				Albumin agglutinating				Incomplete by Coombs technique			
	1	2	3	4	5	6	7	8	9	10	11	12
(*a*) High grade	V	V	—	V	V	V	V	—	V	V	V	V
(*b*) Low grade	—	—	V	—	—	V	—	—	V	V	V	V
(*c*) Low grade	—	—	—	—	—	—	—	—	V	V	V	V
(*d*) Low grade	V	—	—	—	—	—	—	—	V	—	V	V
(*e*) High grade	w	(+)	w	(+)	w	+	(+)	w	V	V	V	V

existence of D^u presents a problem when typing red cells using two anti-D sera; some red cells will be typed falsely as Rh negative when they are in fact D^u (*see* Chapter 12).

The D^u antigen if injected into individuals lacking D (*e.g.* cde.cde individuals) stimulates the production of normal anti-D antibodies which are in no way distinguishable from such antibodies which have been produced in response to a normal D.

The possible production of anti-D antibodies in a D^u individual has been widely considered and many D^u individuals, particularly of the low grade type, have had their serum examined for anti-D. It is unlikely that the true D^u is capable of being immunised by the D antigen. D positive people, who are found to have anti-D are most often those with a part of the D antigen missing who have formed an antibody against the missing fraction (*see* Chapter 33). These people are usually discovered through having the antibody in their serum rather than showing anything unusual in their red cell reactions. Only a study of their cells with many unpooled anti-D typing sera reveals their particular antigenic structure. It is usual to regard all D^u individuals as Rh positive for all practical purposes. (*See also* Chapter 33.)

CHAPTER 12

Rh SUB-TYPING

THE simple division of the Rh system into Rh positive (D positive) and Rh negative (D negative) using anti-D sera only, can now be extended by the use of the other Rh sera (anti-C, anti-E, etc.). These sera are not, however, in sufficiently good supply to allow of their routine use in Rh testing, nor indeed would the knowledge of the Rh sub-type be any real advantage for most purposes. This means that we have to consider how much testing is really necessary and the most economical way of using the available sera. The first step is always the division into D-positive and D-negative, therefore the further divisions and their appropriate techniques will be described under three headings: (1) subdivisions of D-negative; (2) subdivisions of D-positive ("genotyping"); (3) further investigation of anomalous results with anti-D.

Subdivision of D-negative

The subdivisions of the D-negative individuals are: (1) cde.cde (rr); (2) Cde.cde (R′r); (3) Cde.Cde (R′R′); (4) Cde.cdE (R′R″); (5) Cde.CdE ($R'R_y$); (6) cdE.cde (R″r); (7) cdE.cdE (R″R″); (8) cdE.CdE ($R''R_y$); (9) CdE.cde (R_yr); (10) CdE.CdE (R_yR_y).

Most of the foregoing subdivisions are very rare and thus seldom encountered. The most important is, of course, No. (1) cde.cde, after which (2) Cde.cde and (6) cdE.cde are the most frequent. Individuals of these sub-groups are all capable of making anti-D if stimulated by the D antigen and should, if in need of a blood transfusion, receive blood which is either Rh negative (cde.cde) or of their own genotype. Since the latter alternative is impracticable all of these must be regarded as Rh negative recipients.

It can be seen that all but the true Rh negatives (cde.cde) have either C or E or both of these antigens and if they are used as Rh negative donors for transfusion they may stimulate the production of anti-C or anti-E in the recipient. This means that every donor who is negative to anti-D serum must be tested further with anti-C and anti-E. Whenever time allows it is advisable to test all D negative patients also with anti-C and anti-E.

In practice it is recommended that this testing is carried out, not with pure anti-C and anti-E sera but with mixtures which contain anti-D as well. As will be seen in Chapter 14 sera which contain anti-D and anti-C (called for convenience anti-C+ D or anti-CD sera) and those which contain anti-D and anti-E (called for convenience anti-D + E or anti-DE sera) are much more readily obtainable than the pure sera and are just as suitable, if not more so, for the testing of red cells which have already been shown to be D negative. A possible error which has continually to be guarded against if Rh typing is to be done accurately is the designation Rh negative, R′ or R″ to red cells which are in reality Rh positive but of the very low grade D^u type. It is not dangerous to mistake low grade D^u individuals for R′ or R″ since they will then be regarded as Rh positive if they are donors of blood and Rh negative if they themselves are recipients. It is very fortunate that in the white population D^u is usually associated with C or E, cD^ue being very rare indeed. However, with the increase in the number of non-white races in Britain now, it is becoming essential to test all anti-D negatives for D^u. If several different anti-D sera are used to test any samples which appear to be D negative the chance of failure in detecting a low grade D^u is lessened, hence the advantage of using anti-C + D and anti-D + E mixtures in the further testing of D negatives. Moreover in this way two birds are killed with one stone! A test is made for the antigen C or E and D^u at the same time. A further method for the detection of low grade D^u is the indirect anti-human globulin test, with a powerful incomplete anti-D.

If there is still any doubt papain treated cells are tested with pure incomplete anti-D sera; almost all D^u cells give strong positive reactions by this technique.

The exact routine adopted for the confirmation of D negative blood samples is influenced by one or both of two main considerations: (*a*) whether the samples to be tested are from prospective donors or from patients who are, therefore, potential recipients; (*b*) the actual number of samples with which the laboratory has to deal. With regard to (*a*) it will by now have been appreciated that it is far more important to diagnose accurately the "D" position of donors than of patients. If a patient's blood is found to be negative with two anti-D, one anti-CD and one anti-DE or even merely with two anti-D sera then they are called Rh(D) negative and receive Rh negative blood. Donors, however, whose blood is negative with two anti-D sera should be tested more extensively. At this point consideration (*b*) arises, for, on the whole, samples from prospective donors are dealt with in large numbers by the serological laboratories of the Transfusion Service so that the routine selected must of necessity be related to the problem of coping with large numbers of tests. We recommend that donors' samples be tested with four additional anti-D sera. This can be done either by using two anti-D, one anti-CD and one anti-DE or, rather than rely on one serum for C and one for E, with two anti-CD and two anti-DE sera (provided sufficient sera of these types are available). By this means adequate tests for D can be carried out simultaneously with tests for C and E. The indirect anti-human globulin test is too involved and time-consuming a technique for the detection of D^u in large-scale testing unless the staff position and time factor will allow for the careful and meticulous handling that is needed for this test. The papain technique is a slightly more convenient technique which will detect all but a very few low grade D^u samples. If only one anti-CD and one anti-DE serum are used, further tests are necessary when a positive reaction is obtained with either the anti-CD or the anti-DE serum. This is for two reasons: (1) as stated above (Chapter 11) the presence of an antigen in the red cells should always be confirmed by testing with more than one anti-serum containing the corresponding antibody and (2) the possibility that the reaction is due to D^u. If two anti-CD and two anti-DE sera are used, providing the results are consistent, the first point is already covered but the second, the possibility of D^u, still remains.

It must be borne in mind that there are two antibodies operating in an anti-C + D or anti-D + E mixture so that any positive reaction obtained, in the one case might be due either to anti-C or anti-D and in the other to anti-D or anti-E. The cells being tested with such sera already will have been found negative with at least two anti-D sera so that any reaction obtained is more likely to be due to a C — anti-C or E — anti-E combination than to D — anti-D. However, there is always the possibility that the blood sample in question may in fact be of a low grade D^u type which happens to react with the particular anti-D which is present in one of the mixtures. In view of this, therefore, it is advisable to confirm samples which appear to be R′ or R″ with at least one if not two further anti-C + D or anti-D + E mixtures where this has not already been done. Moreover, a large number of apparent R′ and R″ cells are in fact of the low grade D^u type which only reveals its D antigen by indirect anti-human globulin test. Any samples which give positive reactions with either the anti-CD or anti-DE mixtures should be tested against incomplete anti-D sera by the anti-human globulin and papain techniques. If pure anti-C, and anti-c sera are available R′ cells can be checked with these, similarly R″ cells with anti-E and anti-e. We do not describe the use of these sera in techniques 12.1–4 but reference can be made to technique No. 12.5.

Before describing details of techniques the choice of controls for anti-CD and anti-DE sera must be mentioned. (*See* Table 21.) These are selected to test the satisfactory working of each antibody *independently*. In effect this means that any red cell containing C and not D can be used as a positive control for the anti-C component of the anti-CD mixture and any red cell containing D and not C will be suitable as a positive control for the anti-D of the same mixture. The most readily available cells

Table 12.1

Controls for Rh Sub-typing

Anti-serum	Positive controls	Negative controls*
D	R_1r or R_1R_2	rr or R′
CD	R′ and R_2r	rr
DE	R″ and R_1r	rr
C	R_1R_2	R_2r
C (from known D negative)	R_1R_2	R_2R_2
C (from known D positive)	R_1R_2	rr
E	R_1R_2	rr
c	R_1R_2	R_1R_1
e	R_1R_2	R_2R_2

* If group AB red cells of the required Rh sub-type are available, they form the best negative control, as they also control that the sera are adequately absorbed for anti-A and anti-B.

are R′r (Cde.cde) and R_2r (cDE.cde) respectively. Similarly for the proper control of the two components of the anti-DE mixture, red cells containing E and not D and others containing D and not E are suitable. The most easily obtained are R″r (cdE.cde) and R_1r (CDe.cde). For both mixtures the negative control is rr (cde.cde). (Table 12.1.)

All the tests described in this chapter are done by the standard tube method, emergency techniques not being applicable to confirmatory tests. In the case of an urgent blood transfusion, a patient who is negative with one or two anti-D sera is given Rh negative blood.

Techniques

Technique No. 12.1. Testing of samples screened as D-negative

The tests are set up as described for Rh typing by tube technique (technique No. 9.2) except that four rows of tubes will be required in the fifty-holed block so that the samples can be tested with either two anti-D, one anti-CD and one anti-DE 12.1a or alternatively two anti-CD and two anti-DE mixtures 12.1b. The sera used will be either "saline" or "albumin" type according to availability; all the cell suspensions are made in saline, albumin being added to the appropriate tubes at the end of $1\frac{1}{2}$ hours' incubation. Positive and negative controls as described above are included with each batch of tests. The tubes are incubated at 37°C for at least 2 hours and read taking the usual precautions for dealing with delicate agglutination. For interpretation of results and indications for use of techniques Nos. 12.2–4 *see* Table 12.2. If tests have been done with two anti-CD and two anti-DE sera techniques Nos. 12.2 and 12.3 are omitted.

Technique No. 12.2. Further testing of samples found to be negative with anti-D but positive with anti-CD

Two rows of tubes are required for these tests. In each tube of the first row is placed one volume of an anti-CD serum while in each tube of the second row is placed one volume of a second anti-CD serum. The setting up of this test is completed as for Rh typing (techniques No. 9.2 or 9.3). Controls of OR′, OR_2r and Orr cells are set up at the same time. The R′ and R_2r will control the two components of the anti-CD mixture independently. (*See* page 108.) The tests are read in the usual way after 2 hours' incubation at 37°C.

Technique No. 12.3. Further testing of samples found to be negative with anti-D but positive with anti-DE

The pattern of this test is exactly the same as that described immediately above, but instead of anti-CD sera, two anti-DE mixtures are used. Suitable controls are included (*i.e.* OR″, OR_1r, and Orr) and the tests read after 2 hours' incubation.

Technique No. 12.4a. Detection of low grade D^u in red cells apparently D-negative. Indirect anti-human globulin test

The technique is essentially the same as that described in Chapter 10 (technique No. 10.3a). The object of the test is, however, different. The test already outlined is for the detection of incomplete antibodies, using known standard cells. It is used in the present connexion conversely for the detection of the D^u antigen in unknown cells by means of a known incomplete anti-D.

The test is set up in the usual manner mixing two volumes of a potent incomplete anti-D with a half volume of packed cells from

Table 12.2

Subdivision of D-negative Cells. Interpretation of Results

TECHNIQUE No. 12.1a*

Samples tested	Anti-D	Anti-D	Anti-CD	Anti-DE	Further technique	Conclusion
F.G.	−	−	−	−	None†	rr
H.I.	−	−	+	−	12.2 + 4	
J.K.	−	−	−	+	12.3 + 4	
L.M.	+	−	+	−	12.2 + 4	
N.O.	−	+	−	+	12.3 + 4	
P.Q.	−	−	+	+	12.2, 3 + 4	
R.S.	−	−	+	−	12.2 + 4	

TECHNIQUE No. 12.1b

Samples tested	Anti-CD	Anti-CD	Anti-DE	Anti-DE	Further technique	Conclusion
F.G.	−	−	−	−	None†	rr
H.I.	+	+	−	−	} 12.4 (H.I. to R.S.)	probably R′
J.K.	−	−	+	+		probably R″
L.M.	+	+	−	+		
N.O.	−	+	+	+		
P.Q.	+	+	+	+		probably R′R″
R.S.	+	+	−	−		probably R′

TECHNIQUE No. 12.2			TECHNIQUE No. 12.4		Conclusion
Samples tested	Anti-CD	Anti-CD	Incomplete D	Incomplete D	
H.I.	+	+	−	−	R′
L.M.	+	+	+	+	D^u
P.Q.	+	+	−	−	see below
R.S.	+	+	+	+	D^u
TECHNIQUE No. 12.3					
Samples tested	Anti-DE	Anti-DE			
J.K.	+	+	−	−	R″
N.O.	+	+	+	+	D^u
P.Q.	+	+	see above		R′R″

* Depending upon availability of sera, Technique 12.1(a) or (b) will be used, not both.
† If negroid, Technique 12.4 must be included.

the sample to be tested. The anti-human globulin (Coombs reagent) must be used at the optimum dilution for the detection of IgG (*see* Appendix I). The controls and subsequent procedure are the same as in technique No. 10.3a.

Technique No. 12.4b. Detection of low grade D^u in red cells apparently D-negative. Papain treated cells technique

The cells are papain treated using Löw's enzyme, by incubating at 37°C for 20 minutes. They are then washed and made up to a 2 per cent solution with saline. The cells are tested with three different pure anti-D sera and with AB serum as a negative control, one volume of cells is added to one volume of serum and the mixture incubated for 30 minutes.

The tests are read macro- and microscopically. Controls of Rh positive, Rh type D^u, R′r, R″r and rr cells are included in each batch of tests.

This test will detect almost all examples of D^u but the occasional cell will be encountered which is negative by this test but positive by the anti-human globulin technique (No. 12.4a).

Interpretation of Results

A summary of most of the various results which may be obtained from the above tests is shown in Table 12.2.

Although the testing of these D negative samples and the variety of possible results may seem confusing, it should be realised that in the majority of cases straightforward negative results will be obtained with anti-sera D, CD, and DE and the red cells will be designated Rh negative (cde.cde) accordingly.

In a few cases a positive result may be obtained with either anti-CD or anti-DE which on confirmation will show the red cells to be R′ or R″, or low grade D^u if the indirect Coombs test is positive.

Occasionally a D^u type will be encountered which is of slightly higher grade. This may manifest itself by giving a positive reaction with one or more of the anti-D sera as shown in Table 12.2 although not all the alternative patterns that might be given by D^u are depicted. (*See also* Table 11.6.)

Very rarely indeed the R′R″ (which cannot be distinguished from the even more rare R_yr) may be found. This shows up as D negative but positive with both anti-CD and anti-DE mixtures. Its occurrence should be established carrying out a combination of techniques Nos. 12.2–4, wherein it will be found to be positive with all anti-CD and anti-DE sera but consistently negative with all examples of anti-D. Its distinction from R_y can only be made through family studies.

Subdivision of D-positive

It is only in special circumstances that a subdivision of D-positive red cells is required. This is fortunate because the sera necessary for such subdivision (commonly misnamed "genotyping") are comparatively rare. There are situations, however, in which it is very useful to obtain as accurate an idea as possible of the actual Rh genotype of an individual. Cases in point are D positive persons suspected of having had a hæmolytic transfusion reaction, infants suffering from hæmolytic disease of the newborn, cases receiving multiple transfusions, persons whose sera contain atypical antibodies thought to belong to the Rh system, husbands of Rh negative women whose sera contain atypical antibodies, etc.

Before the actual technique of Rh sub-typing is described the choice of standard cells for controls on the anti-sera used must be discussed. (*See* Table 12.1.) The positive controls must be chosen bearing in mind that the strength of a positive reaction with anti-C, anti-E, anti-c, and anti-e is often considerably weaker with cells of a genotype containing only one "dose" of the corresponding antigen than with cells containing two "doses". This is particularly true of anti-c; cells containing a "double dose" of c through inheriting it from both parents (*e.g.* cde.cde) react more strongly with anti-c than do cells of genotype R_1r (CDe.cde) which contain only one c. A satisfactory positive control is one which corresponds to the weakest positive expected to be found in the tests. Accordingly, cells that are heterozygous for each antigen tested are used. R_1R_2(CDe.cDE) cells are obviously the convenient choice for a positive control which satisfies the foregoing criterion for all anti-sera except anti-D for which R_1r (CDe.cde) cells are the best control. The negative control for each anti-serum has to be selected with the possible contaminants of that serum in mind. (*See* Chapter 14.)

Very strong anti-C, anti-E, and anti-c sera are rare and so weaker examples of them may have to be chosen for test sera than if the selection were wider. In spite of their rarity it is still recommended, therefore, that two examples of sera of each specificity be employed if available. It is essential to conserve stocks as much as possible so the unit volume for the test should not be greater than 0·01 ml.

Technique No. 12.5. Further testing of samples found to be positive with anti-D—Rh "genotyping"

The wooden fifty-holed block should be turned so that a row of seven precipitin tubes and one cell suspension tube can be placed in it for each sample to be tested.

Row 1	contains	anti-C (1)
Row 2	,,	,, (2)
Row 3	,,	anti-E (1)
Row 4	,,	,, (2)
Row 5	,,	anti-c (1)
Row 6	,,	,, (2)
Row 7	,,	AB serum

The unit volumes of each serum, being smaller than those usually handled, must be delivered very carefully to the bottoms of the tubes using a Pasteur pipette specially graduated to deliver these small volumes (Fig. 2.1D). To prevent wetting the side of the tube which may result in loss of such a small quantity, it is advisable to touch the bottom of the tube with the tip of the pipette before the volume of fluid is expelled.

After the tubes have been checked for the presence of serum in each, an equal micro-volume of a 2 per cent red cell suspension in saline is added to each one. This is also delivered to the bottom of the tube without touching the serum with the pipette; carrying out this manœuvre with such a small volume necessitates lifting the tubes from the block so that the contents can be seen. The tubes are then flicked to ensure good mixture and capped, to prevent evaporation; this can be conveniently done with the larger diameter cell suspension tubes. The tests are incubated for at least 2 hours and then read with even more care than usual owing to the small volume of fluid available for spreading on the slide. No reaction should be scored as definitely positive unless at least of "+" strength. Any discrepancy occurring between the results obtained with two sera of the same specificity necessitates repeating the test. If the anomalous results are confirmed the sample is tested with as large a panel of sera of the requisite specificity as is available. Typing sera containing incomplete antibodies should be used by albumin addition technique (9.3) or Löw's papain technique (10.5) whichever is appropriate.

Interpretation of Results

Each possible pattern of reaction with the four anti-sera (including anti-D) will be discussed separately and in conjunction with Table 11.3. A step by step method of deducing the genotypes from first principles is given with the first set of reactions discussed. It should be pointed out that in this table (11.3) the frequency of each genotype is expressed as a percentage of the total population in Column 5 and as a percentage of the particular phenotype in Column 6:

Anti-D	Anti-C	Anti-E	Anti-c
+	+	−	−

This is the easiest pattern to interpret and therefore is dealt with first. Table 11.3 gives the two possible genotypes showing this pattern of reaction. The knack of working out the different alternatives without the aid of a table should be acquired.

A convenient line to adopt is given below.

Taking the result with anti-D first, the positive reaction obtained with this serum shows that at least one D occurs in the genotype. Whether the genotype is DD or Dd cannot be certainly determined because there is no antibody for the detection of "d."

So far then the genotype can be written:

D/D or D/d

The result found with anti-C should be considered together with that for anti-c since these anti-sera are detecting antigens arising from allelomorphic genes. In this case the reaction with anti-C is positive and with anti-c is negative so the genotype must be CC which can now be included thus:

CD/CD or CD/Cd

Lastly the anti-E result must be assessed. This is negative which indicates the absence of E so the genotype can be completed thus:

CDe/CDe or CDe/Cde

i.e. the alternatives are R_1R_1 (CDe.CDe) or R_1R' (CDe.Cde).

From Table 11.3 it can be seen that the genotype R_1R_1 forms 95·5 per cent of the phenotype R_1R_1.

It is, therefore, correct to conclude that the probable genotype of an individual whose cells give this pattern of agglutination reaction is R_1R_1. The fact that the "improbable" genotype R_1R' will occur in 4·5 per cent of the phenotype must not be overlooked!

Anti-D	Anti-C	Anti-E	Anti-c
+	+	−	+

Table 11.3 shows that there are three possible genotypes giving these reactions, but again the odds are overwhelmingly in favour

of one; in this case R_1r. The probable genotype of such an individual is, therefore, R_1r.

Anti-D	Anti-C	Anti-E	Anti-c
+	+	+	+

A positive reaction with all four sera indicating the presence of all four antigens, D, C, E, and c gives rise to many more alternatives. From the table it can be seen that there are nine; R_1R_2, the probable genotype, comprising 88·4 per cent of the whole phenotype.

Anti-D	Anti-C	Anti-E	Anti-c
+	−	+	+

In the phenotype patterning as above there are five alternative genotypes of which the most common is R_2r (77·9 per cent) followed by R_2R_2 14·1 per cent.

It is often an advantage when it is realised that the blood under test falls into this category to expend a little of the rare anti-e and test the blood with this. If a positive reaction is obtained with this serum the probable genotype is R_2r (93·3 per cent) and if a negative reaction is obtained the probable genotype is R_2R_2 (85·6 per cent) (*see* Table 11.3). If no anti-e is available a titration with an anti-E known to show a marked dosage effect may be used instead although the results may not be so clear cut.

Anti-D	Anti-C	Anti-E	Anti-c
+	−	−	+

In this phenotype there are two alternative genotypes R_0r and R_0R_0. The probable genotype in this case is R_0r (96·8 per cent):

Anti-D	Anti-C	Anti-E	Anti-c
+	+	+	−

Although this phenotype is rare, occurring in only 0·2 per cent of the total population, it comprises no less than five genotypes. The probable genotype is R_1R_Z (97·1 per cent).

The circumstances in which it is of value to know the sub-group to which a D positive red cell belongs have already been listed and it will be seen that these differ widely. They must, therefore, be taken into account in the interpretation of results. For the identification of atypical antibodies which may be of the Rh system, a knowledge of the antigens lacking in the patient is more useful than assembling the results for the purpose of postulating a probable genotype. If, on the other hand, the blood of a husband whose wife's serum contains Rh antibodies is being considered, the important point is whether he is homozygous or heterozygous for the antigen corresponding to the antibody in her serum. Most commonly the antibody is anti-D. A knowledge of the husband's antigenic make-up may also be of help in confirming the identity of a maternal antibody. A more detailed discussion of the Rh genotypes of these husbands will be found in Chapter 25.

CHAPTER 13

THE DETECTION AND IDENTIFICATION OF Rh ANTIBODIES, INCLUDING MIXTURES

THE emphasis of this chapter is on specificity, as it is important not only to detect but also to identify any of the Rh antibodies which may be present in a serum. Herein is also included the less straightforward identification of mixtures of Rh antibodies of different specificities occurring in one serum.

Choice of Standard Red Cells

The first step is the selection of suitable standard cells of known Rh sub-types for the routine testing of sera which may contain Rh antibodies. The object is to be able to detect any of the Rh antibodies with cells of a few readily available sub-types.

The trio R_1R_1 (CDe.CDe), R_2R_2 (cDE.cDE), and rr (cde.cde) are the genotypes of choice. Table 13.1 shows not only that these detect any of the antibodies but also that they give a different pattern of reactions with each. A further advantage of using these genotypes is that they have two "doses" of those Rh antigens which show a "dosage" effect. R_1R_1 (CDe.CDe) has a double dose of C and e, R_2R_2 (cDE.cDE) has a double dose of c and E. These two also have a double dose of D but in R_1R_1 the D is partially suppressed by the C; R_2R_2 (cDE.cDE) is the best cell for the detection of anti-D. The third cell rr (cde.cde) has a double dose of c and e. This means that if any of the antibodies anti-C, anti-E, anti-c, or anti-e are present they will be able to react to their maximum capacity with cells containing the double dose of antigen. Thus they are more readily detected. Indeed, when the antibody is weak the use of red cells containing only a single dose of the antigen would probably result in failure to detect the antibody.

In practice, red cells of groups R_1R_1 and rr should be easily available, but R_2R_2 may have to be replaced by R_2r (cDE.cde) or even R_1R_2 (CDe.cDE). If this is done, the antigen E will only be represented in single dose. Since E does not show dosage quite as markedly as c this is not too great a disadvantage, particularly if the technique of handling the cell sediments gently, while reading the tests, is strictly adhered to, so that weak agglutination is not missed. It should be noted that if R_1R_2 replaces R_2R_2, anti-C and anti-D give the same pattern.

Many laboratories favour the use of R_1R_2 and rr red cells only for Rh antibody detection tests, but these represent the absolute minimum. If these are used, the antigens C and E will be present in single dose. As anti-C and anti-E antibodies, in the main, occur as saline agglutinins, it is felt that R_1R_2 should not be substituted for R_1R_1 and R_2R_2 in the saline technique. Moreover, using R_1R_2 and rr cells the pattern of reaction given by anti-C, anti-D and anti-E will be identical, as will that given by anti-c and anti-e. Positive reactions with either or both of these red cells will require further investigation. However, even if a characteristic pattern is obtained with the ideal red cell combination R_1R_1 (CDe.CDe), R_2R_2 (cDE.cDE), and rr (cde.cde) further tests are necessary with a larger panel of cells before the identity of the antibody can be established.

Choice of Techniques

Having selected the most satisfactory set of standard cells from those available it has to be decided which techniques to use. These, of course, must allow for the detection of antibodies occurring in either the complete or incomplete forms (or mixtures of both).

If only a few tests are being performed, saline (technique No. 10.1) indirect anti-human globulin (technique No. 10.4a), and papain (technique No. 10.6) or one of the other enzyme techniques should be chosen. Where the number of sera to be examined for antibodies is very large a method using albumin (techniques No. 10.2 or No. 10.3) can be substituted for the indirect anti-human globulin in spite of its slightly lower sensitivity.

It may be asked whether a saline technique is necessary at all if albumin or indirect anti-human globulin tests are to be included. Will these not also detect saline agglutinins? Saline agglutinins will often agglutinate red cells suspended in bovine albumin, but usually this agglutination is much weaker than when the red cells are suspended in saline. Occasionally, agglutination of cells by saline agglutinins is entirely inhibited by bovine albumin. The anti-human globulin test is not a satisfactory method of detecting saline agglutinins. If the latter are potent the cells are obviously agglutinated at the end of the incubation stage of the test and it is therefore unnecessary to add anti-human globulin reagent. If the agglutinins are less potent they may be entirely removed from the cells at the washing stage of the test so that a false negative is obtained.

On the other hand, agglutination which has already taken place will often be enhanced by the addition of anti-human globulin reagent. This is almost certainly because the red cells have incomplete antibodies attached to them also.

At this point it would seem appropriate to give a short account of the characteristics and method of identification of each Rh antibody separately, although a great deal about anti-D and a few facts about the others will have been dealt with in previous chapters.

Anti-D

Anti-D is the most frequently occurring Rh antibody and presents the greatest clinical problem. The fact that it occurs in both complete and incomplete forms has already been discussed in Chapter 10.

It is produced by D-negative individuals in response to stimulation by the D antigen. The majority of people who form anti-D antibodies are rr (cde.cde), but those who belong to any Rh sub-type which lacks D are equally liable to produce them; it is merely that the other D-negative sub-types are much less common than rr (cde.cde).

If an individual lacks antigen D and his serum gives the pattern of reaction (1) in Table 13.1, then the antibody present in the serum is probably anti-D. However, to confirm the specificity it is essential to test with a different set of known D positive and D negative cells by the techniques with which the antibody was detected. At least three examples of D positive cells and two of D negative must be used; if the serum is consistently positive with the D positive cells and negative with the D negative, then the serum certainly contains anti-D antibodies. Other antibodies may possibly be present but masked by the anti-D; for instance, anti-CD or anti-DE mixtures would give the same pattern of reaction as pure anti-D. Antibodies may also be present but undetected because no cell containing the corresponding antigen has been used in the test. The most common antibody which may be missed in this way is anti-Kell. It is recommended, therefore, that in addition to the test with D positive and D negative cells the serum should also be tested with R′r (Cde.cde), R″r (cdE.cde), and rr (cde.cde) Kell positive cells. A further fairly common antibody is anti-Wr^a (*see also* Chapter 14).

Anti-D usually agglutinates equally well cells which are DD or Dd. It therefore does not normally show dosage. However, D is modified by its accompanying antigens (*see* Chapter 33) and the anti-D titre against D-positive cells of differing Rh genotypes will reflect this, the greatest titre being obtained with R_2R_2 (cDE.cDE) red cells.

Anti-C

Pure anti-C, *i.e.* unmixed with other Rh antibodies (No. 2 in Table 13.1) rarely occurs. Occasionally, however, it is formed by a D-positive, C-negative individual, *e.g.* R_2R_2 (cDE.cDE) or R_2r (cDE.cde) but not as often as might be expected from the number of opportunities for its production that arise. More often it occurs in a mixture with anti-D (*see* below) and has been found associated with anti-e (*see* below). If a serum gives the pattern of reaction characteristic of anti-C, the specificity must be checked by the use of three R′r, two R_2r and two rr samples of red cells. The patient's own cells must be "genotyped", or at least tested and shown to be negative with anti-C.

Anti-C occurs in both complete and incomplete forms, but the complete form is more common.

The antibody sometimes shows a dosage effect, but not markedly.

There is a further discussion of various types of anti-C sera in Chapter 33; before any serum is used as an anti-C typing serum it should be fully investigated along the lines suggested there by a laboratory having available cells of the various rare Rh sub-types necessary.

Anti-E

Pure anti-E occurs more frequently than pure anti-C, being found in general in the serum of R_1R_1 (CDe.CDe) or R_1r (CDe.cde) individuals.

The pattern of reaction it gives is No. 3 in Table 13.1. Confirmatory tests must be carried out to establish the specificity, using three R″r, two R_1R_1, and two rr samples of red cells; the individual's own cells must be tested with anti-E. Anti-E sometimes displays the dosage effect, occasionally to such an extent that it is as reliable as anti-e in distinguishing between EE and Ee cells.

Anti-E is quite often present as an antibody detectable only by an enzyme technique, in which case it is probably naturally occurring. As such it has little clinical significance but may, upon stimulation, develop into a clinically significant antibody.

Anti-c

The pattern of agglutination reaction characteristic of anti-c is No. 4 in Table 13.1.

Table 13.1

Identification of the Five Main Rh Antibodies

Antibody	Standard cells			Mixtures giving same pattern of reaction
	R_1R_1 (CDe.CDe)	R_2R_2 (cDE.cDE)	rr (cde.cde)	
(1) Anti-D	+	+	−	Anti-CD, anti-DE, anti-CDE, and anti-CE (v. rare)
(2) Anti-C	+	−	−	
(3) Anti-E	−	+	−	
(4) Anti-c	−	+	+	anti-Ec
(5) Anti-e	+	−	+	anti-Ce

The antibody is almost always found in D positive persons, since D negatives lacking the antigen c are very rare indeed. The phenotype in which the antibody occurs is R_1R_1 (CDe.CDe), which includes the genotype R_1R' (CDe.Cde). The antigen c, however, seems to be comparatively weak, and most people, even after a number of exposures to it, do not make the corresponding anti-c.

It is important to confirm its specificity by testing against two rr (cde.cde), two R_1r (CDe.cde), and two R_1R_1 (CDe.CDe) cell samples. It should also be tested with R_1R_Z (CDe.CDE) cells, if these are available as anti-c, anti-E mixtures are common (*see* below).

Anti-c is found in both complete and incomplete forms and almost always shows dosage to a high degree. Titres with cc (*e.g.* cde.cde cells) and Cc (*e.g.* CDe.cde) cells will help to confirm the identity of the antibody.

It is essential if it is proposed to use it for Rh typing purposes that it should give a satisfactory titration value with single dose c cells.

Anti-e

This is a very rare antibody, partly because the e antigen seems to be a weak one, but mostly because there are very few individuals who lack it and are, therefore, capable of forming anti-e. The calculated total percentage of the population lacking e is 2·4 per cent, and of these the commonest genotype is R_2R_2 (cDE.cDE), which is 2·0 per cent.

The pattern of reaction of anti-e in number 5 in Table 13.1. It has been found in both complete and incomplete forms and usually displays marked dosage. When it occurs it is often in the form of a papain type antibody. If a serum is suspected to contain anti-e, the red cells should be fully Rh typed, including testing with anti-e. Of the relatively common genotypes R_2R_2 (cDE.cDE) is the only one that will give a negative reaction with anti-e, and this will only occur once in fifty times among random samples. It is, therefore, a good plan to test the suspected anti-e against as many known R_2R_2 (cDE.cDE) red cells as can be procured. It should also be tested with R_2R_z cells (cDE.CDE) for the possible presence of anti-C (*see* below). Dosage titrations can also be performed, using rr (cde.cde) and R_2r (cDE.cde) or R_1R_2 (CDe.cDE) cells as an added confirmation of the specificity.

Anti-CD, Anti-DE, and Anti-CDE Mixtures

These mixtures do not occur in all cases in which they are a theoretical possibility. Rather less than half the Rh antibodies

Table 13.2

Differentiation of Anti-D, Anti-CD, Anti-DE, Anti-CDE and Anti-CE

	R′r (Cde.cde)	R″r (cdE.cde)	R_0r (cDe.cde)
Anti-D	−	−	+
Anti-CD	+	−	+
Anti-DE	−	+	+
Anti-CDE	+	+	+
Anti-CE	+	+	−

found in Rh negative persons are mixtures of anti-D and anti-C, a much smaller number are anti-D + anti-E, and a very few are mixtures of all three antibodies. D is strongly antigenic and it is very rare indeed for anti-C or anti-E to be present and yet anti-D absent in D-negative individuals who are exposed to D as well as C or E.

As already stated above, the panel of red cells recommended for routine antibody testing will not reveal the presence of anti-C and/or anti-E mixed with anti-D. These mixtures will give the same pattern as anti-D alone (Table 13.1). If anti-D is discovered in a serum, a further test is therefore necessary, using R′r (Cde.cde) cells by saline, albumin and papain techniques, which will detect anti-C, and R″r (cdE.cde) by the same techniques, which will detect anti-E (Table 13.2). In the apparent anti-CDE mixture the presence of anti-D must be confirmed with R_0r (cDe.cde) cells.

The quantities and forms of the antibodies in these mixtures vary considerably. Anti-D is normally present in higher titre

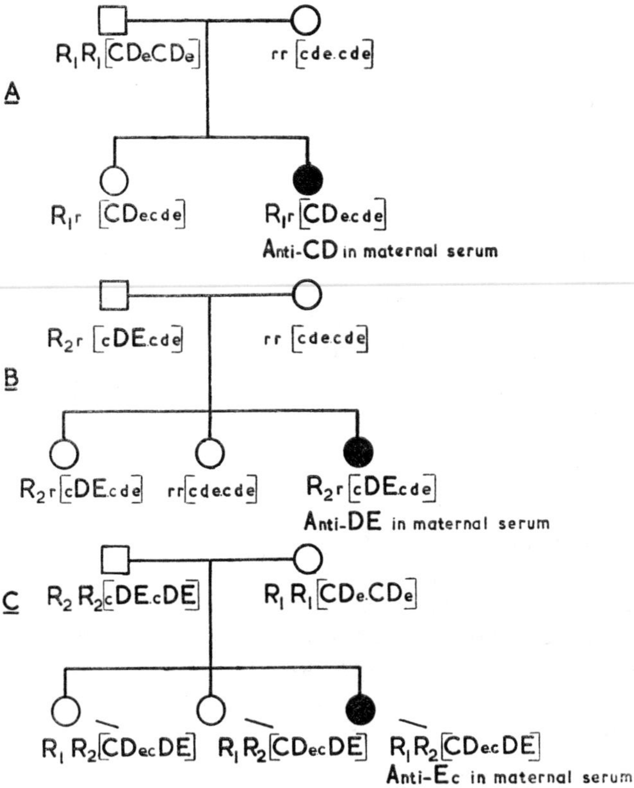

FIG. 13.1. A–C
Families showing how mixtures of Rh antibodies may arise.

than the others. Indeed, anti-C and anti-E are often only found in trace amounts. Sometimes both antibodies occur in the complete form, or one will be complete and the other incomplete. The anti-C and anti-E components are more often of the complete type and are occasionally accompanied by anti-D in the incomplete form only. This is useful, for such sera can be used as pure anti-C or anti-E if the saline technique is employed.

Examples of families in which these mixtures have occurred are shown in Fig. 13.1A and B. In Fig. 13.1A an Rh negative (cde.cde) woman married to an R_1R_1 (CDe.CDe) man was found to have anti-C and anti-D antibodies in her serum during her second pregnancy. Both children possessed the antigens C and D which the mother lacked, thus stimulating her to produce both anti-C and anti-D. In Fig. 13.1B where the mother was Rh negative (cde.cde) and the father R_2r (cDE,cde), the first and third children inherited the paternal D and E antigens, causing the formation of anti-D and anti-E in the mother.

Anti-CDE mixtures can occur in families where all three antigens are found among the children, *e.g.* if the mother is Rh negative (cde.cde), the father R_1R_2 (CDe.cDE), some of the children R_1r (CDe.cde) and others R_2r (cDE.cde).

Mixtures of antibodies also arise as a result of transfusions. Indeed, there is more opportunity for a mixture of two or more antibodies to be produced as a result of multiple transfusions than as a result of pregnancy.

Some anti-CD "mixtures" are in reality anti-G, an antibody reacting with part of the D and C antigens. Such "mixtures" are not separable into anti-D and anti-C components (*see also* Chapter 33).

Anti-Ec Mixtures

Another not uncommon mixture of antibodies is anti-E + anti-c. Fig. 13.1C is an example of a family in which this mixture was found.

The identification of the components of mixtures discussed so far has been relatively simple because it has been possible to choose standard red cells specific for each separate component (*e.g.* the case of the anti-CD mixture, R′r (Cde.cde) for the anti-C component and R_0r (cDe.cde) for the anti-D component). This is not always possible for an anti-Ec mixture, for although E-negative c-positive red cells (*e.g.* rr (cde.cde)) are readily available, E-positive c-negative red cells are very rare indeed. Fortunately, the anti-E component is often present in higher titre than the anti-c, so that comparison of titration values against R_1r (CDe.cde), rr (cde.cde), R_2r (cDE.cde), and R_2R_2 (cDE.cDE) will clearly reveal the presence of both antibodies. Where a serum appears to contain anti-c and is known to have arisen as the result of stimulation by cells containing E as well as c, then it is essential to test for the possible presence of anti-E with cells of one of the rare E-positive c-negative genotypes, *e.g.* R_1R_z (CDe.CDE). If necessary, the serum must be sent to a reference laboratory for this purpose.

Anti-Ce Mixtures

Another mixture which has been found on several occasions is that of anti-C + anti-e. The anti-e in such a mixture can be readily identified by the use of rr (cde.cde) and R_2R_2 (cDE.cDE) without interference from the anti-C. The presence of anti-C can be revealed by a comparison of titration values against R_1r (CDe.cde), R_1R_1 (CDe.CDe), R_2r (cDE.cde), and rr (cde.cde) red cells if the titre of anti-C is greater than that of anti-e. Otherwise, the only alternative is the testing with red cells of the very rare genotype R_2R_z (cDE.CDE) which is C-positive but e-negative.

The identification of the components in anti-Ec and anti-Ce mixtures may sometimes be facilitated by absorption and elution experiments. Absorption of both these mixtures with cdecde cells may leave behind identifiable anti-E or anti-C components. Anti-c can be recovered from the cdecde cells if desired (*see* technique 21.3) and identified.

Sometimes the individual antibodies may be tested for separately by the use of two different antibody detection techniques, *e.g.* anti-E or anti-C by saline and anti-c and anti-e by anti-globulin methods.

If the above treatment is unsuccessful it will be necessary to locate cells of the rare genotypes mentioned above.

Antibodies to Compound Antigens

Rh antibodies can also be made to compound antigens, *e.g.* cE, and they will only react with cells that have cE on the same chromosome, *i.e.* in the cis position. In normal tests such antibodies can be mistaken for mixtures of antibodies. They are discussed further in Chapter 33.

Techniques

There are no new techniques mentioned in this chapter, but there are a few points which should be mentioned about the adaptation of already described methods.

Saline, Albumin or Anti-human Globulin and Enzyme Techniques in Parallel

The test serum required for all three techniques should be run out in one operation. This reduces handling to a minimum and saves many rinses of the pipette. The standard cells can be run out in rows after checking that each tube contains serum.

The reading of a block full of saline or albumin antibody tests takes some time, since the contents of every tube have to be examined microscopically. It is therefore inadvisable to remove from the incubator more than one block at a time.

Titration of Mixtures

The technique for titration of mixtures of antibodies is the same as those described in Chapter 10 for the titration of complete and incomplete anti-D. The standard cells used, however, must be selected with the purpose of estimating the strength of each antibody in the mixture independently. Thus for an anti-CD mixture R′r (Cde.cde) cells must be used to estimate the anti-C content, and R_0r (cDe.cde) or R_2r (cDE.cde) cells the content of anti-D.

CHAPTER 14

SELECTION AND PREPARATION OF Rh TYPING SERA

THERE are two main essentials for a satisfactory Rh typing serum:

(1) It must be of sufficient strength to detect the corresponding antigen even when this is weak.

(2) It must be specific for its corresponding antigen.

Selection

A serum is earmarked as useful for typing purposes because its titration value reaches or exceeds a required minimum and because it is sufficiently avid. Either saline agglutinins or incomplete antibodies or a mixture of both can be used equally well.

The various Rh antisera each present individual problems when being selected for typing purposes; they are, therefore, considered separately from this point of view although subsequently they are dealt with together.

Anti-D

Since anti-D is the most frequently encountered of the Rh antibodies there should be plenty from which to choose if all cases are followed up assiduously. The main source of supply is, of course, the Rh negative mother with antibodies who has recently been delivered of an Rh positive infant.

Samples of sera should first be titrated according to the methods given in Chapter 10 (techniques Nos. 10.9 and 10.10). No anti-D with a titre of less than 64 with R_1r red cells should be selected. In addition there should be macroscopic readings at least to a dilution of 1 in 8. These criteria are the minimum required for typing by tube methods (techniques Nos. 9.2 or 9.3). For other techniques, Slide, Chown, etc., the criteria are the same but the titrations must be carried out by the particular technique for which it is proposed to use the serum.

The antibody is suitable whether in the complete or incomplete form or a mixture of both, except for those techniques for which a particular type of serum has been specified. In practice it will be found that potent incomplete anti-D sera are fairly easily obtainable, titres of 512 or over being by no means uncommon. Such a serum of high titre can be used very economically since it will withstand considerable dilution. It is recommended that AB serum (for preparation of suitable AB serum *see* Appendix I) should be used as the diluting fluid.

The importance of checking the specificity of the selected anti-D cannot be over-emphasised. It has already been seen that anti-D is often mixed with anti-C or anti-E or even with both. If serum containing these antibodies is inadvertently used as an anti-D typing serum R′ and R″ patients will be incorrectly typed as D positive. This can have dangerous consequences.

To check the purity of the anti-D, saline and albumin tests against R′r (Cde.cde) and R″r (cdE.cde) are made with at least five examples of each kind of red cell. This will ensure that any anti-C or anti-E which would give positive reactions with such D negative cells will not go undetected. If the serum is to be used for any but the standard techniques, in particular for the very sensitive Löw's papain technique it must be examined for anti-C and anti-E by the appropriate method.

Anti-CD and Anti-DE Mixtures

The suitability of mixtures for Rh typing purposes depends on the strength of each antibody in the mixture reaching a required minimum standard. While it is not difficult to find sera in which the anti-D reaches the minimum requirements laid down above, it is not so easy to find anti-C or anti-E antibodies that do so. The standard, therefore, unavoidably, has to be lowered by one or two dilutions for the anti-C or anti-E component. Nevertheless if titres of sixteen are accepted care must be taken that the serum chosen is avid and gives macroscopic readings to at least a dilution of 1 in 4. It is obvious that the foregoing remarks with regard to choice of serum for a particular method apply also to anti-CD and anti-DE mixtures.

Anti-C (*see also* Chapter 33)

The pure anti-C which is produced by an Rh positive individual, *e.g.* of genotype R_2r, providing the titre is at least sixteen against R′r cells with two or more macroscopic readings, is the most satisfactory source of this reagent. Unfortunately anti-C is only rarely so produced and even when it is the titre is often inadequate. Anti-C sera are, therefore, usually prepared from specially selected anti-CD mixtures. Suitable mixtures are either those in which the anti-C titre greatly exceeds the anti-D or those in which the anti-C antibodies are complete and the anti-D mainly incomplete. In either case it is usually possible to choose a dilution of the serum at which it will behave as pure anti-C. The alternative course of preparing pure anti-C by removing the anti-D with R_2R_2 red cells is seldom successful (*see* below). Such an absorbed serum, however, gives more consistent and reliable results since absorption, in contrast to dilution, actually removes the anti-D component from the serum.

It should be noted that Ce mixtures are not used for the preparation of anti-C as they are more valuable for the e typing of C negative individuals.

Anti-E

As anti-E is fairly readily available it is often possible to choose sera with minimum titration values of sixty-four with R_2r red cells. Even if this standard cannot be maintained it should at least reach that required for anti-C, namely a titration value of sixteen with macroscopic readings at least as far as the 1 in 4 dilution.

The best source of anti-E is the serum of an R_1r individual where it occurs unmixed with other Rh antibodies. The other source of anti-E is from an individual of genotype R_1R_1, in which case it is usually mixed with anti-c. Such a mixture has been discussed in the previous chapter. Since the anti-E is usually considerably more potent than the anti-c the latter is often diluted out, or removed from the serum by absorption with Rh negative red cells. The absorption, however, will almost certainly reduce the titre of the anti-E as well as removing the anti-c so that only those sera having titres which will allow for a reduction are suitable for this treatment.

Anti-c

Anti-c to be suitable for typing purposes must have a minimum titration value of sixteen with R_1r red cells with macroscopic readings at least as far as a dilution of 1 in 4.

As mentioned above (*see also* Fig. 13.1C) anti-c may occur in the same serum as anti-E, but usually such a serum is used as an anti-E rather than anti-c since the anti-E is almost always present in far greater titre. If it is desired to use an anti-Ec mixture as an anti-c typing serum, it must be reserved for the testing of cells which are E negative.

Anti-e

Owing to the great rarity of this antibody, almost all examples of it, however weak, are used for typing purposes, even if this necessitates the adaptation of one of the very sensitive antibody detection techniques such as indirect anti-human globulin or papain.

When an anti-Ce mixture is found it is always used as anti-e for typing red cells which are C negative.

Preparation

Collection and Separation of Serum

A donor found to have suitable antibodies for the preparation of an Rh typing serum will donate from 100 to 480 ml. of blood according to his or her clinical condition. The blood is taken into a dry bottle and allowed to clot. Although clot retraction is slower in the cold the antibody may deteriorate slightly if the blood is allowed to clot at 37°C; it is preferable, therefore, to leave the bottle at 4°C for 24 hours by which time the serum will be well separated. After this as much serum as possible is collected, cell free, taking aseptic precautions if the serum is not for immediate preparation. A further yield can almost certainly be obtained by centrifuging the clot. The separated serum is stored in bulk at – 20°C until it is processed.

Pooling of Sera

With anti-D, anti-CD and anti-DE sera it is often an advantage to make a pool of sera from four or five donors. A serum which is just below the minimum standards can be included in a pool with stronger sera, and thus increase the total amount of reliable serum available. Moreover such pools of sera are more likely to detect the D^u antigen than a serum from a single donor. Another advantage of a pool is that one standard serum can be used for several weeks or even months thus giving results which are strictly comparable.

It is not recommended, however, that the rarer sera should be pooled. Any laboratory will only have a limited number of anti-C, anti-E, anti-c, etc., sera available and more reliable results are obtained by using them in parallel rather than mixed in a pool.

When it is decided to make a pool it should be done before the absorption and sterilisation stage. If the sera are of differing ABO groups this is an advantage as the pool will then be easier to absorb for anti-A and anti-B. If possible at least one very good serum (titre 512 or over) should be included in each pool. The pooled serum should be tested to see that it fulfils the criteria; if the constituents have been well chosen it will usually have a titre considerably above the minimum in spite of the inclusion of one weaker serum. On the other hand the final titre is occasionally disappointingly low and the pool will need the addition of a further very potent serum.

Pooled serum is processed as for single sera except that for the absorption of anti-A and anti-B agglutinins the quantity of red cells can be reduced by half if the pool is made from sera of differing ABO blood groups as the A and B substances in the sera will neutralise some of the anti-A and anti-B agglutinins.

Removal of Unwanted Antibodies

Unwanted antibodies fall into three classes; (*a*) other Rh antibodies; (*b*) anti-A and anti-B agglutinins; (*c*) antibodies of other blood group systems.

(*a*) **Removal of Other Rh Antibodies.** It has already been seen that Rh antibodies often occur as mixtures so that a serum chosen for typing purposes may have a component which it is desirable to remove.

A trace of unwanted antibody can be diluted out if by so doing the titre of the required antibody is not reduced below the minimum. A satisfactory dilution is one which goes well beyond the range of activity of the antibody which is being diluted out. For example, if the titre of an unwanted anti-C in an anti-CD mixture is two, then the serum must be diluted at least to 1 in 10 before it can be used with safety as pure anti-D; this means that the initial anti-D titre would have to be at least 2,000. The best diluting fluid to use is specially prepared AB serum (for preparation *see* Appendix I).

The alternative method of ridding the serum of unwanted Rh antibodies is that of absorption. The serum is mixed with cells which will specifically combine with the unwanted antibodies. After a suitable time interval the serum-cell mixture is centrifuged and the supernatant serum collected while the cells are discarded and with them the unwanted antibodies. This is the method of choice for the removal of anti-A and anti-B agglutinins (*see* below) but a complication often arises if it is used for the removal of one Rh antibody from another which it is desired to retain in the serum. It would seem that in many instances when antibodies of different specificities yet of the same blood group system co-exist in a serum, some of the antibody molecules have double specificity. For example, if R_2R_2 (cDE.cDE) cells are used to remove anti-D from an anti-CD mixture in an attempt to make the serum a pure anti-C some of the anti-C also will be removed from the serum. This is mainly due to the presence of anti-G, an antibody which reacts with C and D and which is removed by absorption with D positive C negative cells (*see also* Chapter 33). Absorption is not, therefore, advisable unless the titre of the required antibody is sufficiently great to withstand a certain reduction without rendering it unfit for use. The titre of the component that is to remain in the serum should well exceed the titre of the antibody that is to be removed. Before the absorption of the main bulk of serum is undertaken pilot tests, using small quantities of cells and serum, should be carried out. These will show whether it is possible to prepare a pure reagent from the selected mixture and also the optimum proportion of cells to serum for the bulk absorption.

It is sometimes useful to absorb with papain-treated red cells by technique No. 14.2 to remove traces of unwanted antibody. Here again pilot absorptions will give an indication as to whether it is possible to prepare a pure reagent.

When the titres of the separate antibodies making up a given mixture approximate each other it is almost always impossible to prepare a pure reagent from the serum.

(*b*) **Removal of Agglutinins Belonging to the ABO Blood Group System.** In any serum selected as a suitable typing reagent there are almost always unwanted ABO agglutinins present. It is a very worth while procedure to remove these from the serum which otherwise can only be used for the typing of cells of compatible ABO group.

Anti-A (including anti-A_1) and anti-B agglutinins are removed by absorption with red cells of the appropriate group. The most useful red cells to use are those of group A_1B. These will remove anti-A, anti-A_1 and anti-B agglutinins if present. If A_2B cells are used, the anti-A_1 fraction will remain in the serum. It is, of course, possible to use group B cells to absorb anti-B from a group A serum or group A_1 cells to absorb anti-A from a group B serum. Nevertheless, if these are used they require an extra wash as they contain anti-A or anti-B agglutinins which it is obviously undesirable to add to the serum being absorbed.

The Rh sub-type of the cells chosen will of course depend upon the specificity of the anti-serum being prepared. Anti-D, anti-CD, and anti-DE mixtures will be absorbed by A_1B rr (cde.cde) cells; these are often the cells of choice for the absorption of anti-C and anti-E sera also, unless considerations dealt with in section (*a*) indicate the use of cells of a different Rh sub-type. Absorption of anti-c requires cells of genotype A_1B R_1R_1 (CDe.CDe) and anti-e of A_1B R_2R_2 (cDE.cDE).

The red cells used for absorption can have been stored up to fourteen days provided they have been preserved in the standard acid-citrate-dextrose anti-coagulant solution (A.C.D. *see* Appendix I). They must be washed free of their own plasma, for this would, on mixture with the serum to be absorbed, form a plasma clot which could make the subsequent handling of the mixture extremely difficult.

The quantity of red cells required for the removal of anti-A and anti-B agglutinins will naturally vary according to the potency of these agglutinins. It is advisable to aim at excess. It will usually be found that a volume of packed washed cells equal to the volume of serum to be absorbed is satisfactory. If the agglutinins are immune and of exceptionally high titre a larger quantity of cells may be needed. If the serum is freshly bled it is advisable to inactivate it to prevent hæmolysis of the absorbing red cells by any anti-A or anti-B hæmolysins which may be present. The serum-cell mixture is left at 4°C for at least 2 hours or preferably overnight.

In order to confirm that the anti-A and anti-B agglutinins have been removed from the serum, tests should be made against red cells from a number of group A and/or group B individuals. Red cells from different individuals vary in their reactivity to traces of antibody remaining in a serum and it is not uncommon to find that small quantities of antibody are detected by some cells but not by others. If even small quantities of anti-A or anti-B agglutinins remain in the serum after absorption it is advisable to reabsorb unless it is proposed to use the serum considerably diluted. If, for any reason, absorption of the serum with red cells is impracticable, the unwanted agglutinins can be "neutralised" by the addition of A or B group specific substances either in saliva or purified. This method of suppressing their activity is not recommended since the agglutinins are not actually removed from the serum. Neutralised sera should not be stored.

The use of enzyme techniques is so widespread that it is advisable that sera should have a final absorption with one-quarter volume of papain-treated red cells to remove the last traces of anti-A and anti-B (technique No. 14.2).

(*c*) **Removal of Antibodies of Other Blood Group Systems.** Antibodies belonging to other blood group systems may occur in a serum chosen for Rh typing. The range and characteristics of these are described in Chapters 16 to 20. If present it is advisable to remove them with appropriate red cells containing their corresponding antigen. This can usually be combined with the absorption of anti-A and anti-B agglutinins, *e.g.* if the serum also contains an unwanted anti-P_1 agglutinin A_1B cells of suitable Rh genotype which are also P_1 positive can be selected.

Standardisation

Having selected and absorbed a serum, it must be standardised. At this stage the two main essentials for a satisfactory anti-serum mentioned at the outset, namely potency and specificity, should more than ever be borne in mind.

The serum must first be re-titrated although normally the titration value will not have altered appreciably during the absorption process. If the titre is well above the minimum with red cells containing a single dose of the corresponding antigen, the serum can be tried out at several different dilutions.

The serum, both undiluted and suitably diluted if strong enough, must then be tested against at least thirty random red cell samples in parallel with a known typing serum of the same specificity. In addition it should be tested against a number of specially selected samples of appropriate ABO groups and known Rh genotype to find out whether or not all unwanted antibodies have been successfully removed. In fact the final tests must be so designed to ensure that the typing serum will detect the presence of the corresponding antigen, however weak, and that it will be specific for it.

Panels of cells containing rare antigens Wr^a, By^a, Vw, etc. (*see* Chapter 15) should be available for the final checking of all standard sera as although the antigens are rare the corresponding antibodies are more common.

Sterilisation and Storage

It is strongly recommended that Rh typing sera should be stored in a sterile condition. This is particularly important if such sera are ever distributed by post.

The titres of Rh antibodies are not often reduced by Seitz filtration of the serum, therefore this method of sterilisation can be adopted. It should be remembered that at least 5 ml. of serum will be lost in the Seitz filtration process. For very small quantities (up to 4 ml.) the Hemmings* filter can be used—this is a small filter which uses a Ford sterimat of 1·375 sq. cm. in area, *i.e.* of $\frac{11}{16}$ inch diameter—the loss of serum will not be more than 0·4 ml. Alternatively it is suggested that small amounts of a rare serum are apportioned out in such small quantities that sterility will

* The Hemmings filter is manufactured by H. A. Jones, of Beaumaris, Anglesey.

not be so important. The method of sterilisation by heating at 56°C for 30 minutes on three successive days while the serum stands at room temperature between the applications of heat is definitely detrimental to Rh antibodies. A small knife-point of sodium azide can be added after the individual containers have been opened and taken into use. Rh typing sera should be stored frozen solid at approximately −20°C. At higher temperatures than this, although the serum may appear to be completely frozen, the potency of the antibody may decrease quite rapidly. If kept under satisfactory conditions the sera will usually remain efficient for several years. However, some sera do not maintain their properties as well as others, so that if sera are kept for a long time they should be restandardised at regular intervals.

Techniques

Technique No. 14.1. Absorption of ABO agglutinins from an Rh typing serum

If the serum has been frozen it is thawed out gradually at room temperature or 37°C but not more rapidly than this. It is then inactivated by heating at 56°C for 30 minutes. While the serum is being thawed and inactivated, the red cells for the absorption can be washed, twice if they are of group AB or three times if of groups A or B. The proportional volume of saline to cells for washing should be at least 4 to 1. It is convenient to use a centrifuge specially designed for M.R.C. transfusion bottles, but in the absence of this convenience the washing can be carried out in universal containers or large test-tubes. Sterile precautions are not essential. The red cells used should be well sedimented so that most of the supernatant plasma can be sucked off before the first aliquot of saline is added. If it is not possible to select blood that has settled, one extra washing of the cells must be included.

The serum to be absorbed and an equal volume of well packed, washed cells are mixed and left at 4°C for 2 hours or preferably overnight.

The serum-cell mixture is centrifuged and the supernatant absorbed serum collected. This is then standardised and if found satisfactory, Seitz-filtered. If, however, more than trace amounts of ABO agglutinins remain after absorption, the serum must be re-absorbed. For a re-absorption, an amount of red cells equal to a quarter of the volume of serum to be absorbed should be sufficient. Alternatively an absorption using a quarter volume of papain treated cells may be more efficient. The sera should be bottled in quantities which are related to the normal turnover. Large laboratories will find 10 ml. amounts of anti-D sera convenient. On the other hand rare sera which are used slowly should be stored in quantities not greater than 0·25 ml. to avoid continual alternate freezing and thawing which is detrimental to the serum.

Technique No. 14.2. The use of papain-treated red cells for absorption of sera

The last traces of anti-A and anti-B (and indeed of other unwanted antibodies) are often best removed with papain-treated red cells.

A_1B Rh negative* cells are papain-treated either by mixing two parts of Löw's papain solution or alternatively two parts of a 1 per cent solution of papain (without activator) to one part of packed washed red cells, and the mixture incubated for ½ hour at 37°C. The red cells are then washed twice in a large volume of saline and packed. The serum to be absorbed is mixed with one-quarter of its volume of papain-treated cells and incubated for ½ hour at 37°C, spun and separated. The process is repeated until there is no agglutination of the papain-treated cells. The separated serum is then tested for complete absorption with a panel of A and B Rh negative cells.

Technique No. 14.3. Standardisation of an Rh typing serum

Tests to Show that the Serum is Free from ABO Agglutinins. The serum is tested by saline tube technique against ten red cell samples of each appropriate ABO group and Rh type at 4°C, R.T. and 37°C. The tests are left for 2 hours and read in the usual way. In addition the serum is tested against the same red cell samples at 37°C by albumin technique and also by any method by which it is proposed to use the serum. If any appreciable reaction is obtained the residual antibody should be titrated; according to the titre it is decided whether to re-absorb or rely upon diluting out the antibody.

Tests to Show that the Serum is Free from Other Contaminants. The serum is tested by saline, albumin and any other appropriate techniques at room temperature and 37°C against at least five red cell samples which are chosen because they contain the antigen corresponding to the contaminating antibody. It is particularly

* For anti-D; for other antibodies the absorbing cells will be suitably chosen, *e.g.* A_1 B R_1 R_1 for anti-c.

important that if possible some of them should contain the appropriate antigen in "double dose". Any residual contaminant is titrated and if present in appreciable amount removed by re-absorption.

Selection of Dilution for Use. The following tests will be done by the method by which it is proposed to use the serum, usually saline or albumin but occasionally others, *e.g.* indirect anti-human globulin for a serum which is to be used to detect D^u.

Table 14.1

Red Cell Samples Required for the Standardisation of the Various Rh Anti-sera

Anti-serum	Red cell samples needed					
	Random	R′	R″	R_2	Arr	Brr
Anti-D	30	5	5		10	10
Anti-CD	30	8	5	10	10	10
Anti-DE	30	5	8		10	10
Anti-C	30	8	5	10	10	10
Anti-E	30	5	8	10	10	10
					AR_1R_1	BR_1R_1
Anti-c	30				10	10
Anti-e	This presents a particular problem, but as many R_2R_2 and R_2r samples as possible must be included.					

Each component of the serum is titrated separately. The serum is tested at one or more dilutions, each of which must fulfil the criteria for the antibody or antibodies concerned. Table 14.1 shows the number and type of red cell samples with which each typing serum should be tested. The neat serum, or a dilution, is regarded as being satisfactory for use when all the positive reactions are V or ++ and there is no reaction whatever in the negative controls.

BIBLIOGRAPHY FOR Rh SECTION*

LEVINE, P., and STETSON, R. E. (1939), "An unusual case of intragroup agglutination." *J. Amer. med. Ass.*, **113,** 126.

WIENER, A. S., and PETERS, H. R. (1940), "Hemolytic reactions following transfusions of blood of the homologous group, with three cases in which the same agglutinogen was responsible." *Ann. int. Med.*, **13,** 2306.

LANDSTEINER, K., and WIENER, A. S. (1940), "An agglutinable factor in human blood recognised by immune sera for rhesus blood." *Proc. Soc. exp. Biol. N.Y.*, **43,** 223.

LANDSTEINER, K., and WIENER, A. S. (1941), "Studies on an agglutinogen (Rh) in human blood reacting with anti-rhesus sera and with human iso-antibodies." *J. exp. Med.*, **74,** 309.

LEVINE, P., KATZIN, E. M., and BURNHAM, L. (1941a), "Iso-immunisation in pregnancy, its possible bearing on the etiology of erythroblastosis fetalis." *J. Amer. med. Ass.*, **116**, 825.

LEVINE, P., VOGEL, P., KATZIN, E. M., and BURNHAM, L. (1941b), "Pathogenesis of erythroblastosis fetalis: statistical evidence." *Science*, **94,** 371.

LEVINE, P., BURNHAM, L., KATZIN, E. M., and VOGEL, P. (1941c), "The role of iso-immunisation in the pathogenesis of erythroblastosis fetalis." *Amer. J. Obstet. Gynec.*, **42,** 925.

RACE, R. R., and TAYLOR, G. L. (1943), "A serum that discloses the genotype of some Rh positive people." *Nature, Lond.*, **152,** 300.

RACE, R. R., TAYLOR, G. L., BOORMAN, KATHLEEN E., and DODD, BARBARA E. (1943), "Recognition of Rh genotypes in man." *Nature, Lond.*, **152,** 563.

RACE, R. R. (1944), "An 'incomplete' antibody in human serum." *Nature, Lond.*, **153,** 771.

RACE, R. R., TAYLOR, G. L., CAPPELL, D. F., and MCFARLANE, MARJORY N. (1944), "Recognition of a further common Rh genotype in man." *Nature, Lond.*, **153,** 52.

COOMBS, R. R. A., MOURANT, A. E., and RACE, R. R. (1945), "A new test for the detection of weak and 'incomplete' Rh agglutinins." *Brit. J. exp. Path.*, **26,** 255.

MOURANT, A. E. (1945), "A new rhesus antibody." *Nature, Lond.*, **155,** 542.

WIENER, A. S. (1945), "Conglutination test for Rh sensitization." *J. Lab. clin. Med.*, **30,** 662.

HILL, J. M., HABERMAN, S., and JONES, FRANCES (1946), "Hemolytic Rh immune globulins: evidence for a possible third order of antibodies incapable of agglutination or blocking." *Blood, Special Issue*, No. 2, 80.

PICKLES, MARGARET M. (1946). "Effects of cholera filtrate on red cells as demonstrated by incomplete Rh antibodies." *Nature, Lond.*, **158,** 880.

STRATTON, F. (1946), "A new Rh allelomorph." *Nature, Lond.*, **158,** 25.

MORTON, J. A., and PICKLES, M. M. (1947), "Use of trypsin in the detection of incomplete anti-Rh antibodies." *Nature*, **159,** 779–789.

RACE, R. R., SANGER, RUTH, and LAWLER, SYLVIA D. (1948), "Allelomorphs of the Rh gene C." *Heredity*, **2,** 237.

LÖW, B. (1955), "A practical method using papain and incomplete Rh antibodies in routine Rh blood grouping." *Vox Sang.*, **5,** 94–97.

LEVINE, P., CELANO, M. J., WALLACE, J., and SANGER, R. (1963) "A human D-like antibody." *Nature Lond.* **198.**

* These are mostly papers of historical interest. They are arranged in date order. See also bibliographies chapters 25 and 33.

Section 4—Other Blood Group Systems

"And thick and fast they came at last,
And more, and more, and more——"

Lewis Carroll, THROUGH THE LOOKING GLASS

CHAPTER 15

GENERAL INTRODUCTION TO OTHER BLOOD GROUP SYSTEMS

WE now approach a number of blood group systems which are of great interest and importance to the genetically minded blood group serologist but their practical aspects are by no means as far reaching as those of the ABO and Rh groups. This does not mean that they are entirely without clinical significance, indeed some of their antibodies have proved to be "killers". Nevertheless, the occurrence of these antibodies is comparatively rare. For this reason, routine antibody detection tests are not undertaken for each system individually. The identification of any atypical antibody that may be detected during routine ABO and Rh testing, and the full investigation of any serum suspected to contain atypical antibodies is described in Chapter 21.

The discovery of a blood group system is made through the finding of an antibody either accidentally or through the deliberate immunisation of animals, carried out in the hope that hitherto unknown antibodies will be produced as a result. The MN system (*see* next chapter) is, like the Rh system, an example of one which was disclosed by animal antibodies, although other antigens connected with the system were revealed later by antibodies of human origin.

Occasionally the discovery of a new system follows on the heels of the discovery of a new antibody detection technique. For example, the Kell groups were discovered within a few weeks of the development of the anti-human globulin technique. Not every new antibody heralds a new system. Some are found to detect antigens belonging to systems already described. Nor is it always at first easy to see the connexion between new antibodies and their antigens and old systems. Very often relationships only fall into place after thousands of tests have been performed or after inspection and correlation of the results of several teams of workers. Family studies also provide valuable evidence as to whether or not a "new" antigen belongs to one of the known blood group systems. These are undertaken both to see whether a newly-found antigen is travelling with a known antigen of one of the established systems (in which case the genes are said to segregate together) and to determine whether the antigen detected could be the product of a gene allelomorphic to one already known.

The MN system, as we shall see in the next chapter, was extended in both ways, a gene S was found to segregate with the M or N gene, MS being more common than NS; later an antiserum was found which reacted with s, a product of a gene allelomorphic to S.

New antigens are thus divided into three categories, those that belong to previously discovered systems; those that can be shown to be segregating independently of all previous known systems and therefore comprise new systems; and a large category where their precise position has not been determined.

Family studies are obviously difficult where the antigen is either very frequent or very rare and it is no wonder that there are many blood group antigens which are not yet accorded system status as it has not been possible to show their complete independence of all known systems.

In the P system, the antigen Luke falls into a new category in that it is a genetically independent part of the system—this is discussed in more detail in Chapter 34.

H, in the ABO system and LW in the Rh system are also genetically independent; these antigens are discussed in Chapters 32 and 33 respectively.

The frequencies of the blood group antigens vary from being so infrequent that they seem to be confined to the members of one family (private antigens) to being so common that they seem to be "non specific" and require long, patient testing before a pattern of reaction for them can be worked out. Of the first category the factor Di^a is an example, being found in four members of one family while 2,600 random bloods were negative and of the second anti-k of the Kell system where in the original tests of 2,500 blood specimens only five were negative with the new antibody.

Racial variations in antigen frequency very often occur; these may be striking and result in interesting findings. A comparison between the bloods of negroid and white races yields many instances of differences in antigenic frequencies, *e.g.* in the Duffy system the sub-group Fy(a-b-) is rare in whites but common in negroes. These racial distinctions occasionally account for the finding of apparent "private" antigens when mixed marriages occur.

The Di^a antigen mentioned above is a case in point. Admixture of white with native Indian blood accounted for the appearance in the family of what seemed to be a rare antigen. Subsequent studies of North and South American Indians, Chinese and Japanese bloods showed an incidence of Di^a of 3 to 45 per cent. There are other examples of this.

It would seem that mixed marriages and the transfusion of blood from members of one race to another should be a rich field for the study of new antigens and antibodies.

The progress of all blood group systems, following their discovery, seems to be through a period of clarity into the fog of increased complications as new alleles are discovered and afterwards, emergence, still in many cases partial, into a new understanding of the ramifications of the system in question. And how is all this related to routine work? As stated earlier, the antibodies of the blood groups to be described below have little practical importance owing either to their infrequent occurrence or their low potency.

As expected, it is the warm antibodies that cause hæmolytic disease or transfusion reactions. However, potent cold antibodies may work at 37°C either as agglutinins or as incomplete antibodies requiring complement, *e.g.* anti-P, anti-Le^a, or even if reactive below 37°C, may be stimulated to become active at 37°C by the corresponding antigen. This means that for transfusion purposes it is better not to use blood containing antigens corresponding to antibodies reactive at room temperature.

The practical importance of a blood group system is not only related to the efficiency of its antigens in the production of warm antibodies, but also upon their opportunity for stimulating antibody formation; this is related to their frequency. For example, the k antigen is so common that only 1 in 500 people lack it, so inevitably, however good an antigen k may be, the antibody will always be one of the rarest in existence.

At the other end of the scale are very rare antigens, *e.g.* Mg, V^w, Wr^a, etc., for which the antibodies are comparatively common. These antibodies are usually of the "cold" type and occur in the sera of people who have not been stimulated to produce them by the corresponding antigen. A serum, which is found to agglutinate only one red cell sample when tested with many, thus merits special investigation. The possibility of standard sera

Table 15.1

Antigens & Antibodies of the Established Blood Group Systems

Blood group system	Antigens	Clinical significance of antibodies*		
		Hæmolytic transfusion reactions	Hæmolytic disease of the newborn	Other clinical association
ABO	$A_1A_2A_3A_x$, B, H. Rare A and B variants	Anti-A, anti-B	Anti-A, anti-B (usually when Mother Group O)	
MNSs	M, N, S, s, U'M^c'M_1, Tm'M^k Hu, He, Mi^a, Vw Mur-Hil'Vr, Ri^a, St^a, Mt^a, Cl^a, Ny^a'Sul'Sj, M_2'N_2'M^c'M^a-M^r' S_2	Anti-S, anti-s. Rarely anti-M, anti-N, anti-U	Anti-S, anti-s. Very rarely anti-M. Anti-U	
P	P_1, P^k, P_2. Luke	Anti-PP_1, P^k. (Originally called anti-Tja). Very rarely anti-P_1		Anti-Tja may be related to abortion. Anti-P can occur as a cold auto-ant in P.N.H. Donath-Landsteiner antibody
Rh	D, D^u, C, C^u, C^w, C^x, c, E, e, e^s (VS)'hr_s, E^w, E^u, G, ce, ce_s (V), Ce, CE, cE, D^w, E^T, LW and rare variants Go^a, Go^b	Anti-D most important but all Rh antibodies can cause transfusion reactions	Anti-D most important together with anti-CD and anti-DE. Other Rh antibodies also cause hæmo-disease. Severity of the disease is roughly related to the anti-human globulin titre of the serum. Antibodies only detected by enzyme techniques rarely cause hæmolytic disease	Anti-e is a common auto-antibody in the "warm" type hæmolytic anæmias. Other Rh antibodies also found as auto-antibodies in this disease

Blood group system	Antigens	Clinical significance of antibodies		
		Hæmolytic transfusion reactions	Hæmolytic disease of the newborn	Other clinical association
Lutheran	Lu^a, Lu^b	Anti-Lu^b has caused mild transfusion reaction	Very rarely anti-Lu^b	
Kell	K, k, $Kp^aKp^bJs^aJs^b$Ula	Anti-K, anti-k; probably the other rare antibodies also	Anti-K, anti-k. Anti-Ku also in one case	
Lewis	Le^a, Le^b	Rarely anti-Le^a		
Duffy	Fy^a, Fy^b	Anti-Fy^a, anti-Fy^b	Rarely anti-Fy^a	
Kidd	Jk^a, Jk^b	Anti-Jk^a, anti-Jk^b	Rarely anti-Jk^a, anti-Jk^b	
Diego	Di^a, Di^b	Anti-Di^a, anti-Di^b	Anti-Di^a	
Yt	Yt^a, Yt^b	Antibodies very rare but could cause hæmolytic transfusion reaction		
I	Ii			Auto anti-I in acquired hæmolytic anæmia of the cold antibody type. Anti-i in various hæmatological disorders and associated with infectious mononucleosis.
Xg	Xg^a			
Dombrook	Do^a	Antibody rare but can destroy transfused red cells		

* Antibodies not listed here have little or no known clinical importance.

Table 15.2

Antigens Other than those Known to Belong to the Major Blood Group Systems

Antigen	Clinical significance	Associations excluded	Frequency of antigen	References
Au^a (Auberger)		ABO, MNSs, P, Rh., Duffy, Kidd and Le^a. For relationship with Lutheran, *see* Chapter 34	82%	Salmon *et al.* (1961) Tippett, P. (1963)
At^a (August)	One example Direct, A.h.g. of baby weakly positive	MNSs, Rh, Kidd, Xg	Almost universal	Applewhaite *et al.* (1967)
By (Batty)	Doubtful case of very mild hæmolytic disease. Antibody found in a few cases hæmolytic anæmia	Levay, Mi^a, Be, Ven, Wr^a, Lutheran, Le^a, Duffy, Sex, ABO, Rh, Ca, Diego, Vw, Rm	Very rare	Simmons and Ware (1959) Cleghorn (1960)
Becker	Hæmolytic disease		Very rare	Elbel and Prokop (1951)
Be^a (Berrens)	Hæmolytic disease	Ca, By, Good, Yt, ABO, Duffy, MNSs, Sex	Very rare	Davidson *et al.* (1953)
Bi^a (Biles)	Stimulated by pregnancy	Rh, Sex	Very rare	Wadlington *et al.* (1961)
Bp^a (Bishop)		ABO, MNSs, P, Rh, Duffy, Kidd, Sex	Very rare	Cleghorn (1964) unpublished
Bg^a, Bg^b, Bg^c(Ho)(Ot) (Bennett-Goodspeed, Donna, Sturgeon)		ABO, MNSs, P, Rh, Duffy, Kidd, Secretor, Sex, Lutheran, Kell	29% Bg^a, Bg^b Rare	Buchanan and Afganis (1963) Chown *et al.* (1963) Dorfmeir *et al.* (1959) Van der Hart *et al.* (1961) Seaman *et al.* (1967)
Bu^a (Probably allelic to Sm)	Mild transfusion reaction	ABO, MNSs, P, Rh, Lu, Duffy, Kidd, Dombrock, Wr^a, Sex	Rare	Anderson *et al.* (1963)
Bx^a (Box)		ABO, MNSs, P, Rh, Duffy, Kidd, Lutheran, Kell	Very rare	Jenkins and Marsh (1961)
Cavaliere	Hæmolytic disease, 1 case	Be^a	Rare	Wiener and Brancato (1953)
Chido			Very frequent	Harris *et al.* (1967)
Chr^a			Very rare	Kissmeyer-Nielsen (1955)
Co^a	Found on direct match	ABO, MNSs, P, Rh, Duffy, Kidd, Do, Sex	Very frequent	Heistö *et al.* (1967)

(contd.)

Antigen	Clincial significance	Associations excluded	Frequency of antigen	References
Cs^a	Active 37°C	Rh, MNSs, Duffy, Kidd, Sex	98 %	Giles *et al.* (1965)
Dp		MNSs, Rh, Secretor, Duffy, Sex	Very frequent	Schmidt *et al.* (1967)
El			Very frequent	Schmidt *et al.* (1967)
En	Anti-Eh^a active at 37°C	ABO, MNS_s, Rh, Duffy, Sex	Almost universal	Furuhjelm *et al* (1969)
Evans	One case hæmolytic disease	Possibly belongs to Rh system	Rare	Weiner (1966)
Ge		ABO, MNSs, P, Rh, Kell, Kidd, Sex	Very frequent (Two types of anti-Ge sera known)	Rosenfield *et al.* (1960)
Gf		MNSs, Rh, Dombrock, Sex	Very rare	Cleghorn *et al.* (1966) unpublished.
Good	Hæmolytic disease	ABO, MNSs, Rh, Kell, Levay, Wr^a, Be^a, By, Sw^a	Very rare	Frumin *et al.* (1960)
Heibel	Hæmolytic disease	Most known	Very rare	Ballowitz *et al.* (1968)
Ho (*see* Bg^b)		As for Bg^b	Rare	Van der Hart *et al.* (1961) Seaman *et al.* (1967)
Ht^a (Hunt)	Hæmolytic disease	MNSs, Rh, Sex	Very rare	Jahn and Cleghorn (1962) unpublished
Jn^a			Very rare	Kornstad *et al.* (1967)
Kamhuber	Transfusion reaction	Most	Very rare	Speiser *et al.* (1966)
Lan	Transfusion reaction	None (Lan negative probably recessive)	Very frequent	Van der Hart *et al.* (1961)
Levay		MNSs, Sex, By, Good, R^m, Js, Yt	Rare	Callender and Race (1946)
Ls^a		ABO, MNSs, P, Rh, Lutheran, Kidd, Sex	Very rare	Cleghorn and Dunsford (1963) unpublished
Marriott		ABO, P, Rh		Zeitlin *et al.* (1960) unpublished
Or (Orriss)		ABO, Rh, Sec, Sex	Rare	Cleghorn *et al.* (1964) unpublished
Ot (*see* Bg^c)	Found at direct match	MNSs, P, Rh, Duffy, Kidd, Sec, Sex	2 in 300	Dorfmeier (1959)

Table 15.2 (*contd.*)

Antigen	Clinical significance	Associations excluded	Frequency of antigen	References
Raddon	Found at direct match		Rare	Lockyer and Tovey (1967) unpublished
Rd		ABO, MNSs, Rh, Kell, Kidd, Sex	Rare	Rausen *et al.* (1967)
Rm	Hæmolytic disease	Levay, Wr^a, By, Be^a	Rare	Van der Hart *et al.* (1954)
Sd^a		ABO, MNSs, P, Rh, Lu, K, Lewis, Duffy, Kidd, Yt, and Xg	91%	Macvie *et al.* (1967) Renton *et al.* (1967)
Sm		All save Diego and Yt	Extremely frequent	Schmidt, R., *et al.* (1962)
		Related to Bu^a		Lewis *et al.* (1964)
Stobo		Probably part of Bg antigen complex	Very rare	Wallace and Milne (1959)
Sw^a (Swann	Found at direct match; occurs in some hæmolytic sera	ABO, MNSs, P, Rh, K, Duffy, Kidd, Sec, Sex, and many rare antigens	Very rare	Cleghorn (1960)
To^a (Torkildsen)		MNSs, P, Sec, Sex	Very rare	Kornstad *et al.* unpublished
Tr^a (Traversu)		ABO, MNSs, P, Rh, Duffy, Kidd, Sec, Sex	Very rare	Cleghorn (1962) unpublished
Ul^a (Karhula) (see Kell)		ABO, MNSs, P, Rh, Lu, Duffy, Kidd, Dombrook, Sec, Sex	Up to 5% in Finns; otherwise rare	Furuhjelm *et al.* (1968)
Vel.	Transfusion reaction	ABO, MNSs, Rh, Lewis, Duffy, Lu, Kidd	99·9%	Sussman and Miller (1952)
Ven.	Hæmolytic disease	By, R^m, Wr^a	Very rare	Van Loghem *et al.* (1952)
Wb (Webb)		ABO, MNSs, Rh, 23 rare antigens, Sex	Very rare	Simmons and Albrey (1963)
Wr^a (Wright)	Hæmolytic disease and transfusion reactions	ABO, MNSs, P, Rh, Kell, Duffy, Kidd, Sex	0·3% Dutch 0·1% English	Holman (1953)
Wu (Wulfsberg)			Very rare	Heistö (1966) Kornstad and Wolthuis (1967) unpublished

containing such antibodies and therefore giving a false positive with blood containing the rare antigen is an extra reason why two sera of the same specificity should be used for all testing. Wherever possible, of course, the laboratory preparing the serum will have checked it against cells containing the known rare antigens but they may not possess a "full set" and new rare antigens with common antibodies will probably continue to be found for many years to come.

Most blood group antigens show "dosage" so that wherever possible the "double dose" cell (*e.g.* KK, Fy^aFy^a) should be used for antibody detection techniques. The distinction between the homo- and heterozygote is not usually sufficiently clear cut however for genotyping to be done on "dosage" alone.

Table 15.1 summarises the blood group systems, including ABO and Rh and gives an idea of their clinical importance. These systems are further discussed in the next three chapters.

Table 15.2 deals with the other blood group antigens which have not, as yet, attained the status of independent systems. It will be realised that these also may be of clinical importance.

In Chapter 21, Table 21.2(I), (II) and (III) blood group antibodies, whether relating to known systems or to unclassified antigens, are arranged in three sections according to the frequency of the antigen they are detecting (I) those giving almost 100 per cent positives, (II) 95 per cent to 1 per cent positives, and (III) <1 per cent including those so rare as to be found only in the family of the propositus. This table also gives the systems, if any, to which the antibodies belong, the approximate frequency with which the antibody is found and the usual technique and temperature for its detection.

BIBLIOGRAPHY

ANDERSON, C., HUNTER, J., ZIPURSKY, A., LEWIS, M., and CHOWN, B. (1963), "An antibody defining a new blood group antigen Bu^a." *Transfusion*, **3**, 30.

APPLEWHAITE, F., GINSBERG, V., GERENA, J., CUNNINGHAM, C. A. and GAVIN, JUNE (1967), "A very frequent red cell antigen At^a." *Vox Sang.*, **13**, 444.

BALLOWITZ, L., FIELDER, M., HOFFMAN, C., and PETTENKOFEN, H. (1968), "'Heibel' a new rare human blood group antibody, revealed by hæmolytic disease of the new born." *Vox Sang.*, **14**, 307–309.

BUCHANAN, D. I., and AFAGANIS, A. (1963), "The Bennett–Goodspeed–Sturgeon or 'Donna' red cell antigen and antibody." *Vox Sang.*, **8**, 213.

CALLENDER, SHEILA T., and RACE, R. R. (1946), "A serological and genetical study of multiple antibodies formed in response to blood transfusion by a patient with lupus erythematosus diffusus." *Ann. Eugen. Lond.*, **13**, 102.

CHOWN, B., LEWIS, M., KASTIAN, H. (1963), "The Bennett–Goodspeed antigen or antigens." *Vox Sang.*, **8**, 281.

CLEGHORN, T. E. (1959), "A 'new' human blood group antigen, Sw^a." *Nature*, **184**, 1324.

CLEGHORN, T. E. (1960), "The inheritance of the antigen Sw[a] and evidence for its independence of other blood group systems." *Brit. J. Hæm.*, **6,** 433.

CLEGHORN, T. E. (1960), "The frequency of the Wr[a], By and Mg blood group antigens in blood donors in the South of England." *Vox Sang.*, **5,** No. 6.

DAVIDSOHN, I., STERN, K., STRAUSER, E. R., and SPURRIER, WILMA (1953), "Be, a new 'private' blood factor," *Blood*, **8,** 747.

DORFMEIER, HANNY, HART, MIA VAN DER, NIJENHUIS, L. E., and LOGHEM, J. J. VAN (1959), "A 'New' blood group antigen of rare occurrence (Ot)." *Proc.-7th Cong. int. Soc. Blood Transf.* 608.

ELBEL, H., and PROKOP, O. (1951), "Ein neues erbliches Antigen als Ursache gehäufter Fehlgeburten." *Zeitschr. f. Hygiene*, **132,** 120.

FRUMIN, A. M., MCKEE, PORTER, M., and EICHMAN, M. F. (1960), "The Good factor as a possible cause of hæmolytic disease of the newborn." *Blood*, xv, **5,** 681–682.

FURUHJELM, U., NEVANLINNA, H. R., NURKKA, RÜTTA, GAVIN, JUNE, TIPPETT, PATRICIA, GOOCH, ANN, and SANGER, RUTH (1968), "The Blood Group Antigen Ul[a] (Karhula)." *Vox Sang.*, **15,** 118.

FURUHJELM, U., MYLLYLǍ, G. NEVANLINNA, H. R., NORDLING, S., PIRKOLA, ANNA, GAVIN, JUNE, GOOCH, ANN, SANGER, RUTH, and TIPPETT, PATRICIA (669) "The red cell phenotyre En(a—) and anti-En[a]; serological and physico-chemical aspects" *Vox Sang.*, **17,** 256.

GILES, CAROLYN M., HUTH, M. C., WILSON, T. E., LEWIS, H. B. M., and GROVE, G. E. B., (1965) "Three examples of a new antibody, anti-Cs[a] which reacts with 98 per cent of red cell samples." *Vox Sang.*, 10, 405.

HARRIS, JEAN P., TEGOLI, J., SWANSON, JANE, FISHER, NATHALIE, GAVIN, JUNE, and NOADES, JEAN (1967), "A nebulous antibody responsible for cross-matching difficulties (Chido)." *Vox Sang.*, **12,** 140.

HART, MIA VAN DER, BOSMAN, HÉLÈNE, and LOGHEM, J. J. VAN (1954), "Two rare human blood group antigens." *Vox Sang.*, **4,** 108.

HART, MIA VAN DER, MOES, MEIKE, VEER, MARGA V D. and LOGHEM, J. J. VAN (1961), "Ho and Lan—two new blood group antigens." *Proceedings of VIIIth European Congress Hæmatology*.

HEISTÖ, H., HART, MIA VAN DER, MADSEN, GRETHE, MOES, MEIKE, NOADES, JEAN, PICKLES, MARGARET M., RACE, R. R., SANGER, RUTH, and SWANSON, JUNE (1967), "Three examples of a new red cell antibody, anti-Co[a]." *Vox Sang.*, **12,** 18–24.

HOLMAN, C. A. (1953), "A new rare human blood-group antigen (Wr[a])." *Lancet*, ii, 119.

JENKINS, W. J., and MARSH, W. L. (1961), "Auto immune hæmolytic anæmia; three cases with antibodies specifically active against stored red cells." *Lancet*, **2,** 16–18.

KISSMEYER-NIELSEN, F. (1955), "A new rare blood group antigen Chr[a]." *Vox Sang.*, **5,** 102.

KORNSTAD, L., KOUT, M., LARSEN, A. M. J., and ØRJASACTER, H. (1967), "A rare blood group antigen, Jn[a]." *Vox Sang.*, **13,** 165–170.

LEWIS, MARION, CHOWN, B., SCHMIDT, R. PAULINE, and GRIFFITHS, J. T. (1964), "A possible relationship between the blood group antigens Sm and Bu[a]." *Amer. J. hum. Genet.*, **16,** 254.

LOGHEM, J. J. VAN, and HART, MIA VAN DER (1952), "Een zeldzaam voorkomende bloedgroep (Ven)." *Bull. van het Centraal Laboratorium van de Bloedtransfusiedicast van het Nederlandse Rode Kruis*, **2,** 225.

MACVIE, S. I., MORTON, J. A., and PICKLES, M. M. (1967), "The reactions and inheritance of a new blood group antigen Sd[a]." *Vox Sang.*, **13,** 485.

RAUSEN, A. R., ROSENFIELD, R. E., ALTER, A. A., HAKIM, S., GRAVEN, S. N., APPOLLON, CORA J., DALLMAN, P. R., DALZIEL, JOAN C., KONUGRES, ANGELYN, A., FRANCIS, BETTY, GAVIN, JUNE, and CLEGHORN, T. E. (1967), "A 'new' infrequent red cell antigen Rd (Radin)." *Transfusion, Philad.* **7,** 336.

RENTON, P. H., HOWELL, P., IKIN, ELIZABETH, W., GILES, CAROLYN, M., and GOLDSMITH, K. L. G. (1967), "Anti-Sd^a, a new blood group antibody." *Vox Sang.*, **13,** 493.

ROSENFIELD, R. E., HABER, GLADYS V., KISSMEYER-NIELSEN, F., JACK, J. A., SANGER, RUTH, and RACE, R. R. (1960), "Ge a very common red-cell antigen." *Brit. J. Hæm.*, **6,** No. 4, 344–349.

SALMON, C., SALMON, D., LIBERGE, G., ANDRE, R., TIPPETT, P., and SANGER, R. (1961), "Un nouvel ontigene de groupe sanguin erythrocytaire present chez 80 per cent des sujets de race blanche." *Nouv. Rev. France Hemat.*, **1,** 649.

SCHMIDT, R. P., GRIFFITHS, J. J., and NORTHMAN, F. F. (1962), "A new antibody anti-Sm reacting with a high incidence antigen." *Transfusion*, **2,** 338.

SCHMIDT, R. PAULINE, FRANK, SALLY, and BAUGH, MARIE (1967), "New antibodies to high incidence antigenic determinants (anti-So, anti-El, anti-Hy and anti-Op)." *Transfusion, Philid.*, **7,** 386.

SEAMAN, M. J., BENSON, R., JONES, M. N., MORTON, J. A., and PICKLES, M. M. (1967), "The reactions of the Bennett-Goodspeed group of antibodies with the Auto-Analyser." *Brit. J. Hæmat.*, **13,** 464.

SIMMONS, R. T., and ALBREY, J. A. (1963), "A new blood group antigen Webb (Wb) of low frequency found in two Australian families." *Med. J. Aust.*, **1,** 8.

SIMMONS, R. T., and WERE, S. O. M. (1955), "A 'new' family blood-group antigen and antibody (By) of rare occurrence." *Med. J. Aust.*, ii, 55.

SPEISER, P., KÜHBÖCK, J., MICKERTS, D., PAUSCH, V., REICHEL, G., LAUER, D., POREMBA, I., DOERING, I., and HAMACHER, H. (1966), " 'Kamhuber' a new human blood group antigen of familial occurrence, revealed by severe transfusion reaction." *Vox Sang.*, **11,** 113.

SUSSMAN, L. N., and MILLER, E. B. (1952), "Un nouveau facteur sanguin, 'Vel'." *Rev. d'Hem*, **7,** 368.

SWANSON, JANE, POLESKY, H. F., TIPPETT, PATRICIA, and SANGER, RUTH, "A 'new' blood group antigen Do^a." (1965) *Nature*, 206, 313.

TIPPETT, PATRICIA (1963), "Serological Study of the Inheritance of Unusual Rh and other Blood Group Phenotypes." Ph.D. Thesis, University of London.

WADLINGTON, W. B., MOORE, W. H., and HARTMANN, R. C. (1961), "Maternal sensitisation due to Bi, a preserved 'new private' red cell antigen." *Amer. J. Dis. Ch.*, **101,** 623.

WALLACE, J., and MILNE, G. R. (1959), "A 'new' human blood group antigen of rare frequency." *Proc. 7th., Congr. Int. Soc. Blood Transf.*, 587.

WIENER, A. S., and BRANCATO, G. J. (1953), "Severe erythroblastosis fetalis caused by sensitization to a rare human agglutinogen." *Amer. J. Hum. Genet.*, **5,** 350.

WEINER, W. (1966). Unpublished observations quoted Race R. and Sanger, R. *Blood Groups in Man.* Fifth Edition (1968).

CHAPTER 16

THE MNSs SYSTEM

THE MN groups were discovered by Landsteiner and Levine (Landsteiner and Levine, 1927, 1928) when experimenting with rabbit sera after the animals had received injections of human red cells. Two antibodies, called anti-M and anti-N, were identified and these were found to divide the human population into three groups:

(1) Persons whose red cells were agglutinated only by anti-M —group M.

(2) Persons whose red cells were agglutinated only by anti-N—group N.

(3) Persons whose red cells were agglutinated by both anti-M and anti-N—group MN.

No persons were found whose cells did not agglutinate with either of the two anti-sera.

The frequency of the three groups in the English population has been found to be:

Group M	About 28 per cent
Group N	About 22 per cent
Group MN	About 50 per cent

The two antigens have been shown to be derived from a single pair of genes which are allelomorphic and co-dominant. Chromosomes, therefore, can only be of two kinds M or N with three ways of pairing:

(*a*) M can pair with M giving rise to genotype MM—phenotype or group M.

(*b*) N can pair with N giving rise to genotype NN—phenotype or group N.

(*c*) M can pair with N giving rise to genotype MN—phenotype or group MN.

Thus it can be seen that given suitable anti-M and anti-N antisera three phenotypes can be differentiated.

The possible matings and the children that may arise from

them are shown in Table 16.1. The last column in the table sets out the MN groupings that cannot arise from each given mating.

The clinical significance of MN groups is slight. One or two cases of transfusion reaction have been reported, a single case incriminating anti-M as the cause of hæmolytic disease of the newborn and one relating its presence in a serum to the occurrence of stillbirths. The system is helpful in cases of disputed paternity since the genotypes are easily determined and for the most part unequivocal. In addition the MN groups are often used when it is desired to trace the survival *in vivo* of transfused red cells.

Table 16.1

Matings within the MN System

MN group of parents	Possible MN groups of children	Impossible MN groups of children
M × M	M	N MN
M × N	MN	M N
M × MN	M MN	N
N × N	N	M MN
N × MN	N MN	M
MN × MN	M N MN	

The antigens are so weakly antigenic in Man that it is perfectly safe, for example, to transfuse type N blood to type M patient.

The production of good anti-sera for MN typing purposes is by no means easy. Anti-M and anti-N antibodies are of comparatively rare occurrence in human sera. They are neither regularly present in individuals lacking the antigen as in the ABO system nor are they fairly readily produced in response to stimulation by the appropriate antigen as in the Rh system. When they are found anti-N are almost invariably rather weak naturally occurring cold antibodies; anti-M antibodies tend to be stronger and can often be used for MN typing by technique 16.1.

Anti-sera for MN typing are most satisfactorily made in rabbits in similar fashion to those of the original experiments which disclosed the existence of the system.

The main problem with regard to the production of good anti-sera is that of satisfactory absorption. The production of a potent specific anti-serum from the raw material is by no means easy and not comparable with the simple process of absorption which is adequate for most Rh sera. The serum of any rabbit normally contains various agglutinins for human red cells, in particular one which reacts preferentially with human group A red cells; these agglutinins are collectively known as "anti-Man". When human red cells of type M or type N are injected for the purpose of producing anti-M or anti-N agglutinins, the "anti-Man" antibodies rise in titre as might be expected. Moreover, unless group O red cells are used immune anti-A and/or anti-B agglutinins may be produced in the rabbit, and these also must be removed. The amount of red cells required for absorption is very critical—too few red cells leave a serum which is not specific and gives false positive reactions—too many red cells cause a "non-specific" absorption of the anti-M or anti-N agglutinins which may make the serum too weak for typing purposes. In this respect anti-N agglutinins are more readily non-specifically absorbed by type M cells than are anti-M agglutinins by type N cells (*see* below).

The seeds of the plant Vicia graminea on extraction with saline in a similar manner to technique 6.3 yield a potent anti-N reagent although this may require some adjustment of dilution to give a specific reaction. This reagent is suitable for use by either technique 16.1 or 16.2.

For the accurate MN typing of red cells at least three examples of both anti-M and anti-N* sera should be used. The anti-sera usually show quite marked dosage effect giving stronger results with genotypes MM or NN than with MN; no typing therefore should be done without a control of MN cells. Rare forms of M and N have been described which are agglutinated by some anti-sera but not others. These have been designated M_2 (Friedenreich and Lauridsen, 1938) and N_2 (Friedenreich, 1936) but they are hardly ever encountered. Another antigen M^c which appears to be intermediate between M and N has been discovered more recently (Dunsford *et al.*, 1953). Other rare alleles are given in Chapter 35.

The Ss System and its Association with MN

In 1947 a new antibody was discovered which defined an antigen in human red cells associated with the MN groups (Walsh and Montgomery, 1947; Sanger and Race, 1947). The newly discovered antigen and its corresponding antibody were termed S and anti-S. In the English population the proportion of blood samples agglutinated by anti-S is approximately 55 per cent.

* Extract of Vicia graminea can be substituted for one of the anti-N sera.

However, this proportion varies if the three groups M, N, and MN are considered separately. Of M samples about 73 per cent are agglutinated by anti-S, of N samples 32 per cent are agglutinated and of MN samples 54 per cent are agglutinated. These figures show that S occurs in association with M rather than with N which suggests that there is some relationship between the MN system and S. This relationship can be confirmed using statistical methods.

In 1951 (Levine *et al.*, 1951) another antibody was found which was shown to detect the product of a gene allelomorphic to S. This antibody, therefore, was designated anti-s and the antigen detected by it, s. The discovery of this second antibody makes the existence of a pair of genes, separate from M and N but closely associated, the most likely explanation of the connexion between MN and Ss.

Individuals can be of genotype SS, Ss, or ss. The frequencies of these are as follows:

Genotype SS	About 11 per cent
Genotype Ss	About 44 per cent
Genotype ss	About 45 per cent

Anti-S and anti-s, therefore, agglutinate the red cells of about 55 per cent and 89 per cent of the population respectively. Unlike anti-M and anti-N, these antibodies are usually active at 37°C. Anti-S has been shown to be responsible for both hæmolytic disease of the newborn and hæmolytic transfusion reactions and so has the rarer anti-s. In routine work anti-S may be available, although it is rare, but not anti-s. Typing of red cells with anti-S is carried out by saline or albumin tube technique, usually at 37°C, or the indirect anti-human globulin test may have to be used. The method chosen will depend on the optimum for each individual anti-serum.

The various phenotypes and genotypes are shown in Table 16.2. Results of large numbers of family studies have shown that each M or N gene has S or s closely related to it, so closely in fact that no crossovers have been discovered and they segregate as though they were one gene. This means, as can be seen in Table 16.2, there are 10 ways in which the four genes can be arranged. Since anti-s is so rare and only available to a few serologists the phenotypes given in this table are those defined by the anti-sera M, N, and S.

In spite of the association between the MN and Ss genes, which has led to their being regarded as belonging to the same blood group system, for most practical purposes they can be considered quite separately. Indeed their antibodies have widely diverse characteristics. Anti-M and anti-N are cold agglutinins which rarely become active at 37°C and are of little clinical significance. Anti-S and anti-s are immune antibodies active at 37°C appearing in both complete and incomplete forms and have been responsible for both hæmolytic disease of the newborn and hæmolytic transfusion reactions.

Table 16.2

The MNSs Phenotypes as Defined by Anti-M, Anti-N, and Anti-S, and the Genotypes Comprised

Reactions with			Phenotype	Genotype
Anti-M	Anti-N	Anti-S		
+	−	+	MS	MSMS MSMs
+	−	−	Ms	MsMs
+	+	+	MNS	MSNS MSNs MsNS
+	+	−	MNs	MsNs
−	+	+	NS	NSNS NSNs
−	+	−	Ns	NsNs

Cross Reactions between M and N

There is often marked cross-reactivity between anti-N and M cells. In fact continual absorption of rabbit anti-N with human M cells may result in almost complete uptake of the anti-N although there is little or no uptake of anti-M by N cells. Cross reactions between M and anti-N are increased by lowering the temperature or by treatment of the cells with trypsin (but not papain). The plant anti-N from Vicia graminea also cross reacts. The cross reactions are thought to be due to an N-like receptor on M red cells.

In practice, the tendency for cross reactivity means that care has to be taken in the absorption of sera when preparing anti-M and anti-N grouping reagents and in the carrying out of the M and N typing tests.

The Effect of Enzymes

Papain, trypsin, ficin and bromelin inhibit MNSs reactions, though the cross reaction of anti-N with M cells is enhanced by trypsin.

Further Ramifications of the MNSs System

In this chapter we have described the simple MNSs relationships. Rare alleles exist and the genetic background is more complicated than the above description implies.

Those interested, will find a section of Chapter 34 which deals with these further ramifications which add considerably to our understanding of this important system.

For most practical work, however, the simple MNSs system will be found to be adequate. Only when apparent anomalies arise or an unusual antibody, which seems to be related to MNSs, is encountered need the possibility of, for example, a rare MN allele be considered.

Techniques

Technique No. 16.1. Typing of red cells for M and N-tube technique

At least two and preferably three anti-M and the same number of anti-N typing sera are used at the recommended dilution in saline (*see* technique No. 16.5). One unit volume (approximately 0·03 ml.) of each serum is delivered into the required number of precipitin tubes including three tubes for each serum with control cells of types M, N, and MN.

To each tube is added an equal volume of the red cells to be tested made up to a 2 per cent suspension in saline (judged by eye). The tests are left at 20°C (room temperature) for two hours.

The tests are then read as for ABO grouping, including gentle tapping of the tube as false positive results may be obtained if the cell sediment is not agitated.

The controls must be read first. The results obtained with an antiserum which is giving more than a weak (w) reaction with cells with which it should be negative must be discarded.

Technique No. 16.2. Typing of red cells for M and N—tile technique

Two or preferably three examples of each anti-serum are used at a dilution suitable for tile grouping (*see* technique No. 16.5).

The test is performed on a white opalescent glass tile appropriately marked out in squares. One drop of antiserum is placed in each square of a row of the required length, allowing for controls of M, N, and MN cells. One drop of a 5 per cent suspension of the red cells to be tested (previously washed in saline) is added to each drop of antiserum. The serum and cells are mixed thoroughly with the corner of a microscope slide or with a glass rod. After standing for two or three minutes, the tile is gently rocked. When the MN control is giving a good reaction and while the negative controls are still completely clear, the results are read.

Technique No. 16.3. Typing of red cells with anti-S

Anti-S is rare so that small unit volumes of the order of 0·01 ml. of one antiserum only should be used. Negative reactions should, wherever possible, be confirmed with a second anti-S serum.

The method of testing will depend upon the nature of the antibody.

If the anti-S is an agglutinin the saline tube technique as for Rh typing is employed (technique No. 9.2) incubating either at 37°C or room temperature according to the reactivity of the particular antibody. The reading is also done in the manner recommended for Rh tests. An incomplete anti-S is best used by anti-human globulin technique (technique No. 12.4a) although bovine albumin methods (technique No. 9.3) may occasionally be found satisfactory.

With each batch of tests known S positive and S negative red cells are included as controls.

Technique No. 16.4. Preparation of anti-M and anti-N typing sera

The following account is based on the methods used by Dr. E. W. Ikin of the Medical Research Council Blood Group Reference Laboratory.

Injection of Rabbits. To obtain several satisfactory sera, at least six rabbits should be used to produce anti-M sera, and at least six to produce anti-N sera. Cells of the type OM are given to the "anti-M" rabbits, and ON cells to the "anti-N" rabbits. A course consists of injecting 0·5 ml. washed packed cells from an OM (or ON) person into each rabbit, intraperitoneally on the first day and intravenously on the five successive days. The intraperitoneal dose is given on the first day to prevent anaphylactic shock. The vein most easily used is the posterior peripheral auricular vein. On the ninth or tenth day after the last injections the rabbits are bled about 30–40 ml. from the peripheral auricular vein.

Absorption of Anti-M Sera. Rabbits sometimes possess a

naturally occurring anti-A and thus it is best to use group A_1 rather than group O blood for absorption. Very rarely they possess a naturally occurring anti-B which may necessitate a special absorption with group BN red cells. Alternatively if available, group A_1BN cells can be used routinely for these absorptions. The sera are always absorbed after dilution with saline, and trial 2 ml. absorptions will show whether $\frac{1}{10}$, $\frac{1}{20}$, $\frac{1}{30}$, $\frac{1}{40}$, or even $\frac{1}{80}$ is the optimum dilution. The following is a suggestion for preliminary trial absorption of an unknown rabbit serum:

Formula	Amount of blood for absorption (washed packed cells), ml.	Amount of saline, ml.	Amount of serum, ml.
2 ml. dil. $(\frac{1}{10}) \times A_1N\ \frac{1}{4}$	0·5	1·8	0·2
" " $(\frac{1}{10}) \times A_1N\ \frac{1}{2}$	1	1·8	0·2
" " $(\frac{1}{20}) \times A_1N\ \frac{1}{4}$	0·5	1·9	0·1
" " $(\frac{1}{20}) \times A_1N\ \frac{1}{2}$	1	1·9	0·1
" " $(\frac{1}{40}) \times A_1N\ \frac{1}{4}$	0·5	1·95	0·05
" " $(\frac{1}{40}) \times A_1N\ \frac{1}{2}$	1	1·95	0·05
" " $(\frac{1}{40}) \times A_1N\ 1$	2	1·95	0·05

The absorptions are carried out at room temperature for 1 hour. The absorbed sera are then titrated with M, MN, and N cells. An absorption will be regarded as satisfactory if the titre against M cells is at least thirty-two, against MN cells sixteen and there is no reaction at 1 in 2 with N cells.

If none of the absorptions give entirely satisfactory results further trial absorptions can be attempted according to the titrations on the first trial sera. For example, in the above case, supposing that the most satisfactory trial serum was $(\frac{1}{20}) \times A_1N\ \frac{1}{2}$ and the titration with the three standard cells (M, MN, and N) was as follows:

DILUTIONS OF SERUM

Type of red cell	1	$\frac{1}{2}$	$\frac{1}{4}$	$\frac{1}{8}$	$\frac{1}{16}$	$\frac{1}{32}$	$\frac{1}{64}$
M	C	C	V	V	++	+	w
MN	C	C	V	++	+	w	—
N	+	w	—	—	—	—	—

Then a satisfactory serum could probably be prepared with the following formula—($\frac{1}{20}$) × A_1N $\frac{5}{8}$; and this might have the titration:

DILUTIONS OF SERUM

Type of red cell	1	$\frac{1}{2}$	$\frac{1}{4}$	$\frac{1}{8}$	$\frac{1}{16}$	$\frac{1}{32}$	$\frac{1}{64}$
M	C	C	V	++	+	(+)	w
MN	C	V	V	++	(+)	w	—
N	w	—	—	—	—	—	—

It is advisable not to over-absorb sera as this tends to remove some of the required anti-M. Moreover, a second absorption following an insufficient first absorption is often most unsatisfactory, much of the anti-M also being removed. It has been found worth while to experiment until a good formula has been obtained and then to do a large absorption (say 50 ml.) with this formula.

Successive bleedings after further course of injections of the same rabbit will usually yield sera to which the same or a very similar formula can be applied. For example, a further bleeding from the rabbit above whose optimum formula was ($\frac{1}{20}$) × A_1N $\frac{5}{8}$ might work best at the formula ($\frac{1}{20}$) × A_1N $\frac{3}{4}$. As a rule, later bleedings from the same rabbit require slightly more absorption.

Absorption of Anti-N Sera. These are carried out exactly as for the anti-M sera except that the sera from rabbits which have been injected with ON cells are absorbed with cells from an A_1M person. As seen above, there is a greater tendency for the titre of the anti-N to be reduced by absorption with the heterologous (M) cells.

Technique No. 16.5. Standardisation of anti-M and anti-N typing sera

After absorbing the main portion of serum, it must be retitrated with appropriate red cells since the values obtained at this stage may not be quite the same as those for the serum absorbed in the pilot experiment. It will usually be found that, however successful the absorption, small amounts of "anti-Man" antibodies will remain in the serum and cause agglutination of the heterologous red cells. It is more satisfactory to dilute these out than to embark upon a reabsorption, providing the specific titre after the necessary dilution still reaches the required minimum. As seen above (technique No. 16.1) trace amounts of anti-Man antibodies can be dispersed when handling the tests at the reading stage since the specific agglutination is usually so firm that it is not appreciably broken down, whereas the agglutination caused by residual anti-Man antibodies is eliminated. When using the tile method (technique No. 16.2) the careful timing of the tests will avoid slight reaction caused by traces of anti-Man antibodies.

The next step is to run the serum in parallel with known sera against at least thirty random red cell samples and in addition to include red cells of types AM, AN, BM, and BN. With these additional samples it is possible to detect any residual antibody in the rabbit specific for A and B red cells. If this antibody is too potent to be diluted out a further absorption with red cells of the appropriate ABO and MN type may be necessary, but this should be avoided if possible.

Detection of Antibodies

The detection of anti-M, anti-N, anti-S, and anti-s in human sera is discussed in Chapter 21.

BIBLIOGRAPHY

DUNSFORD, I., IKIN, ELIZABETH W., and MOURANT, A. E. (1953), "A human blood group gene intermediate between M and N." *Nature, Lond.*, **172**, 688.

FRIEDENREICH, V. (1936), "Ein erblicher defekter N Receptor, der wahrscheinlich eine bishe unbekannte Blutgruppeneigenschaft, innerhalb des MN-systems darstellt." *Dtsch. Ztschr. gerichtl. Med.*, **25**, 358.

FRIEDENREICH, V., and LAURIDSEN, A. (1938), "On a variety of human type antigen M and its relation to other M antigens." *Acta path. microbiol. Scand.*, supp. 38, 155.

LANDSTEINER, K., and LEVINE, P. (1927), "A new agglutinable factor differentiating individual human bloods." *Proc. Soc. exp. Biol., N.Y.*, **24**, 600.

LANDSTEINER, K., and LEVINE, P. (1928), "On individual differences in human blood." *J. exp. Med.*, **47**, 757.

LEVINE, P., KUHMICHEL, A. B., WIGOD, M., and KOCH, ELIZABETH (1951), "A new blood factor, s, allelic to S." *Proc. Soc. exp. Biol., N.Y.*, **78**, 218.

SANGER, RUTH, and RACE, R. R. (1947), "Subdivisions of the MN blood groups in man." *Nature, Lond.*, **160**, 505.

WALSH, R. J., and MONTGOMERY, CARMEL (1947), "A new human isoagglutinin subdividing the MN blood groups." *Nature, Lond.*, **160**, 504.

CHAPTER 17

THE KELL, DUFFY AND KIDD SYSTEMS

(1) The Kell System

THIS system was first described in 1946 (Coombs *et al.*, 1946); the antibody being found in the serum of a mother whose infant suffered from hæmolytic disease of the newborn. The antigen K was found to occur in 10 per cent of the British population and it was postulated that the system was governed by a pair of allelomorphic genes called K and k which controlled the production of the corresponding antigens K and k. The groups, therefore, are as follows:

Phenotype as defined by anti-K	*Genotype*		
Kell positive	KK	about	0·2 per cent
	Kk	,,	10 per cent
Kell negative	kk	,,	90 per cent

There is evidence supporting the view that K is rather strongly antigenic, but since it occurs in only 1 in 10 of the population, the opportunity for sensitisation is small. When the antibody does occur it is almost invariably active at 37°C and often associated with a hæmolytic transfusion reaction or hæmolytic disease of the newborn. If the ABO and Rh systems cannot be incriminated in such clinical conditions it is well worth considering the possibility of Kell being the cause of the hæmolysis. Anti-K is most readily detected by the indirect Coombs test. Some anti-K antibodies are detectable only by the indirect Coombs technique while others are detectable by cells suspended in group AB serum, in bovine albumin or even occasionally in saline. Group AB serum appears to be a better medium for anti-K than bovine albumin. However, whatever the medium in which the antibody is detectable, the indirect Coombs test is the most reliable way of detecting the presence of the antibody and of Kell typing unknown red cells.

Anti-k originally called anti-Cellano(Levine *et al.*, 1949) has been found but owing to the rarity of KK (the only genotype in which it can occur), anti-k will always be one of the rare antibodies.

The phenotype K-k- was found in a case investigated by Chown *et al.* (1957). The propositus had an antibody which reacted with all cells except that of her sister; both sisters were found to be K-k- (*and also* Kp^a-Kp^b- *see below*). The antibody was designated anti-K^u (*see also* Corcoran *et al.*, 1961).

Kp^a and Kp^b

A new antigen in the Kell system was reported by Allen and Lewis in 1957. The antigen Kp^a occurred in about 2 per cent of the population and family studies suggested that it was associated with the Kell system.

Later, the same workers described an anti-Kp^b (Allen *et al.*, 1958). All five Kp^b negatives were Kp^a positive. Only two Kp^b negatives were found in testing 5,500 unrelated people. It was realised that these two antigens were almost certainly produced by a further pair of allelomorphic genes within the K system.

Js^a and Js^b

Giblett in 1958 described an antibody anti-Js^a which reacted with about 20 per cent of negro donors and not with 240 white persons. (Subsequently, only one white person has been found to be positive among some hundreds tested.)

An antibody, giving antithetical results to anti-Js^a was found by Walker *et al.* (1963).

In 1965 Stroup *et al.* showed that K-k-Kp^a-Kp^b-persons were also Js^a and Js^b negative. It seems certain that Js^a and Js^b are also part of the Kell system or very closely related to it.

The inheritance of the Kell system is discussed further in Chapter 34 and the 1 antibodies are included in Table 15.1 in Chapter 15 and Table 21.2 in Chapter 21.

Techniques

Technique No. 17.1. Typing of red cells with anti-K. It will be found that anti-K sera are individual in their behaviour and, therefore, the optimum working conditions for any given anti-serum must be found by trial and error. For instance, the optimum time required for the sensitisation stage of the test may vary. Better results are obtained sometimes when the test cells and anti-serum are incubated together for not more than 1 hour. The following is an anti-human globulin technique which usually works satisfactorily.

Two anti-K sera should be used. Two volumes of each anti-K are mixed with a half volume of packed thrice washed test cells and incubated at 37°C for 1–2 hours. Alternatively 4 volumes of

5 per cent cells may be used; this can be measured more accurately than a half volume of packed cells which depends on the tightness of the packing, the extra diluent is unimportant, possibly even aiding sensitisation. It is important to include known K positive and known K negative controls. After incubation, the cells are washed carefully at least three times in a large volume of saline, and then mixed with an anti-human globulin serum on an opalescent tile in exactly the same manner as described for indirect anti-human globulin technique. (Technique No. 10.3a.) When the agglutination of the known K positive cells has developed fully the tests are read. For the choice of Coombs reagent (anti-human globulin serum) for the various blood group systems *see* Chapter 21 and Appendix I.

(2) The Duffy System

The Duffy blood group system was discovered in 1950 (Cutbush and Mollison, 1950). The new antibody was found in the serum of a man suffering from hæmophilia who had had a number of blood transfusions. The antigen which the new antibody detected was found in the red cells of about 65 per cent of the English population. It was called Fy^a, and the antibody anti-Fy^a, in accordance with the plan adopted for some other blood group systems. The phenotypes and genotypes of the system as defined by anti-Fy^a are as follows:

Phenotype as defined by anti-Fy^a	*Genotype*	*Occurrence*
Fy(a+)	Fy^aFy^a	About 17 per cent
	Fy^aFy^b	About 49 per cent
Fy(a−)	Fy^bFy^b	About 34 per cent

The anti-Fy^a antibody has been shown to cause hæmolytic transfusion reactions, one of which was fatal, and hæmolytic disease. The first anti-Fy^a antibodies discovered were only detectable by the indirect anti-human globulin technique but later ones were found which reacted by saline, albumin and trypsin techniques. In fact, if an antibody is detectable only by anti-globulin technique, it may well be anti-Fy^a. The antibody does not react in papain; agglutination caused by anti-Fy^a can be dispersed by addition of papain. However, the indirect anti-human globulin method is by far the most reliable way of detecting and using this antibody. Some eighteen months after the discovery of Fy^a and anti-Fy^a the expected allelomorph Fy^b was found when a "new" antibody proved to be anti-Fy^b (Ikin *et al.*, 1951). This antibody was found in the serum of a woman who had had three children and no history of blood transfusion. None of the children had suffered from hæmolytic disease.

Recently the phenotype Fy (a− b−) has been discovered in 85 out of 125 New York negroes tested, and in 33 out of 37 West Africans (Sanger *et al.*, 1955). This suggests that there may be a third allele at the Duffy locus which is at present designated Fy; if the corresponding antibody is found it will be called anti-Fy^{c} and the allele Fy^{c}. The Fy (a− b−) phenotype seems to be confined to and very common in negroes (*see also* Chapter 34).

Techniques

Technique No. 17.2. Typing of red cells with anti-Fy^{a}. Anti-Fy^{a} is not in sufficiently good supply to allow the use of two antisera in parallel. If possible negative reactions should be confirmed with a second anti-serum. It is usually found most satisfactory to use an indirect anti-human globulin method (technique No. 10.3a), even though the particular antibody selected for typing purposes may react by other methods. Two volumes of anti-Fy^{a} serum are mixed with a half volume of packed cells or preferably 4 volumes of 5 per cent cells and incubated at 37°C for 1–2 hours. Known Fy^{a} positive and Fy^{a} negative controls are included. Anti-Fy^{a} usually needs a broad-spectrum reagent, *i.e.* reacting well with both γG and γM immuno-globulins; care should be taken to use this at the correct dilution.

(3) The Kidd Blood Group System

The Kidd blood group system was discovered in 1951 (Allen *et al.*, 1951), the antibody being found in the serum of a woman whose sixth child suffered from hæmolytic disease of the newborn. The role of the new antibody in connexion with this disease could not be assessed because the maternal serum also contained anti-Kell. Since this time a few cases have been reported where the Kidd antibody has been stimulated either by transfusion, or pregnancy or both. In most instances this antibody has been accompanied by other blood group antibodies; a case in which it caused kernicterus has been reported.

The antibody was called anti-Jk^{a} and phenotypes and genotypes were postulated as follows:

Phenotype as defined by anti-Jk^{a}	*Genotype*	*Occurrence*
Jk(a+)	Jk^{a}Jk^{a}	About 25 per cent
	Jk^{a}Jk^{b}	About 50 per cent
Jk(a−)	Jk^{b}Jk^{b}	About 25 per cent

Later anti-Jk^b (Plaut *et al.*, 1953) was discovered. This antibody was found in association with anti-Fy^a and seemed to have been stimulated by transfusion. Several other examples of anti-Jk^b have since been found.

Later still the phenotype Jk(a− b−) was found through detection of an antibody following a transfusion reaction (Pinkerton *et al.*, 1959). The antibody reacted with all cells tested except the patient's own and was found to contain anti-Jk^a and anti-Jk^b which consisted of separable anti-Jk^b and inseparable anti-Jk^aJk^b. The phenotype was found in a Filipina with Spanish and Chinese ancestry. It has not yet been detected in negroes or whites. *See also* Chapter 34.

The original anti-Jk^a serum worked at first as a saline agglutinin but later it became necessary to use the anti-human globulin test. Most Kidd anti-sera seem to give the best reactions by anti-human globulin technique, particularly if this is performed on trypsin-treated red cells or in the presence of complement. The sera at the present time are too rare for routine use.

Techniques

Technique No. 17.3. Typing of red cells with anti-Jk^a by indirect anti-human globulin on trypsin treated cells. This is a two-stage method involving the performance of an indirect anti-human globulin test on trypsin treated red cells. The unknown cells together with known Jk^a positive and negative controls are trypsin treated (technique No. 10.4) and then incubated with anti-Jk^a serum for 30–45 minutes in the proportion of two volumes of serum to a half volume of packed trypsin treated red cells. The subsequent procedure is identical with the indirect anti-human globulin technique (No. 10.3a) from the washing stage onwards.

Technique No. 17.4.* Typing of red cells with anti-Jk^a by anti-human globulin with the addition of complement. E.D.T.A. two-stage method for complement-binding antibodies and the anti-human globulin test.

(*a*) *Inactivation of Complement and Complementoid with E.D.T.A. Diaminoethanetetra-acetic Acid*

A neutral solution of E.D.T.A. is prepared:

14·8 gm. E.D.T.A. (dipotassium salt)
1·1 gm. NaOH
333·3 ml. water
} pH 7·0–7·4

* For a description of this technique we are indebted to Miss Caroline Giles of the Blood Group Reference Laboratory.

This solution is placed in tubes in proportionate amounts and allowed to evaporate at 37°C; *e.g.* 0·1 ml. of E.D.T.A. solution for 1·0 ml. of serum.

It has been estimated that 4 mgm. of E.D.T.A. should be added to 1 ml. of serum to inactivate it completely. Inactivation is immediate and permanent, and no dilution of antibody in the serum takes place since the serum is added to a dry tube.

(*b*) *Two-stage Technique with Fresh Human Complement and Anti-human Globulin*

(i) The serum to be tested is transferred to the dry E.D.T.A. tube for inactivation.
(ii) Two volumes of this serum (i) are incubated with 1 volume of washed packed red cells for 1½ hours at 37°C.
(iii) The cells are washed four times with a large excess of saline to remove all traces of anti-complementary E.D.T.A.
(iv) The washed cells (iii) are packed and incubated with 2 volumes of fresh human complement at 37°C in a *water bath* for 15–20 minutes.
(v) The cells (iv) are again washed four times.
(vi) The washed cells (v) are tested as a 50 per cent suspension with an A.H.G. diluted optimally for anti-β_1. (The fraction of globulin involved for complement.)

Notes

(i) Fresh human complement will retain its activity for two weeks when stored at −20°C. Storage at −50°C or lower is advisable for longer periods.
(ii) The anti-human globulin (A.H.G.) reagent must contain anti-β_1; a broad spectrum reagent is recommended. It should have been standardised by this technique and found satisfactory. The dilutions used would probably be in the range of 1 in 8 to 1 in 60.
(iii) This technique is ideal for incomplete Lewis antisera, good for many Kidd antisera and possibly helpful with some Kell and Duffy antisera that will bind complement.
(iv) Hæmolysis may occur with very potent antibodies on addition of complement to the sensitised cells. This can be overcome by dilution of the antiserum.

BIBLIOGRAPHY

ALLEN, F. H. Jr., and LEWIS, S. J. (1957), "Kp^a (Penney) a New Antigen in the Kell Blood Group System." *Vox Sang.*, **2**, No. 2, 81.

ALLEN, F. H. Jr., and LEWIS, S. J., and FUDENBERG, H. (1958), "Studies of anti-Kp^b, a New Antibody in the Kell blood group system." *Vox Sang.*, **3**, No. 1.

ALLEN, F. H., DIAMOND, L. K., and NIEDZIELA, BEVELY (1951), "A new blood group antigen." *Nature, Lond.*, **167**, 482.

CHOWN, B,. LEWIN, MARION, and KAITA, HIROKO (1957), "A 'new' Kell Blood Group Phenotype." *Nature, Lond.*, **180**, 711.

COOMBS, R. R. A., MOURANT, A. E., and RACE, R. R. (1946), "In vivo iso-sensitisation of red cells in babies with hæmolytic disease." *Lancet*, **i**, 264.

CORCORAN, PATRICIA A., ALLEN, F. H., Jr., LEWIS, MARION, and CHOWN, B. (1961), "A new antibody, anti-Ku (anti-Peltz), in the Kell Blood-Group System." *Transfusion*, **1**, No. 3, 181.

CUTBUSH, MARIE, and CHANARIN, I. (1950), "The Duffy blood group." *Heredity*, **4**, 383.

GIBLETT, ELOISE R. (1958), "Js, a 'new' blood group antigen found in Negroes." *Nature, Lond.*, **181**, 1221.

IKIN, ELIZABETH W., MOURANT, A. E., PETTENKOFER, H. J., and BLUMENTHAL, G. (1951), "Discovery of the expected hæmagglutinin, anti-Fy^b." *Nature, Lond.*, **168**, 1077.

LEVINE, P., WIGOD, M., BACKER, A., MAY, and PONDER, RUTH (1949), "A new human hereditary blood group property (Cellano) present in 99.8 per cent of all bloods." *Science*, **109**, 464.

PINKERTON, F. J., MERMOD, L. E., LILES, B. A., JACK, J. A. Jr., and NOADES, J. (1959), "The phenotype Jk(a−b−) in the Kidd Blood Group System." *Vox Sang.*, **4**, No. 2, 155.

PLAUT, GERTRUDE, IKIN, ELIZABETH, W. MOURANT, A. E., SANGER, RUTH, and RACE, R. R. (1953), "A new blood-group antibody, anti-Jk^b." *Nature, Lond.*, **171**, 431.

SANGER, RUTH, RACE, R. R., and JACK, J. (1955), "The Duffy blood groups of New York negroes: The phenotype Fy(a−b−)." *Brit. J. Hæm.*, **1**, 370.

STROUP, MARJORY, MACILROY, MIJA., WALKER, R., and AYDELOTTE, JANE V. (1965), "Evidence that Sutter belongs to the Kell blood group system." *Transfusion Philad.*, **5**, 309.

WALKER, R. H., ARGALL, C. I., STEANE, E. A., SASAKI, T. T., and GREENWALT, J. J. (1963), "Js^b of the Sutter blood group system." *Transfusion*, **3**, 94.

WALKER, R. H., ARGALL, C. I., STEANE, E. A., SASAKI, T. T., and GREENWALT, T. J. (1963), "Anti-Js^b, the expected antithetical antibody of the Sutter blood group system." *Nature, Lond.*, **197**, 295.

CHAPTER 18

LUTHERAN, LEWIS, P, I

(1) Lutheran

This system was first defined in 1946 when a hitherto unknown antibody appeared in the blood of a patient who had received many blood transfusions. (Callender and Race, 1946.) The antibody was immune, the stimulating antigen being present in one of the donors whose name was Lutheran; thus the antibody was called anti-Lu^a and the phenotypes Lu(a+) and Lu(a−).

Experiment has shown that anti-Lu^a can be produced as a result of transfusion of Lu(a+) blood into Lu(a−) persons; Mainwaring and Pickles (1948) found antibodies in two out of eight Lu^a negative patients who had received Lu^a+ blood.

Anti-Lu^a has not been incriminated in hæmolytic disease of the newborn and has not so far produced a hæmolytic transfusion reaction of any degree of severity. The anti-Lu^a antibodies are characteristically saline agglutinins and are usually more reactive at room temperature than at 37°C, although some examples have been found which have given stronger agglutination reactions at 37°C. The optimum temperature of reactivity has been shown in some cases to vary with the Lu(a+) cells used.

Later, anti-Lu^b was found in an individual who proved to be of the very rare genotype Lu^aLu^a Cutbush and Chanarin (1956). The antibody was a saline agglutinin. Only one or two anti-Lu^b antibodies have been discovered since. None of them have had great clinical significance.

The phenotypes and genotypes can be summarised as follows:

Phenotypes defined by anti-Lu^a	*Genotypes*	*Occurrence*
Lu(a+)	Lu^aLu^b	About 8 per cent
	Lu^aLu^a	About 0·2 per cent
Lu(a−)	Lu^bLu^b	About 92 per cent

Technique No. 18.1. Lutheran typing of red cells. One unit volume of anti-Lu^a serum is mixed with one unit volume of a 2 per cent suspension of test cells in a precipitin tube. It is advisable to use microvolumes of about 0·01 ml. since the anti-serum is rare. A positive and a negative control consisting of known Lu(a+) and

Lu(a−) red cells must be included with each batch of tests. After 2 hours' incubation at the optimum temperature for the anti-Lu^a serum being used (usually 15°C) the contents of each tube are pipetted gently on to a microscope slide and read for presence or absence of agglutination.

Lutheran agglutination is characteristic, being composed of loose clumps (morulæ) in a field of free cells.

(2) The Lewis Blood Group System

A hitherto unknown antibody, believed to be naturally occurring, was found by Mourant in samples of blood from two different persons (Mourant, 1946). This antibody recognised an antigen present in about 22 per cent of the English population. The system was called Lewis after one of the two individuals in which it was first found. In accordance with the adopted convention the antigen is now designated Le^a and the antibody anti-Le^a.

Le^a typing of red cells can be carried out quite satisfactorily by tube technique in saline or papain at room temperature or 15°C. More than one example of anti-Le^a should be used. Occasionally an anti-Le^a antibody is found which reacts well by indirect anti-globulin technique especially in the presence of complement.

Anti-Le^a sera will sometimes hæmolyse Le^a positive cells in the presence of complement. Hæmolysis is a regular feature if ficin enzyme technique is used; this is a helpful fact in the the identification of these antibodies. Hæmolysis also occurs using papain treated Le^a positive cells with many but not all anti-Lewis antibodies.

Le^a has been found to be unique among blood groups in several respects. Firstly, there is a connexion between Le^a and the secretion of A, B, and H substances. All Le^a positives are non-secretors of the blood group substances A, B, and H, but secretors of Le^a substance, *see* Chapter 32. The associations between Le^a positives and non-secretors of A, B, H substances is caused by an interaction at the phenotypic level. The Lewis and secretor genes are inherited quite independently of each other (*see* Fig. 32.3, Chapter 32).

The frequency of Le^a positives in infants up to eighteen months is higher than in adults. The reason for this is probably best accounted for by the fact that infants' plasma contains Le^a substance which is taken up on to the red cells (*see* below).

Antibodies have been found, indeed they are not uncommon, whose reactions with red cells are to a great extent antithetical to those of anti-Le^a. These antibodies, therefore, have been designated anti-Le^b and the corresponding antigen Le^b. It is now known that the Le^b antigen does not arise from a separate gene Le^b but is a product of interaction between the Le^a and H genes (*see* Chapter 32). Four to six per cent individuals are both Le^a negative and Le^b negative. Moreover, most anti-Le^b sera do not give the same number of positive reactions in all ABO groups, in particular in groups A_1 and A_1B which contain a far higher proportion of Le^b negatives than groups O, A_2, B, and A_2B; in addition Le(b−) × Le(b−) parents may have Le(b+) children.

The inheritance of the Lewis system is now becoming better understood in the light of work by Sneath and Sneath 1955 which shows that the system is primarily composed of soluble antigens existing in the serum and body fluids and is not an erythrocyte blood group system at all. Thus, the most reliable way of determining the Lewis status of an individual is by testing the saliva by inhibition technique against appropriate antisera. The presence of the antigen on the red cells depends on there being a sufficient quantity in the serum for it to be taken up by the cells.

The great importance of the Lewis system in the understanding of the development of the ABO blood group antigens is discussed in Chapter 30.

Most anti-Le^a sera originate from people of the phenotype Le(a− b−) and very often contain weak anti-Le^b. Anti-Le^b sera are also usually made by people of phenotype Le(a− b−) but they are the non-secretors of ABH, Le^a and Le^b substances. Anti-Le^b sera often contain anti-H. It is obvious therefore that these sera need to be carefully controlled if used for typing.

Technique No. 18.2. Typing of red cells with anti-Le^a. At least two anti-Le^a sera should be used. Equal volumes of serum and a 2 per cent suspension of the red cells to be typed are mixed in precipitin tubes and left for 2 hours at room temperature or 15°C. Known Le^a positive and Le^a negative red cells are included as controls.

The tests are read taking the same precautions that are necessary for Rh typing.

(3) The Blood Group System P

This was one of the earlier known blood group systems, being discovered during the same experimental immunisation of rabbits with human red cells which led to the finding of M and N (Landsteiner and Levine, 1927).

The serum of one rabbit after absorption with certain human

red cells was found to contain an antibody which did not appear to belong to the ABO or MN systems, the only two known at the time. The human red cells which were positive with the rabbit anti-P, now called anti-P_1 (*see* p. 164), were designated P positive and those which were negative with it, P negative. Anti-P_1 frequently occurs in the serum of P_1 negative individuals as a naturally occurring cold agglutinin and also in the serum of some animals, in particular horses, rabbits, pigs and cattle. Unfortunately these anti-P_1 sera are usually of low titre.

The estimation of the frequency of P_1 is difficult owing both to the rarity of potent anti-sera and to the existence of individuals whose red cells only react weakly even with the best available anti-sera. Among the P_1 positives, three classes can be distinguished according to their strength of reaction with anti-P_1 sera: (1) P_1 strong; (2) P_1 medium; (3) P_1 weak. There is no evidence, to date, that there is any qualitative difference between them. In fact the result of absorption tests with P_1 weak cells and anti-P_1 sera show that these cells are as efficient in removal of anti-P_1 from a serum as are cells which are P_1 strong. Much of the variation in agglutinability of P_1 positive red cells seems to depend upon their genotype.

Anti-P_1 is rarely of importance from the clinical viewpoint. One case of hæmolytic disease has been attributed to it and only one or two transfusion reactions. The absence of clinical significance is undoubtedly due to the fact that anti-P_1 is characteristically a cold agglutinin of the saline agglutinating type. Nevertheless, a few anti-P_1 antibodies have been found active at 37°C and such antibodies are potential causes of hæmolytic reactions. Moreover, some anti-P_1 sera in which the antibody is not active at 37°C by a saline technique can be shown to react at this temperature if the indirect anti-human globulin plus complement method is used. (Technique No. 21.5.) However, it is as a cold agglutinin that anti-P_1 will be encountered by those who do routine blood grouping tests. Henningsen (1949) by the use of delicate techniques has demonstrated the presence of anti-P_1 active at 4°C in a high proportion of P_1 negative individuals. Anti-P_1 reacting at room temperature is comparatively rare but when it does occur it often produces anomalous results in ABO serum grouping tests. These anomalous results due to anti-P_1 can only be avoided if P_1 negative A and B red cells are chosen as standard cells. This choice is not usually convenient. When the occasion arises it is advisable to carry out tests which will establish the cause of the anomalous results. (*See* Chapter 21.) In the event of an anti-P_1 agglutinin being identified it should be secured as an anti-P_1 typing serum if sufficiently potent since those that can be relied upon to detect all P_1 weak cells are rare. Accurate P_1 typing of red cells is not easily accomplished and should always be performed with at least two, preferably more, anti-P_1 sera. P_1 weak cells should always be included among the positive controls.

In December 1955 (Sanger, 1955) the P system which had remained undisturbed since its discovery in 1927 was shown to be directly related to the Jay system of blood groups (Levine *et al.*, 1951).

The Jay system was defined by an antibody called anti-Tj^a reacting with an antigen Tj^a found in almost all human red cells. The anti-Tj^a was characterised by its power to hæmolyse red cells strongly at room temperature. Only fourteen persons belonging to the Tj^a negative group (members of only eight families) were found between 1951 and 1962. The anti-Tj^a sera have all contained potent antibodies active at room temperature and at 37°C, and have been incriminated as causing miscarriages; the antibodies are probably naturally occurring, no case of a Tj^a negative person without anti-Tj^a in their serum has so far been encountered.

The antibody contained in the Jay blood groups previously called anti-Tj^a was shown by Sanger to be composed of two antibodies, one the well-known anti-P and the other an antibody reacting with all P positive and P negative individuals except those P negative persons who are Tj^a negative and whose sera contain anti-Tj^a (anti-P + P_1).

The expanded P system is therefore as given below:

Antibodies Anti-P_1 (previously anti-P)
Anti-P + Anti-P_1 (previously anti-Tj^a)

Antigens P_1 (previously P) } previously Tj^a
P_2 (previously p) }
p (previously Tj^b)

Therefore the old P positive group (including P strong, P medium and P weak) contains three genotypes P_1P_1 (29 per cent), P_1P_2 (50 per cent) and P_1p (v. rare). The P negatives can be split into 3 genotypes P_2P_2 (21 per cent), P_2p (v. rare) and pp (v. rare).

A helpful analogy with the A_1 and A_2 sub-groups can be drawn. P_1 is regarded as having two antigens, namely P_1 and P, and P_2 as having one, namely P, just as A_1 is made up of A_1 and A, and A_2 made up of A. Anti-P reacts with P_1 and P_2 cells by virtue of the common antigen P, similarly pure anti-A (without anti-A_1) reacts with A_1 and A_2 by virtue of the common antigen A. Anti-P_1 corresponds to anti-A_1 and reacts only with P_1 cells.

For further antigens of the P system, Table 15.2 and Chapter 34 should be consulted.

Technique No. 18.3. Typing of red cells with anti-P_1. The standard tube technique is used. Equal volumes of a suitable anti-P_1 anti-serum and a 2 per cent suspension of red cells to be tested are mixed and left for 2 hours. Known P strong, P weak and P negative cells are included with each batch of tests. Each sample is tested with three different anti-P_1 anti-sera whenever possible. The temperature at which the tests are incubated will depend upon the particular anti-sera used. It is preferable to choose anti-sera which will work well at a cool room temperature, *e.g.* 15°C. At 4°C other cold agglutinins may interfere with the results although with well tried and well controlled anti-sera this temperature may be found to be satisfactory.

The tests are read in the same manner as for Rh typing since the agglutinated clumps are often fragile.

(4) The I Blood Group System

This system is complicated and interesting and is of practical importance because the blood group serologist is unlikely to be able to avoid encountering anti-I antibodies.

In 1956 Wiener *et al.* gave the name anti-I to an antibody found in the serum of a patient suffering from hæmolytic anæmia of the "cold" antibody type. Of 22,000 donors tested, only five were negative and therefore designated i.

In 1960 Jenkins *et al.* described a blood donor whose cells were i and whose serum contained anti-I. With the cells of this donor it was possible to show that a number of cases of acquired hæmolytic anæmia of the cold type have anti-I and in addition many so-called non-specific antibodies in normal sera are anti-I. This work led to the recognition of two types of anti-I, one called "natural" which occurs regularly in the serum of i individuals and one called "auto anti-I", as found associated with hæmolytic anæmia.

The differences between I and i are not completely clear-cut in that using special techniques (*e.g.* ficin) it can be shown that i cells react with anti-I, although to a lesser degree than the cells from I individuals. Moreover, there is a great range of I activity in I positive people. Cord cells give relatively very weak reactions with potent anti-I and fail to react at all with most anti-I sera, but they are strongly i-positive. The I antigen reaches adult strength approximately 18 months from birth and at the same time the amount of i falls.

Marsh, 1960, described the finding of two examples of anti-i with reactions antithetical to anti-I but also having the characteristic of not making clear-cut differentiation between I and i since some adult I cells reacted weakly with them.

Two types of i have been distinguished; i_1 is the weaker and so far found only in whites, i_2 is a little stronger and found in negroes. Both are very rare. They are not identical with i cord.

In 1965 Jenkins *et al.* found an antibody which reacted with O and A_2 adult cells, very weakly with O cord and Oi adult cells and not at all with Oh and Ai cells. They postulated that the antibody reacted with a compound antigen one part of which is O and the other I. They suggest HI and anti-HI.

Since this time an extensive literature has developed on the antibodies related to I and H.

The original anti-HI sera were not inhibited by saliva, but Lodge and Voak (1968) have described one that was inhibitable. Tegoli *et al.* (1967) showed that anti-IB antibodies existed. Voak *et al.* (1968) have amplified the suggested nomenclature of Wiener *et al.* (1966), where H^c represents the H antigen of red cells and H^s the secreted H substance, and have given all these antibodies superscripts based on whether or not they are inhibited by saliva. Thus, for example, the common anti-HI antibodies which are not inhibited by saliva are called anti-HI^c and the rare one which is inhibited anti-HI^s.

Relationship to Disease

Jenkins *et al.* (1965) have investigated a case of leukæmia with weakened A in which I was also depressed. However the i reaction was stronger than in the average adult cell, so that the reciprocal relationship between I and i was maintained.

Schmidt *et al.* (1965) have stimulated the interest of others besides blood group specialists with their experiments on mycoplasma strains. 18 out of 25 strains of these organisms inhibited anti-I agglutination. Agglutination by anti-Le^a, anti-Le^b and anti-A_1 was not so inhibited. Mycoplasma have been demonstrated in association with leukæmia which may explain the inagglutinability by anti-I of red cells of patients with leukæmia.

Anti-I has been shown to be the auto-antibody concerned in most cases of "cold-type" hæmolytoic anæmia (see Chapter 26).

Anti-i has been shown to be the cold auto-agglutinin present in some cases of infective mononeucleosis.

The Identification of Anti-I in Practice

Anti-I is usually detected as a saline cold agglutinin. Its activity is often enhanced by such enzymes as ficin, papain or bromelin, in fact it is sometimes only detectable by enzyme techniques. It is characterised by reacting strongly with adult cells (usually including the patient's own cells) but being negative or at most very weak with cord cells. It is differentiated from other antibodies which are weak or negative with cord cells, *e.g.* anti-H, anti-P_1 and anti-Le^a plus anti-Le^b mixtures, by the fact that it is usually an auto-antibody and also that it is uninhibited by human saliva. If the anti-I is not an auto-antibody the patient's cells will be i-positive. The other similar antibody from which anti-I needs to be differentiated is anti-HI, an antibody which reacts preferentially with O cells (as anti-H) but is not inhibited by human saliva (as anti-I). It is sometimes regarded as "anti-I preferring O cells" but many workers believe that it is detecting a compound antigen and so the designation anti-HI is more correct. It has also been called anti-OI, as it is the antibody which used to be called anti-O. We feel that this is not a good name as it is not detecting a product of the O gene. If the rare i-adult cells are available for testing anti-I will be weak or negative with these [as will anti-H or anti-HI. All i-adult cells so far found are both I and H negative or very weakly positive].

BIBLIOGRAPHY

CUTBUSH, MARIE, and CHANARIN, I. (1956), "The expected blood-group antibody, anti-Lu^b." *Nature, Lond.*, **178**, 855.

JENKINS, W. J., MARSH, W. L., and GOLD, E. R. (1965), "Reciprocal relationship of antigen I and i in health and disease." *Nature, Lond.*, **205**, 813.

JENKINS, W. J., MARSH, W. L., NOADES, J., TIPPETT, P., SANGER, R., and RACE, R. R. (1960), "The I antigen and antibody." *Vox Sang.*, **5**, No. 2, 97.

KORTEKANGAS, A. E., NOADES, J., TIPPETT, PATRICIA, SANGER, RUTH, and RACE, R. R. (1959), "A second family with the red cell antigen P^k." *Vox Sang.*, **4**, No. 5, 337.

LANDSTEINER, K., and LEVINE, P. (1927), "Further observations on individual differences of human blood." *Proc. Soc. exp. Biol., N.Y.*, **24**, 941.

LEVINE, P., BOBBITT, O. B., WALLER, R. K., and KUHMICHEL, A. (1951), "Iso-immunisation by a new blood group factor in tumour cells." *Proc. Soc. exp. Biol., N.Y.*, **77**, 403.

LODGE, J. W., and VOAK, D. (1968), "An example of Inhibitable anti-HI in a group B donor." *Vox Sang.*, **14**, 60–62.

MAINWARING, V. R., and PICKLES, MARGARET M. (1948), "A further case of anti-Lutheran immunisation with some studies on its capacity for human sensitization." *J. Clin. Path.*, **1**, 292.

MARSH, W. L. (1960), "A cold antibody defining the Ii relationship in human red cells." *Brit. J. Hæm.*, **7**, 200.

MATSON, G. A., SWANSON, J., NOADES, J., SANGER, R., and RACE, R. R. (1959), "A 'new' antigen and antibody belonging to the P blood group system." *Amer. J. hum. Genet.*, **11**, 26.

MOURANT, A. E. (1946), "A 'new' human blood group antigen of frequent occurrence." *Nature, Lond.*, **158**, 237.

SANGER, R. (1955), "An association between the P and Jay systems of blood groups." *Nature*, **176**, 1163.

SCHMIDT, P. J., BARILE, M. F., and MCGINNES, M. H. (1965), "Mycoplasma (pleuropneumonia-like organisms) and blood group I. Association with neoplastic disease." *Nature, Lond.*, **205**, 371.

SNEATH, J. S., and SNEATH, P. H. A. (1955), "Transformation of the Lewis groups of human red cells." *Nature, Lond.*, **176**, 172.

TEGOLI, J., HARRIS, J. P., ISSITT, P. D., and SANDERS, C. W. (1967), "Anti-IB, an expected 'new' antibody detecting a joint product of the I and B genes." *Vox Sang.*, **13**, 144.

TIPPETT, PATRICIA, SANGER, RUTH, RACE, R. R., SWANSON, JANE, and BUSCH, SHIRLEY, (1965) "An agglutinin associated with the P and the ABO blood group systems." *Vox Sang.*, 10, 269.

TIPPETT, P., NOADES, J., SANGER, R., RACE, R. R., SAUSAIS, L., HOLMAN, C. A., and BUTTIMER, R. J. (1960), "Further studies on the I antigen and antibody." *Vox Sang.*, **5**, No. 2, 107.

VOAK, D., LODGE, T. W., HOPKINS, JEAN, and BOWLEY, C. C. (1968), "A study of the antibodies of the H"O" I–B Complex with special reference to their occurrence and notation." *Vox Sang.*, **15**, 353.

WIENER, A. S., MOOR, JANKOWSKI J., and GORDON, E. B. (1966), "The relationship of the H substance to the ABO blood groups." *Int. Arch. Allergy.*, **29**, 82.

WIENER, A. S., UNGER, L. J., COHEN, L., and FELDMAN, J. (1956), "Type-specific cold auto-antibodies as a cause of acquired hemolytic anæmia and hemolytic transfusion reactions; biologic test with bovine red cells." *Ann. intern. Med.*, **44**, 221.

Chapter 19

THE DIEGO, YT, DOMBROCK SYSTEMS AND THE X LINKED BLOOD GROUP SYSTEM, XG

Diego

The antigen Di^a (Layrisse *et al.*, 1955) has already been referred to in that when it was first found it was thought to be a very rare antigen; over 2,000 white persons were tested without a further example being found apart from the family of the propositus. When South American Indians were tested, however, as many as 36 per cent of some tribes were found to be Di^a positive. For a review of the antigen distribution, *see* Layrisse *et al.*, 1966. The antigen is found among most Mongolian peoples, but appears to be absent, or almost so, from Eskimos (Lewis *et al.*, 1956).

In 1967, Thomson *et al.* found the antithetical antibody anti-Di^b. So far no Di(a−b−) persons have been discovered.

Diego has been shown to be independent of the other systems with the exception of Lutheran, which awaits the finding of more Lu^a positive Di^a positive persons, and the testing of their families. (Allen and Corcoran, 1960.)

Anti-Di^a is a possible, though rare, cause of hæmolytic disease of the fœtus. In fact the first 3 examples found had been associated with this disease. Anti-Di^b has caused a transfusion reaction. Both are very rare antibodies.

Yt

The Yt system is defined by two antibodies, anti-Yt^a (first described in 1956 by Eaton *et al.*) and anti-Yt^b (Giles and Metaxas, 1964).

Yt^a is a very frequent antigen occurring in about 99·8 per cent of the population; Yt^b occurs in about 8·1 per cent of whom are, of course, Yt(a+b+). So far, no Yt(a−b−) persons have been found.

Yt has been shown to be independent of all the main systems, but not so far of Diego.

The antibodies usually react by the anti-human globulin technique, or by enzyme—anti-globulin test [only certain anti-globulin sera are suitable] and are a possible cause of transfusion reactions. They appear mainly in the sera of much transfused persons, but one anti-Yt^a was found in the serum of a mother whose Yt^a positive child gave a positive direct anti-human-globulin reaction although it was clinically normal.

Dombrock

This is another system where the antibody (anti-Do^a) is very rare, the first example being found by Swanson *et al.* in 1965. Moreover, tests with anti-Do^a need to be performed with specially selected anti-human globulin reagents. Many otherwise excellent reagents are unsuitable for detecting this antibody and it may well be that in cases where an antibody is suspected in the serum on clinical grounds, testing with a suitable reagent might reveal anti-Do^a.

The frequency of Do^a positives is about 66 per cent. This makes Do^a a very useful chromosome marker. The finding of the expected anti-Do^b would make this an exceedingly important blood group system in genetical, medico-legal, and anthropological studies.

This system has been shown to be independent of all the major blood group systems.

Xg

This blood group system which was revealed by the finding of an antibody, anti-Xg^a in 1962 (Mann *et al.*) is unique in that it is controlled by an X-linked locus. The finding of a sex-linked blood group was of great interest and it has caused renewed interest in sex-linked characteristics and has played a large part in mapping the X chromosome.

The first anti-Xg^a was found in a much transfused man (Mann *et al.*, 1962). The antibody was shown to be independent of ABO, MNSs, and Rh, but appeared to be sex-linked. This was recognised as being of great importance and a large number of families were studied to confirm the finding. Xg^a was shown to be an X-linked dominant gene. The genotype frequencies for Britain are:

Males		*Females*	
Xg^a	0·675	Xg^a	0·894
Xg	0·325	Xg	0·106

Of the Xg^a females 0·455 would be Xg^aXg^a and 0·439 Xg^aXg (Noades *et al.*, 1966).

The figures for North America and Canada are very similar but in Northern Europe the frequency of Xg^a positives appears to be somewhat lower.

Figure 19.1 shows how Xg^a can be inherited when (*a*) the father and (*b*) and (*c*) the mother are Xg^a positive.

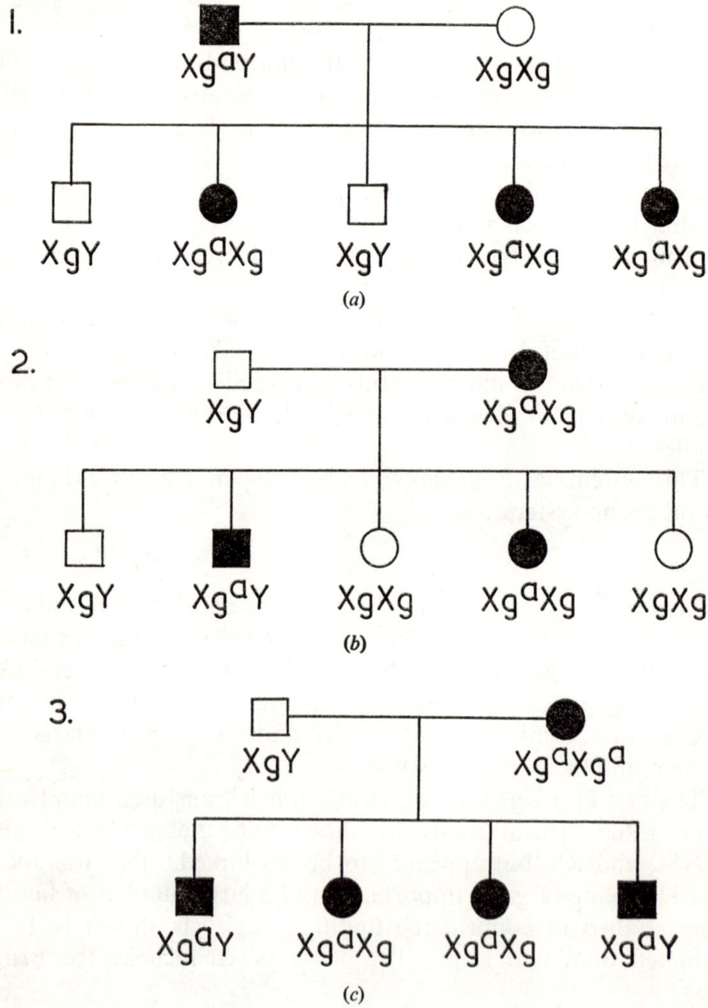

FIG. 19. Families showing inheritance of Xg^a.

Several points about sex-linked inheritance are illustrated in these diagrams.

If the father is Xg^a positive he cannot pass Xg^a on to his sons as they have to inherit his Y chromosome, but he must pass Xg^a on to his daughters as they have to inherit his X chromosome.

If the mother is Xg^a positive she can either be Xg^aXg as in diagram (2) or Xg^aXg^a as in diagram (3).

When she is Xg^aXg she has an equal chance of passing on Xg^a to her sons or her daughters; as her husband is Xg^a negative half the children will be Xg^a positive and half Xg^a negative—if (not shown in diagram) her husband were Xg^a positive the daughters in the family will be Xg^a positive, but the sons would still have an equal chance of being Xg^a positive or Xg^a negative.

When the mother is Xg^aXg^a as in (3), all the chlldren will be Xg^a positive.

The Xg^a typing of individuals with abnormal sex chromosomes and other aspects of Xg^a are reviewed in Chapter 34.

BIBLIOGRAPHY

Cook, I. A., Polley, M., and Mollison, P. L. (1963), "A second example of anti-Xg^a." *Lancet*, **i**, 857.

Eaton, B, R., Morton, J. A., Pickles, Margaret M., and White, K. E. (1956), "A new antibody, anti-Yt^a, characterising a blood group antigen of high incidence," *Brit. J. Hæm.*, **2**, 333.

Layrisse, M., Sanger, R., and Race, R. R. (1959), "The inheritance of the antigen Di^a." *American Journal Hum. Genet.*, **11**, 17–25.

Levine, P., Robinson, Elizabeth A., Layrisse, M., Arends, T., and Dominquez Sisco, R. (1956), "The Diego blood factor." *Nature, Lond.*, **177**, 40.

Mann, J. D., Cahan, A., Gelb, A. G., Fisher, N., Hamper, J., Tippett, P., Sanger, R., and Race, R. R. (1962), "A sex linked blood group gene." *Lancet*, **i**, 8.

Race, R. R., and Sanger, R. (1964), "The X-linked blood group system Xg." *Acta hæmat.*, **31**, 205.

CHAPTER 20

VARIOUS RED CELL AGGLUTINATION PHENOMENA

AGGLUTINATION of red cells is not always caused by antibodies belonging to easily recognisable blood group systems. The phenomenon of agglutination can occur for other reasons. These other kinds of agglutination form the subject of this chapter.

(1) Auto-agglutination

This type of agglutination is caused by auto-antibodies the essential characteristic of which is that they react upon the red cells of the individual in whose serum they occur. In addition they seem to detect an antigen common to all, or almost all, human red cells since they give a positive reaction with the cells of all individuals irrespective of any known blood group system. Both complete and incomplete auto-antibodies are found.

In some cases we can identify the auto-antibody. For instance anti-H and anti-I both occur as cold auto-antibodies; among warm auto-antibodies anti-e is the most common although warm auto-antibodies of the other Rh specificities have been described.

Atypical auto-antibodies in virus pneumonia are usually anti-I, possibly because mycoplasma are also associated with this disease, and are believed to destroy the I antigen.

Complete Auto-antibodies

These are agglutinins and are normally active only in the cold. They occur in the sera of very many healthy individuals as can be readily ascertained by testing 2 per cent suspensions of red cells against an equal volume of serum from the same individuals at 4°C. Very occasionally auto-agglutinins may become active to the extent of having appreciable titres at room temperature. These more potent cold auto-agglutinins can also occur in healthy individuals but are often associated with pathological states, *e.g.* hæmolytic anæmia. Auto-agglutinins having titres at 4°C of 1,000 or over are often associated with virus pneumonia and are of value in differential diagnosis. (*See* technique No. 20.2.)

Auto-agglutination that confines its activity to low temperatures does not interfere with blood grouping tests but that which takes place at laboratory or higher temperatures must be dealt with before blood grouping is attempted. When auto-agglutination is sufficiently strong to interfere with tests it is usually obvious to the naked eye and will be seen during the handling of the sample of the patient's blood. Less strong auto-agglutination may be missed at this stage in which case it may cause anomalous results. Warm washing the red cells in saline at 37°C will usually free them of auto-agglutinins. Occasionally it may be necessary to wash at a temperature higher than 37°C or even allow the cells to remain at a higher temperature for 5–10 minutes in order to break down the auto-agglutination. (Technique No. 20.1.)

Incomplete Auto-antibodies

Incomplete auto-antibodies can be of both "cold" and "warm" types. If clotted or defibrinated normal blood is allowed to stand at 0°–2°C and thereafter an anti-human globulin test carried out on the red cells, the reaction is often positive due to absorption of incomplete cold auto-antibodies from the serum. Blood samples containing anti-coagulant, *e.g.* sequestrine, heparin, citrate, etc., do not give this reaction. This phenomenon does not interfere with most blood grouping tests, but accounts for some anomalous positive anti-human globulin tests, if red cells stored overnight in the refrigerator as clotted samples are used. It is, however, possible to overcome this difficulty by the choice of a suitably diluted anti-human globulin reagent or especially prepared anti-IgG anti-human globulin that does not react with these antibodies of the cold type. (*See* Appendix I.)

The presence of "warm" incomplete auto-antibodies is usually associated with pathological states especially hæmolytic anæmias. For a discussion of these and other auto-antibodies, including the Donath-Landsteiner antibody, which are concerned in the ætiology of hæmolytic anæmia, *see* Chapter 26.

(2) Bacteriogenic Agglutination

This agglutination is unlike any discussed so far in that it is bacteriogenic. It can occur in one of two ways. Either red cells are acted upon by certain bacteria and viruses in such a way that they become agglutinated by all human sera and are, therefore, said to be pan-agglutinable, or a sample of serum may become infected with certain organisms rendering it capable of agglutinating all samples of red cells; in this case the serum is said to be pan-agglutinating.

Poly-agglutinable Cells

Certain bacteria have the power of modifying red cells *in vitro* by causing the exposure of receptors for which there is a corresponding antibody in normal human sera. This is the basis of "T" agglutination. A latent receptor "T" on the human red cell acts as an agglutinogen when exposed by the action of certain bacteria, *e.g. Cl. Welchii, Vibrio choleræ*. A corresponding antibody, anti-T, is present in all human sera (with the exception of the sera of newborn infants) so that cells which have been modified by the bacteria are agglutinated by all sera and are, therefore, said to be pan-agglutinable.* Anti-T can be specifically removed from serum samples with such pan-agglutinable cells.

Pan-agglutinating Serum

Davidsohn and Toharsky showed that when serum became infected with a strain of corynebacterium which they called H, it agglutinated all samples of human red cells. This agglutination was caused by the organism acting upon adult and infant serum *in vitro* to produce "anti-h" agglutinins for which there is a corresponding agglutinogen H in all red cells. The H–anti-h agglutination has been shown to be distinct from T–anti-T. It should not be confused with the H–anti-H which has already been described in connexion with the ABO blood group system. One of the chief dangers associated with a pan-agglutinating serum is an error of blood group caused by a grouping serum becoming infected and thus pan-agglutinating. Such a possibility, however, presents no problem to those who consistently include adequate controls as the phenomenon would be detected in the negative control and the tests repeated with fresh serum.

(3) Poly-agglutination

A few individuals have been described whose red cells are agglutinated by a proportion of normal human sera which are compatible from the point of view of all known blood groups. These cells are said to be poly-agglutinable (agglutinated by many sera) in contradistinction to pan-agglutinable (agglutinated by all sera). This agglutination may also be of bacterial origin but no proof of this exists. Sterile samples taken from the patient are poly-agglutinable and incapable of passing on their agglutinability

* In practice the agglutination is variable according to the degree of bacterial infection in the cells are usually poly- rather than pan-agglutinable.

to normal cells. This is quite different from the *in vitro* pan-agglutination where an inoculum of infected cells will within 24–48 hours infect normal cells causing them to become pan-agglutinable. On the other hand poly-agglutinability is not a constant characteristic of the cells of the individual, persisting for several weeks only in most of the cases described. From a practical point of view cells from such an individual would appear to be group AB while the serum would give the reactions typical of his true ABO group. Tests with AB sera would reveal that the red cells were agglutinated by the majority, proving them poly-agglutinable. The ABO group of the patient can be determined on serum reactions.

The cell typing for ABO, Rh type, etc., can be done in one of two ways.

(*a*) A standard anti-serum can be used to prepare a saline eluate of the required antibody (technique No. 21.3). Such an eluate will not contain the poly-agglutinating antibody whose presence in almost all sera makes their use for typing poly-agglutinable cells impossible.

(*b*) Poly-agglutinable red cells can be typed by inhibition technique, a modification of technique No. 8.2 being used. Briefly an anti-serum (titre approximately 32) is titrated both before and after absorption with an equal quantity of poly-agglutinable red cells. A definite reduction in titration value of the anti-serum indicates that the corresponding antigen is present in the unknown poly-agglutinable red cells.

(4) Pseudo-agglutination

Pseudo-agglutination is the clumping of red cells by other means than antigen-antibody reaction. It is chiefly associated with a protein shift in the serum, *e.g.* in case of multiple myelomatosis or with the addition of certain substances which alter the serum viscosity, *e.g.* dextran (*see* Plate 5(*a*) and (*b*)).

It is mentioned again here because it may easily be confused in practice with auto-agglutination, pan-agglutination, etc. The method by which it may most easily be distinguished from true agglutination is the indirect anti-human globulin technique.

Techniques

Technique No. 20.1. The washing of red cells to free them from auto-agglutinins

Any required quantity of red cells showing auto-agglutination are suspended in saline and allowed to reach a temperature of

37°C, either in an incubator or water bath, and left for 5–10 minutes. They are then centrifuged in warm centrifuge cups and the supernatant saline is quickly removed. The cells are washed twice more in warm saline and allowed to cool to room temperature. If examination under the microscope reveals that they are completely unagglutinated they may be used for grouping purposes. If on the other hand, they still show agglutination the process should be repeated raising the temperature to 45°C or even 56°C if necessary. In cases where a temperature above 37°C is needed it is preferable wherever possible to obtain washed cells from a sample which is not allowed to cool below 37°C from the moment of withdrawal from the patient to the completion of the washing process.

Technique No. 20.2. Titration of a serum containing auto-agglutinins

Serial dilutions of the serum are made in saline in the usual manner, technique No. 4 or by master titre technique No. 6. The number of rows prepared should allow for titrations using the patient's own cells prepared by technique 53 and two standards, one of group O and the other of the same ABO group as the patient, at 4°, 18°, 32°, and 37°C. The serial dilutions and the appropriate cells must be warmed to 32°C and 37°C respectively before they are mixed together. This ensures that agglutination does not begin to take place at a lower temperature. The titrations are left for 2 hours at the various temperatures before being read.

BIBLIOGRAPHY

HÜBENER, G. (1925), "Untersuchungen über isoagglutination, mit besonderer Berücksichtigung scheinbarer Abweichungen vom Gruppenschema." *S. Immun. Forsch.*, **45**, 223.

THOMSEN, O. (1927), "Ein vermehrungsfähiges Agens als Veränderer des isoagglutinatorischen Verhaltens der roten Blutkörperchen, eine bisher unbekannte Quelle der Fehlbestimmung." *S. Immun. Forsch.*, **52**, 85.

FRIEDENREICH, V. (1930), *The Thomsen Hemagglutination Phenomenon.* Copenhagen.

Section 5—Practical Applications of Blood Group Theory

"The knowledge that holds good in working, cleave thou to that."

Thomas Carlyle, PAST AND PRESENT

"Skill to do comes by doing."

Emerson

CHAPTER 21

IDENTIFICATION OF ANTIBODIES AND MIXTURES OF ANTIBODIES

THE various blood group systems have been described separately, but obviously when an unidentified antibody is discovered they must all be considered together, since the antibody may belong to any of them.

Apart from the detection of anti-A and anti-B agglutinins (serum grouping technique No. 3.2) routine antibody tests are designed mainly to detect Rh antibodies. (*See* Chapters 10 and 13.) This is because Rh antibodies are the most common cause of transfusion reaction and hæmolytic disease of the newborn. Nevertheless, in some cases a pattern of reaction which is not characteristic of any of the Rh antibodies will be obtained in the routine testing. Evidence for the presence of other atypical antibodies may also be found in other cases in which it has been deemed necessary, in the absence of any trace of Rh antibodies, to seek further for a serological cause of a clinical syndrome. Cold agglutinins will not normally be detected unless especially sought. However, occasionally their presence will be advertised by an anomalous result occurring in serum grouping tests for ABO agglutinins.

The detection and identification of Rh antibodies has already been considered in detail in Chapter 13. It is, therefore, unnecessary to reconsider them here. In this chapter we are concerned with the detection and identification of other atypical antibodies and also mixtures of antibodies belonging to different blood group systems, including Rh.

Choice of Standard Red Cells

It is essential that any laboratory undertaking the identification of atypical antibodies has a good panel of standard cells which have been tested for as many blood group systems as possible. These, of course, should all be of group O to avoid interference by the reaction of A with anti-A and B with anti-B. It should not be too difficult to select approximately twelve different red cell standards which will not only detect most of the known antibodies but also distinguish between them. An example of a useful panel is shown in Table 21.1. These standard red cells should be used whenever the routine Rh antibody test has given anomalous results or in those cases in which the routine Rh antibody test is negative but there are clinical reasons for suspecting the presence of an atypical antibody. In addition if the antibody is reacting with most or all standard cells the rare homozygotes must be included, *e.g.* Lu^aLu^a, KK, Vel negative, etc. If the antibody reacts with one cell only then knowledge of the rare antigens it contains will be helpful, *e.g.* Wr^a+, Sw^a+ or V^w+, etc.

Investigation of the Serum

It is suggested that the unknown serum be tested with the selected standard cells and the patient's own cells by some or all of the standard antibody detection methods. The investigation of the serum by all these methods in parallel is described in technique No. 21.1.

An idea as to which methods will be the most profitable to use in any particular case may be gained from the results of the routine antibody tests that have already been done. If, for example, the antibody seems to be more readily detectable by albumin technique, then in further tests with the enlarged panel of red cells, saline and papain techniques might well be omitted. Similarly, if the presence of a cold agglutinin is suspected, tests with cells suspended in saline will usually yield satisfactory results.

Interpretation of Results

The temperature of reactivity, the techniques which have to be employed to show the presence of the antibody and the frequency of positive reactions obtained, are all guides to identity *see* Table 21.2. For example, an antibody reacting better at 37°C than at a lower temperature is not a cold antibody. This observation makes it unlikely that the antibody is anti-P_1, anti-H, anti-HI, anti-M, anti-N, anti-Le^a, anti-Le^b, or anti-Lu^a. An antibody reacting by

Table 21.1

(a) Identification of Antibodies by Testing with a Selected Panel of Standard Red Cells

Standard red cells (all group O)	Rh type	Antigens in red cells																Unknown serum St.					Unknown serum Mc.				
		C	D	E	c	d	e	M	N	S	P_1	Lu^a	K	Le^a	Le^b	Fy^a	Jk^a	R.T.	37°C				R.T.	37°C			
																		Sal.	Sal.	Alb.	C	P	Sal.	Sal.	Alb.	C	P
LB	rr	−	−	−	+	+	+	−	+	+	+s	−	−	−	+	+	+	V	w	−	−	−	−	−	−	−	−
ML	rr	−	−	−	+	+	+	+	+	+	+s	+	−	−	+	−	−	V	−	−	−	−	−	−	−	−	−
RS	rr	−	−	−	+	+	+	+	+	+	+w	−	+	+	−	+	−	w	−	−	−	−	−	−	−	+++	−
RL	R_1R_1	+	+	−	−	(−)	+	+	−	+	+s	+	−	−	+	+	+	V	−	−	−	−	−	−	−	−	−
RZ	R_1R_1	+	+	−	−	(−)	+	−	+	−	−	−	−	−	+	+	+	−	−	−	−	−	−	−	−	−	−
BH	R_1r	+	+	−	+	(+)	+	+	+	−	+s	−	−	−	+	+	−	V	w	−	−	−	−	−	−	−	−
LP	R_1r	+	+	−	+	(+)	+	+	+	+	−	−	−	+	−	+	+	−	−	−	−	−	−	−	−	−	−
CL	R_1r	+	+	−	+	(+)	+	+	+	+	+ m	−	−	−	+	−	+	+	−	−	−	−	−	−	−	−	−
RB	R_2R_2	−	+	+	+	(−)	−	+	+	+	+s	−	−	+	−	+	+	V	−	−	−	−	−	−	−	−	−
DM	R_2R_2	−	+	+	+	(−)	−	+	+	+	−	−	−	−	+	−	+	−	−	−	−	−	−	−	−	−	−
MP	R_2r	−	+	+	+	(+)	+	+	−	−	+s	−	−	−	+	+	+	V	w	−	−	−	−	−	−	−	−
JRL	R_2r	−	+	+	+	(+)	+	+	+	+	−	+	+	−	+	+	+	−	−	−	−	−	−	−	−	+++	−
Own St.	R_1r	+	+	−	+	(+)	+	+	+	+	−	−	−	−	+	+	+	−	−	−	−	−					
Own Mc.	rr	−	−	−	+	+	+	+	−	+	+ m	−	−	−	+	−	+						−	−	−	−	−

Table 21.2

Section I. Antibodies for Frequent Antigens

Antibody	Antigen	System	Approximate frequency of antigen	Frequency of antibody	Usual technique and temperature	Remarks
Anti-At^a	August	—	No random At^a negative	One example only so far	a.h.g. 37°C	Probably immune to pregnancy (another At^a negative had no anti-At^a)
Anti-Chido	Chido	—	High	Fairly rare	a.h.g. 37°C	Antibodies known tend to give variable reactions.
Anti-Co^a	Colton	—	99·7%	Four known	a.h.g. or a.h.g.-papain 37°C	
Anti-Cs^a	Cs^a		97·5%	A few known	a.h.g. 37°C	Marked variation of strength of antigen
Anti-Di^b	Di^b	Diego	100% in White and Negroes and Eskimos	Rare	a.h.g. 37°C	See also Section II
Anti-e	e	Rh	97%	Fairly common	a.h.g. and papain 37°C	Also found as auto antibody in some hæmolytic anæmia cases
Anti-En^a	En^a		Almost universal	V. rare	Saline, alb, a.h.g. and enzyme	En(a-) cells give unusual reactions for MN and RL
Anti-Ge	Ge (Gerbich)		Very frequent no random Ge neg found	Rare	Some a.h.g. 37°C others saline RT	Antibodies show slight differences in specificity
Anti-Go^b	Go^b	Rh	Very frequent	One known	a.h.g. 37°C	
Anti-Gy^a	Gy^a (Gregory)		Very frequent	Rare	a.h.g. 37°C	
Anti-H	H	ABO	Very frequent	Common	Saline 4°C or 15°C sometimes Pap. 37°C	Reacts best with GpO cells and least well with Gp, A_1B cells. Weak with cord cells. Usually inhibitable with secretor saliva

Section I. Antibodies for Frequent Antigens (*contd.*)

Antibody	Antigen	System	Approximate frequency of antigen	Frequency of antibody	Usual technique and temperature	Remarks
Anti-HI	HI	ABO and I	Very frequent in adults. Cord cells, weak or negative	Common	Saline 4°C or 15°C	Reactions similar to anti-H. Also negative with Oii and hhI cells. Usually not inhibited by secretor saliva
Anti-I	I	I	Very frequent in adults. Not found in infants	Common	Saline 4°C or 15°C. Can also be a.h.g. or papain 37°C	Often found as auto-antibody in "cold"-type hæmolytic anæmia. Not inhibited by secretor saliva
Anti-I^T	I^T	I		Found as cold auto agglutinin Melanesians	Saline cold	Strong with cord cells. Less strong with adult I cells. Weak with adult i cells
Anti-i		I	Weak with almost all adult cells. Strongly positive with all cord cells.	Rare	Saline cold	Also found as auto-antibody associated with infectious mononucleosis
Anti-Js^b(K7)	Js^b	Kell	100% Whites 99% Negroes	Rare	a.h.g. 37°C	
Anti-k (K2)	k	Kell	99%	Rare	a.h.g. 37°C	
Anti-KL	KL	Kell	Extremely frequent	Very rare	a.h.g. 37°C	KL negative persons lack K and may have traces only of k, Kp^b and Js^{b-}
Anti-Kp^b(K4)	Kp^b	Kell	Extremely frequent	Rare	a.h.g. or papain 37°C	
Anti-KU(K5)	A Kell antigen common to all cells except (K-k-Kpla-b-) Js(a-b-)	Kell	1 in 16,518 negative	Eight known	a.h.g. 37°C	

Section I. Antibodies for Frequent Antigens (*contd.*)

Antibody	Antigen	System	Approximate frequency of antigen	Frequency of antibody	Usual technique and temperature	Remarks
Anti-Lan	Lan		1 in 4,000 negative	One known	a.h.g.	
Anti-Lu^b	Lu^b	Lutheran	99·8 %	Rare	Saline or a.h.g.	
Anti-Lu^aLu^b	Lu^aLu^b	Lutheran	Extremely frequent	Three known	a.h.g.	Reacts with all but the very rare Lu (a-b-) cells
Anti-Luke	Luke	P	98 %	Three known	a.h.g. or a.h.g. on enzyme treated cells	Genetically independent of P
Anti-P	P	P	Very frequent	Rare	Saline R.T. or 37°C	Often occurs with anti-P_1 and P^k, originally called anti-Tj^a
Anti-Sm	Sm	(Sm and Bu^a)	Very frequent	Two known	a.h.g. 37°C	
Anti-So	So		Very frequent	Two known	a.h.g. 37°C	
Anti-T	T		Very frequent	Very frequent	Saline R.T.	Only reacts with cells that have been modified by bacteria to expose T receptor
Anti-U	U	MNSs	Very frequent	Rare	a.h.g. 37°C	All U- persons are S- s-
Anti-Vel	Vel		Very frequent (4 in 16,000 English negative)	Rare	Saline 37°C	May also hæmolyse Vel positive cells
Anti-Yt^a	Yt^a	Yt	99·8 %	Rare	a.h.g. 37°C	

Section II. Antibodies for Antigens of Frequency Less than 95% to about 1%

Antibody	Antigen	System	Approximate frequency of antigen	Frequency of antibody	Usual technique temperature	Remarks
Anti-A	A	ABO	42% (S. England) (A+AB)	Found in sera of all A negative persons	Saline R.T. (also active 37°C)	
Anti-A_1	A_1	ABO	34% (S. England) (A_1 and A_1B)	*Typical* component of all anti-A sera *Atypical*. In about 25% of A_2 and A_2B sera	Saline R.T. (also active 37°C) Saline 4°C may also be active R.T. and very rarely at 37°C)	
Anti-Au^a	Auberger		82% (French and English)	One known	a.h.g. 37°C	Relationship between dominant Lu (a-b-) type and Auberger (*see* Chap. 34)
Anti-B	B	ABO	10% (S. England) (B and AB)	Found in sera of all B negative persons	Saline R. T. (also active 37°C)	
Anti-Bg^a	Bg^a (Bennet–Godspeed–Sturgeon–Donna)		29%	Fairly common	Saline or a.h.g.	Antibodies usually weak and give variable positive frequency
Anti-Bg^b	Bg^b (HO)		23 in 895	Rare	a.h.g. 37°C	Sera may contain mixtures *e.g.* anti-Bg^a and Bg^b
Anti-Bg^c	Bg^c (Ot)		2 positive in 300	A few examples	a.h.g. 37°C	
Anti-C	C	Rh	63·5%	Commonly found with anti-D in Rh negative persons. More rarely in Rh positives and then often in association with anti-e	Saline and papain 37°C (also a.h.g. 37°C)	Anti-D sera should be tested with R′ cells for possible presence of anti-C. (*See also* anti-G.)
Anti-c	c	Rh	80%	Fairly rare	a.h.g. and papain 37°C	Found in R_1R_1 persons often in association with anti-E

Section II. Antibodies for Antigens of Frequency less than 95% to about 1% (*contd.*)

Antibody	Antigen	System	Approximate frequency of antigen	Frequency of antibody	Usual technique temperature	Remarks
Anti-C^w	C^w	Rh	Varies with race from 2–9%	Fairly rare less uncommon as a component of anti-C and anti-CD sera	Saline a.h.g. and papain 37°C	
Anti-Ce	Ce in Cis position	Rh	63%	Rare—pure but a component of many anti-C sera	Saline, a.h.g. and papain 37°C	
Anti-cE	cE in cis	Rh	31%	Rare	a.h.g. or papain 37°C	
Anti-ce	ce in cis	Rh	64%	Rare alone found in many anti-c and anti-e sera	a.h.g. or papain 37°C	
Anti-ce^s	ce^s in cis	Rh	Rare in whites, up to 40% in negroes	Three known	a.h.g. and papain 37°C	
Anti-Ce^s	Ce^s in cis	Rh	Rare in whites, common in negroes	Fairly rare	a.h.g. and papain 37°C	
Anti-D	D	Rh	85%	Common	Saline, alb., a.h.g. and/or papain 37°C	
Anti-Di^a	Di^a	Diego	Found in Mongolian races and South American Indians. Varies 2·5%–36%	Rare	a.h.g. 37°C	
Anti-Di^b	Di^b	Diego	In Mongoloid races allelic to Di^a distribution	Rare	a.h.g. 37°C	
Anti-Do^a	Do^a	Dombrock	Europeans 66% American Negroes and Indians lower. Thais 13%	Rare	a.h.g. 37°C	a.h.g. sera have to be specially chosen
Anti-Donna	Bg^a	(*see* anti-Bg^a)				
Anti-E	E	Rh	30%	Common	Saline, alb., a.h.g. papain 37°C	Often detectable only by pap. tech. especially if naturally occurring
Anti-E^T	E^T	Rh	30% Whites 20% Australian Aborigines	One known	Saline R.T.	

Section II. Antibodies for Antigens of Frequency less than 95% to about 1% (contd.)

Antibody	Antigen	System	Approximate frequency of antigen	Frequency of antibody	Usual technique temperature	Remarks
Anti-e^s	e^s	Rh	35–45% Negroes	Not uncommon often with other Rh antibodies	a.h.g. and papain 37°C	
Anti-f (see anti-ce)	ce	Rh	16%	Rare alone found in most anti-c and anti-e sera	Papain and a.h.g. 37°C	
Anti-Fy^a	Fy^a	Duffy	Whites 66%	Fairly common	a.h.g. 37°C	Inactivated by papain
Anti-Fy^b	Fy^b	Duffy	Whites 34%	Fairly rare	a.h.g. 37°C	Inactivated by papain
Anti-G	G	Rh	85%	Common in anti-CD sera	Saline, alb., a.h.g. and/or papain	
Anti-IP_1	IP_1	I and P	75%	Rare	Saline, cold	
Anti-Jk^a	Jk^a	Kidd	76% (higher in Negroes)	Not uncommon	Saline, cold, a.h.g., and/or a.h.g. on enzyme treated cells	
Anti-Jk^b	Jk^b	Kidd	71% (lower in Negroes)	Rare	As anti-Jk^a	Some sera behave as if they were detecting more than one antigen
Anti-Js^a (K6)	Js^a (Sutter)	Kell	20% in Negroes	Rare	a.h.g. 37°C	
Anti-K (K1)	K	Kell	9%	Common	a.h.g. 37°C	Often found in association with other immune antibodies
Anti-Le^a	Le^a	Lewis	22%	Common	Saline cold and/or a.h.g., a.h.g. and complement and papain 37°C	
Anti-Le^b	Le^b	Lewis	Varies with ABO group and serum used	Common	Saline cold occasionally a.h.g. 37°C (or a.h.g. and complement)	
Anti-Le^X	Probably Le^a	Lewis	90%	Rare	As for anti-Le^a	Positive with cells of all persons who secrete Le^a
Anti-Lu^a	Lu^a	Lutheran	8%	Rare	Saline R.T. or rarely a.h.g. 37°C	

Section II. Antibodies for Antigens of Frequency less than 95% to about 1% (*contd.*)

Antibody	Antigen	System	Approximate frequency of antigen	Frequency of antibody	Usual technique temperature	Remarks
Anti-LW	LW	Rh	85% (give +ve reactions) rr cells are negative but absorb the antibody	Rare	a.h.g. or papain	Genetically independent of Rh
Anti-M	M	MNSs	78%	Common	Saline R.T. can also be a.h.g. 37°C	
Anti-M^1	M^1	MNSs	22·6% of group M 4% of group MN	One known	Saline R.T.	Not identical with anti-M_1
Anti-M_1	M_1	MNSs	About 5% in Whites. About 20% in Negroes	Found in many human anti-M sera	Saline ph 6·5 R.T.	
Anti-N	N	MNSs	72%	Fairly uncommon	Saline R.T.	
Anti-P_1	P_1	P	79%	Very common	Saline or papain R.T.	Can very rarely be active by a.h.g. at 37°C
Anti-Rh	(*See under* anti-D, anti-E, etc.)					
Anti-Rh_A, -Rh_B, etc.	Rh	Rh	Same as anti-D except for very rare cells	Rare	Papain 37°C	
Anti-S	S	MNSs	55% (varies with MN type)	Fairly common	a.h.g. 37°C or saline R.T.	
Anti-s	s	MNSs	98% (varies with MN type)	Rare	a.h.g. 37°C	
Anti-Sd^a	Sd^a		91%	About 1% of normal donors	Saline R.T.	
Anti-S_j	S_j	MNSs	2% Whites 4% Negroes	Very rare (found with anti-Tm)	Saline R.T.	All S_j +ves were Tm+ also
Anti-St^a	St^a	MNSs	Very rare Whites but 14 in 220 Japanese	Rare	Saline R.T.	
Anti-Ul^a	Ul^a (Karhula)		2·6–5% in Finns	One known	a.h.g. 37°C	
Anti-V	V(ce^s)	Rh	Very rare in Whites. Up to 40% in Negroes	Rare	a.h.g. 37°C papain	
Anti-VS	VS(e^s)	Rh	Very rare in Whites reacts with Negroes up to about 60%	Rare	a.h.g. 37°C	React with all V+ and most R^1 Negroes
Anti-Xg^a	Xg^a	Xg	Males 67·5%	Rare	a.h.g. 37°C	Sex linked

Section III. Antibodies for Rare Antigens

Antibody	Antigen	System	Frequency of antigen	Frequency of antibody	Usual technique and temperature	Remarks
Anti-Be^a	Berrens	—	0 in 947 randoms	Rare—but has been produced by immunization of volunteers	a.h.g. 37°C	
Anti-Becker	Becker	—	0 in 122 randoms	One known	a.h.g. 37°C	
Anti-Bi	Biles	—	0 in 1,110 randoms	One known	a.h.g. 37°C	
Anti-Bp^a	Bishop	—	1 in 75,000	Rare	Saline R.T.	Slightly more common in a.h.a. sera than in normal sera
Anti-Bu^a	Bu^a	Bu^a and Sm	1 in 100 to 1 in 1000	Rare	a.h.g. 37°C	Reactions antithetical to Sm
Anti-Bx^a	Box	—	1 in 7,000 approx.	One known		
Anti-By	Batty	—	0 in many thousand	Rare	a.h.g. and papain 37°C	Liable to occur in a.h.a. sera
Anti-C^x	C^x	Rh	4 in 3,931 randoms	Rare in normal sera	Saline and a.h.g. 37°C	Less rare in a.h.a. sera
Anti-CE	CE in cis	Rh	15%	Rare	Saline or papain 37°C	
Anti-Chr^a	Chr^a		1 in 500	Rare	Albumin 37°C	
Anti-Cl^a	Caldwell	MNSs	0 in 11,000	0·45 of normal sera	Saline R.T.	
Anti-D^w	D^w (Wiel)	Rh	Very rare in Whites 9 in 253 Negroes		Papain 37°C	Probably identical with Tippetts Category V
Anti-Di^a	Di^a	Diego	Almost absent in Whites and Negroes (*also* Eskimos)	Rare	a.h.g. 37°C	*See also* Section II
Anti-E^w	E^w	Rh	Rare	Rare	a.h.g. 37°C	
Anti-Evans	Evans	Maybe Rh	Very rare	One known	a.h.g. 37°C	
Anti-Gf	Griffiths		0 in 6,886	Three known	Papain 37°C	
Anti-Go^a	Gonzales	Rh	Very rare	Four known	a.h.g. 37°C	Related to Tippett's category IV O antigen

Section III. Antibodies for Rare Antigens (*contd.*)

Antibody	Antigen	System	Frequency of antigen	Frequency of antibody	Usual technique and temperature	Remarks
Anti-Good	Good		0 in 4,000	Rare	a.h.g. 37°C	
Anti-Gr	Graydon (or V^{w})	MNSs	1 in 1,755	1% of normal sera	Saline R.T.	
Anti-He	Henshaw	MNSs	2·7% West Africans 0% Whites	One known	Saline R.T.	Can be made in rabbits
Anti-Heibel	Heibel		0 in 7,500	One known	a.h.g. 37°C	
Anti-Hill	Hill	MNSs	Very rare. Reacts with Mi^{a+}, Vw-, Mu+, Hill+ cells only	One known	a.h.g. 37°C	
Anti-Ho	Ho now known as Bg^{b}		23 in 895 Dutch	Rare	a.h.g. 37°C	Reactions very variable
Anti-He^{a}	Hunt		0 in 453	One known	a.h.g. 37°C	
Anti-Hu	Hunter	MNSs	Rare in Europe 22% Africans	One human	Saline R.T.	Made in rabbits
Anti-Jn^{a}	Jn^{a}		Very rare	Three known	Saline, cold	
Anti-Js^{a} (K6)	Js^{a}	Kell	Very rare in all but Negroes	Rare	a.h.g. 37°C	(*See also* Section II)
Anti-Kamhuber	Kamhuber		0 in 1,100	One known	a.h.g. 37°C	
Anti-Kp^{a} (K3)	Kp^{a}	Kell	2%	Rare	a.h.g. 37°C	
Anti-Levay	Levay		Very rare	One known	Saline R.T.	
Anti-Ls^{a}	Lewis II		Very rare	One known	Saline R.T.	

Section III. Antibodies for Rare Antigens (*contd.*)

Antibody	Antigen	System	Frequency of antigen	Frequency of antibody	Usual technique and temperature	Remarks
Anti-M^a	M^a	MNSs	Very rare	Very rare	Saline R.T.	M^a may be identical with M
Anti-M^g	M^g	MNSs	Very rare	Common	Saline R.T.	
Anti-M^k	M^k	MNSs	Very rare (cells are M-N-S-s-)	Very rare	Saline R.T.	Antibody very weak
Anti-Marriott	Marriott		Rare	Very rare	Saline R.T.	
Anti-Mi^a	Mi^a	MNSs	Very rare	Fairly common	Saline R.T.	Sometimes found in hæmolytic anæmia sera. Often found as anti-Mi^a+V^w
Anti-Mt^a	Mt^a	MNSs	Very rare	Very rare	Saline R.T.	
Anti-Mur.	Mu^a (Murrell)	MNSs	Very rare	Rare	Saline R.T.	
Anti-Ny^a	Ny^a	MNSs	Rare	Rare	Saline R.T.	
Anti-Or	Or (Orris)		Rare	Rare		
Anti-Ot (anti-Bg^a and Bg^c)	Bg	Bg	Rare (2 in 300)	Very rare	a.h.g. 37°C	
Anti-P^k	P^k	P	Extremely rare	Occurs with anti-P and anti-P_1	Saline R.T. and 37°C	
Anti-Rd	Rd (Radin)		Very rare except 3 in 562 New York Jewish	Very rare	a.h.g. 37°C	
Anti-Raddon	Raddon		Very rare	One known	a.h.g. 37°C	
Anti-Ri^a	Ri^a (Ridley)	MNSs	Very rare	One known	Saline R.T.	
Anti-Rm	R_m		Very rare	One known	a.h.g. 37°C	
Anti-St^a	St^a (Stones)	MNSs	20 in 17,000 Whites. 14 in 220 Japanese	Rare	Saline R.T.	
Anti-Stobo	Stobo		2 in 3,000 Scottish	Fairly rare		May be part of Bg System
Anti-Sul	Sul	MNSs	Rare	Fairly common	Saline R.T.	

Section III. Antibodies for Rare Antigens (*contd.*)

Antibody	Antigen	System	Frequency of antigen	Frequency of antibody	Usual technique and temperature	Remarks
Anti-Sw^a	Sw^a (Swann)		9 in 50,000	Fairly common in pathological sera, aha, etc.	a.h.g. 37°C	
Anti-Tm	Tm	MNSs	Very rare	Rare	Saline R.T.	
Anti-To^a	To^a (Torkildsen)		2 in 3,500	Rare	Saline R.T.	
Anti-Tr^a	Tr^a (Traversu)		2 in 38,000	Rare	Saline R.T.	When antibody found it is usually associated with anti-Wr^a
Anti-Ven	Ven		Rare	One known	a.h.g. 37°C	
Anti-Vr	Vr	MNSs	Rare	Very rare	a.h.g. 37°C	
Anti-Vw	Vw	MNSs	Rare	Common	a.h.g. 37°C	(*See also* Gr)
Anti-Wb	Wb (Webb)		Very rare	Rare	Saline R.T.	
Anti-Wiel	D^w	Rh	Rare	Rare	Papain 37°C	
Anti-Wr^a	Wr^a		Rare	Common	a.h.g. and Papain 37°C often saline R.T. also	
Anti-Wu	Wu		Rare	Rare		

indirect anti-human globulin test at 37°C with approximately 1 in 10 of the samples of red cells used, is most likely to be anti-K. Other similar deductions which give a line on the specificity of an antibody may be made.

A convenient method of recording the results obtained with a panel of known cells is shown in Table 21.1. The arrangement of the results in this fashion makes it easy to see whether the pattern of reactions given by the serum being tested corresponds to a known antigen-antibody system. The findings will fall into one of five categories which will be considered separately; namely (*a*) clear-cut positive and negative reactions; (*b*) indeterminate reactions; (*c*) positive reactions with all standard cells but negative with own cells; (*d*) positive reactions with all cells including own; (*e*) negative reactions throughout.

(*a*) **Clear-cut Positive and Negative Reactions.** When clear-cut reactions are obtained an inspection of a protocol similar to that shown in Table 21.1 will usually suggest the identity of the antibody; but *see also* Table 21.2.II. For example, the unknown serum St. reacts with all P_1 positive cells, giving stronger reactions at room temperature than at 37°C, thus suggesting that the antibody detected as anti-P_1. Its range of reaction is also typical of anti-P_1. The second unknown antibody reacts only by indirect anti-human globulin technique with cells which are K positive, thus suggesting that it is anti-K.

The results of tests with such a known panel of standard cells do not necessarily prove conclusively the specificity of a particular antibody, although the probability that it is of the specificity suggested is high.

A relatively simple statistical method of confirming the specificity of a particular antibody is that of analysing the results by means of Fisher's exact method for 2 × 2 tables to estimate the probability of these reactions occurring by chance.

As an example, the serum St. from Table 21.1 is considered. The results are arranged as follows:

		Serum St		
		+	−	
Known cells	P_1 pos.	8^{a}	0^{b}	8
	P_1 neg.	0^{c}	4^{d}	4
		8	4	12^{N}

If the squares are lettered a, b, c, d, and the total number of red cells tested is N, the probability of the reaction not being due to an anti-P_1 antibody can be determined from the general formula. (This formula is only applicable if b or c = O.)

$$\text{probability} = \frac{(a+b)!\,(c+d)!\,(a+c)!\,(b+d)!}{N!\,a!\,b!\,c!\,d!}$$

$$= \frac{8!\,4!\,4!\,8!}{12!\,8!\,4!\,0!\,0!}$$

$$= \frac{1}{495}$$

This means that the antibody is almost certainly anti-P_1, since a probability of $\frac{1}{20}$ is usually taken as the level of significance for this type of comparison.

Clear-cut results which do not conform to any particular antibody pattern are probably due to the serum containing a mixture of antibodies and it should be investigated as shown below. There is, of course, always the exciting but rather remote possibility that a hitherto undescribed antigen-antibody system is being detected. The establishment of a new system is a long and complicated research project and as such is outside the scope of this book.

(*b*) **Indeterminate Results.** The difficulty of correctly identifying a weakly reacting antibody must be realised. It is nearly always useless to contemplate identification of specificity unless the reactions obtained are in the V to + range. There is also the question of dosage to be considered and the possibility of an antibody reacting only with red cells containing a double dose of the corresponding antigen. It is occasionally possible to identify such an antibody.

Antibodies may increase in titre as the result of immunisation and therefore in certain circumstances (*e.g.* during pregnancy) it is worth testing a later sample in the hope of identifying the antibody.

(*c*) **Positive Reactions with all Standard Cells but Negative with Own Cells.** A positive reaction obtained with all the red cells tested with the exception of the patient's own is indicative of the presence of either: (1) a type of antibody which reacts preferentially with group O cells or (2) an antibody corresponding to an antigen of high frequency, *see* Table 21.2.I, or (3) a mixture of antibodies.

If the antibody is of the cold type it is likely to be anti-I, anti-H or possibly a mixture of anti-Le^a and anti-Le^b. Testing with several examples of group O Le(a− b−) red cells will reveal whether or not the third alternative is correct. If the reactions with these red cells are positive, proving that an anti-Le^a + anti-Le^b mixture is not involved, titrations against red cells in saline of group O, several examples of group A_1 and at least one group A_2 should be performed using the master titre technique (No. 4.5).* If the values obtained are appreciably higher with cells of groups O and A_2 than with cells of group A_1 then the antibody is almost certainly of the anti-HI or anti-H type. A distinction between the two broad classes of such antibodies can be made by the saliva inhibition method, where those inhibited by secretor saliva are said to be anti-H and those not so affected anti-HI, but in routine work this is rarely necessary (*see also* Chapter 30).

Anti-I and anti-HI (sometimes called anti-OI) react in the cold with adult cells, anti-I appearing to be a pan-auto-agglutinin and anti-HI giving similar reactions to anti-H (both anti-I and anti-HI are uninhibited by human saliva), they are characterised by their poor reactivity with cord bloods.

If the unidentified antibody has a wide thermal range yet reacts, better below 37°C, it may be anti-Tj^a (now known to be anti-P + anti-P^k + anti-P_1). This can be confirmed by absorbing a portion of serum with P negative red cells which should then leave an anti-serum specific for all P-positive cells. A potential anti-Tj^a serum should be sent, for further confirmation, to a laboratory known to have the very rare Tj^a negative red cells.

Other rare antibodies, the presence of which might have to be considered, are, anti-U and anti-Vel. This again would mean consultation with a laboratory having the appropriate red cells negative with these antibodies.

The chief "warm" antibodies to be considered are anti-e and anti-k. With the panel of standard red cells shown in Table 21.1, the presence of anti-e would be immediately suggested by the finding of a negative reaction with cells DM and RB which are of genotype R_2R_2 (cDE.cDE). However, the investigator might not be fortunate enough to obtain cells of this genotype, in which case positive reactions would be found in all tests. For further identification of anti-e *see* Chapter 13.

Over 200 random red cell samples might have to be tested before a negative reaction could be obtained if the antibody was anti-k. Therefore, if its presence is suspected, red cells known to be of type KK should be obtained and in addition the cells of the donor of the serum typed with anti-K.

* Anti-H and anti-"HI" agglutinins are usually found in persons of groups A_1 or A_1B but occasionally occur in group B. In the latter eventuality it will only be possible to titrate with red cells of group O and group B, since A_1 and A_2 cells will react with the patient's own anti-A.

The numerous other possibilities can be seen on Table 21.2.I. It should be noted that the sera giving 100 per cent reactions with one ethnic group *e.g.* Whites, may give a quite different frequency if tested with another *e.g.* Negroid.

(*d*) **Positive Reactions with all Cells Including Own.** In this category the following alternatives have to be considered:

(1) Optimum reactions obtained by saline technique at room temperature indicate the presence of cold auto-antibodies or pan-agglutinins (*see* Chapter 20 and techniques 20.1 and 20.2).*

(2) Reactions obtained by indirect anti-human globulin test at 37°C suggest a case of acquired hæmolytic anæmia and tests should proceed as outlined in Chapter 26.

(3) It is by no means unusual to obtain positive reactions with all red cells including the patient's own by papain or trypsin technique. In some cases the phenomenon seems to be associated with the presence of cold auto-antibodies but this is not always so. It is thought that the effect may be due to virus infection in the patient but no clinical significance has as yet been attached to it. Absorption with the patient's own trypsin treated red cells sometimes unmasks an antibody of blood group specificity which is often found to be one of the Rh antibodies. Such an absorbed serum, therefore, should be tested for Rh antibodies (*see* Chapter 13) before embarking upon tests with the enlarged panel of standard cells.

(4) That the reaction may be due to pseudo-agglutination will probably be suspected from the characteristic appearance of the clumps under the microscope. In such circumstances, the anti-human globulin technique is used.

(*e*) **Negative Reactions Throughout** (*see* Tables 21.2 and 3). If the further investigation of the serum was instigated by the occurrence of anomalous results in routine Rh and ABO antibody testing, then the finding of negative reactions with the whole panel of group O red cells is most unlikely, the exception being an anomalous reaction with A_1 cells in routine serum grouping which might be due to anti-A_1 (α_1). This antibody will normally have been identified before tests are made against a panel of group O cells (*see* Chapters 3 and 6) but if not it can now be done.

If the further testing has been undertaken on clinical grounds alone and not because reactions suggestive of atypical antibody formation have been found, then negative results throughout may

* It should be borne in mind that auto-agglutinins may mask the presence of other specific antibodies so that the serum must be re-tested after their removal by absorption with the patient's own cells (technique No. 21.2).

occur. In these circumstances it has to be decided whether the clinical reasons are strong enough for a further investigation to be planned or whether the search for antibodies should be given up at this stage.

Re-testing the serum with the same panel of cells by the papain, the trypsin-Coombs technique (No. 21.4) and/or indirect anti-human globulin plus complement technique (No. 21.5) may be of value. Moreover, if the serum being investigated is the maternal serum in a case suspected to be one of hæmolytic disease of the newborn, it should be tested against the red cells of infant and husband (*see* Chapter 25) or if it is from a suspected case of hæmolytic transfusion reaction, direct matched with the red cells of the donors concerned. (Technique No. 22.4.)

To complete the identification of any atypical antibody the red cells of the patient in whose serum the antibody (or antibodies) occurs should be typed and shown not to contain the corresponding antigen. Indeed it is often worth while, if the necessary typing sera can be spared, to type the patient's cells for as many known blood group antigens as possible at the outset of the investigation (procedure No. 3, Appendix II). A knowledge of which antigens are absent from the red cells will provide a guide to which antibodies can be formed in the serum so that the selected panel of standard cells may be suitably modified.

After the identity of a rare antibody has been established an effort should be made to secure the serum for typing purposes if it is of suitable strength. The principles underlying the selection, standardisation and preparation of such sera are essentially the same as those for Rh typing sera (Chapter 14). The minimum titration values acceptable will depend to a great extent upon the frequency with which a particular antibody is found. Almost any example of a very rare antibody is probably of value for typing although negative reactions will have to be interpreted with caution.

Identification of Mixtures of Antibodies

One of the most difficult serological undertakings is the identification of mixtures of antibodies. These often belong to different blood group systems. It is by no means an uncommon task, since individuals who have reached the stage of producing one atypical antibody readily produce others. If difficulty in identifying the specificity of a serum is experienced, the possibility of the occurrence in it of several antibodies of differing specificity must be considered.

There are several pointers which suggest that more than one antibody has been formed. A different distribution of positive and negative reactions at different temperatures indicates a mixture of "warm" and "cold" antibodies. An example of this might be a serum containing anti-D and anti-P_1. In this case the anti-D would be readily identified by performing the tests at 37°C, for at this temperature anti-P_1 is rarely active. At 37°C, therefore, the reactions would pattern as anti-D. Tests at room temperature would reveal the anti-P_1 but the anti-D might also be active, although not so strongly as at 37°C; therefore it would be essential to confirm the specificity of the anti-P_1 by confining the room temperature tests to red cell samples which were D negative. However, if the anti-D did not react in a saline medium no interference with the anti-P_1 would be experienced since the latter antibody is a saline agglutinin and is tested for by saline technique. Any such mixture of the agglutinin form of one antibody and the incomplete form of another can be readily disentangled and identified even if both have the same temperature range.

Noting the antigens missing from the red cell samples which are negative with the serum under test may aid the detection of the components of a mixture. For instance, a serum containing a mixture of anti-M and anti-P_1 could not be differentiated by testing at various temperatures or by different techniques since both are cold agglutinins and react in a saline medium. Nevertheless a clue to their identity could be obtained by noting that the only red cells negative with the serum in question did not contain either M or P_1. This principle can also be applied to the identification of mixtures containing more than two antibodies. The greater the number of antibodies the larger the panel of known red cells needed.

Titration of the unknown serum against various standard red cells will often reflect a mixture of antibodies since different cells will give different titration values. However, there are other reasons for titration variation of which dosage is a common one. Nevertheless, if the dosage phenomenon can be ruled out, any gross discrepancy in the titre of a serum against different red cells is most likely to be due to the presence of more than one antibody in the serum. An example of this is given in Table 21.3 where the values obtained suggest a mixture of anti-P_1 and anti-M. Note that the titre of the anti-M is that given by the P_1 negative M red cells and that of the anti-P_1 by the P_1 positive N cells. The titration against P_1 negative MN cells suggests that the anti-M may show slight dosage.

If one component of a mixture is very much weaker than another it can probably be diluted out so that the specificity of the stronger component can be directly demonstrated. Alternatively absorption of portions of the serum with various selected red cells may result in a series of absorbed sera containing each of the components separately.

One of the most satisfactory methods of actually isolating and thereafter identifying the individual antibodies in a mixed serum is the elution technique. As mentioned in Chapter 1 antibodies which have been absorbed by red cells can be recovered again if

Table 21.3

Elucidation of a Mixture of Antibodies by Means of Titration

Red cells	Serial dilution						
	1	2	4	8	16	32	64
Type MP_1-	V	+	(+)	−	−	−	−
Type NP_1+	V	V	++	+	(+)	w	−
Type MNP_1-	+	w	−	−	−	−	−
Type MP_1+	V	V	V	+	(+)	w	−
Type NP_1-	−	−	−	−	−	−	−

Protocol of an experiment in which a serum was titrated against various red cells; the results suggest that the serum contains a mixture of anti-M and anti-P_1 antibodies.

the red cells and absorbed antibody are subjected to an increase in temperature for a short time. The selected temperature at which the cells are allowed to absorb antibody from a serum is naturally the optimum for the combination of the particular antigen and its corresponding antibody. Antibodies are usually recovered from the red cells into saline at 56°C, but the optimum temperature for recovery may vary.* The saline containing the recovered antibody is termed the eluate.

The use of the elution technique often makes possible the separation of one antibody from a serum containing a mixture of several. A serum thought to contain anti-S + anti-Fy^a + anti-Kell for example could be divided into three parts and treated as follows:

Part 1 absorbed with S + K − Fy a− red cells and an eluate made in an attempt to obtain pure anti-S.

* There are several more complicated ways of obtaining a saline eluate, most of them involving the making of red cell stromata. For some purposes these are preferable to the straightforward elution technique.

Part 2 absorbed with S − K + Fy a− red cells and an eluate made which would contain any anti-K component.
Part 3 absorbed with S − K − Fy a+ red cells and an eluate made to recover any anti-Fy^a.

The chief drawback to the elution method is that the antibodies may, particularly if they belong to the same blood group system, be removed and recovered together. This is almost certainly because a single antibody molecule can have combining sites of more than one specificity. For example, an eluate made from Rh negative (cde.cde) red cells after incubation with a serum containing anti-c and anti-E would probably have anti-E as well as anti-c specificity, although there are no E receptors on Rh negative (cde.cde) red cells. (*See also* Chapters 32, 33 and 34.)

Techniques

Technique No. 21.1. The full investigation of a serum for atypical antibodies

A full investigation should include the following techniques:

(*a*) Saline, incubating the serum-cell mixtures at room temperature.
(*b*) Saline, incubating the serum-cell mixtures at 37°C.
(*c*) Albumin at 37°C.
(*d*) Indirect anti-human globulin at 37°C.
(*e*) Trypsin and/or Papain.

Techniques (*b*)–(*e*) are carried out in exactly the same manner as for anti-Rh testing (techniques 10.1–5). Technique (*a*) is identical with (*b*), except that the tests are left at laboratory temperature instead of at 37°C.

All the blocks for the entire investigation should be prepared before any serum is run out. Separate blocks will be required for tests by saline technique at room temperature, indirect anti-human globulin and enzyme, but the 37°C saline and albumin tests can, for convenience, be placed on one block.

The serum is tested by each method against a panel of standard red cells and the patient's own cells. (*See* Table 21.1.) A weak incomplete anti-D set up against D positive and D negative cells must be included as a control for albumin, indirect anti-human globulin and enzyme techniques.

The serum to be investigated is then run, in one manipulation, into every tube in which it is required. Löw's papain is added to the appropriate tubes.

The standard cells are washed and each is used as follows:

(*a*) One volume of packed cells is trypsin treated (Technique No. 10.4), or papain treated (Technique No. 10.5b).
(*b*) A 2 per cent suspension of cells in saline is made for the saline, Löw's papain, anti-human globulin and two-stage albumin techniques.
(*c*) If the one stage albumin technique is to be used a 2 per cent suspension of cells in 30 per cent bovine albumin is made. These suspensions are run into the appropriate tubes as soon as they are prepared.

The saline, albumin and indirect anti-human globulin and papain tests are now at the incubation stage from which point the procedure is that appropriate for each technique separately.

The preparation of the trypsin treated and/or papain treated cells is completed while the blocks containing the serum for this technique are warmed to 37°C. The washed enzyme-treated cells are then added and the tests incubated and read 1 hour later.

The results are recorded as shown in Table 21.1.

Technique No. 21.2. The removal of auto-antibodies from a serum

(*a*) *The Removal of Saline Agglutinins.* The red cells used for the absorption are the patient's own red cells. These should be freed from auto-agglutinins (technique No. 20.1) prior to being mixed with the patient's serum. Preferentially "warm separated" red cells may be used.

The serum is then mixed with an equal volume of packed washed red cells and left for at least 2 hours (or overnight) at 0°–4°C.

The mixture is then centrifuged at this temperature and the supernatant absorbed serum collected. This is re-tested against some or all of the panel of twelve standards and the patient's own cells by saline technique at room temperature. If a reaction is obtained with all or almost all of them including the patient's own cells, then the absorption has not been successful and must be repeated. Negative reactions with all red cell samples indicates that the auto-agglutinin has been removed completely and that there was no additional specific antibody present in the serum. Positive reactions with some of the standard cells and not others suggests that a specific antibody has been unmasked and this must be investigated.

(*b*) *The Removal of "Trypsin" or "Papain" Auto-antibodies.* This technique is essentially similar to (*a*) except that packed enzyme treated cells are used for the absorption which, therefore, takes place for 1 hour at 37°C instead of in the cold.

The absorbed serum is tested against selected trypsin treated red cells including the patient's own. If there is still a reaction with the patient's cells a re-absorption may have to be carried out.

Technique No. 21.3. The elution of antibody from the red cell surface

The selected red cells are carefully washed three times in saline and packed as tightly as possible by centrifugation. They are then mixed with the serum in the proportion of 0·2 ml. of packed cells to 1 ml. of serum. This mixture is left for 1½–2 hours at the optimum temperature of reactivity for the particular antibody that it is desired to recover in the eluate (0°–4°C for ABO and cold agglutinins and 37°C for Rh antibodies, etc.).

The red cells are then carefully washed at least four times in a large volume of saline (6–8 ml.) maintaining as far as possible the temperature at which the absorption has taken place. If this temperature is 0°–4°C the cells must be washed in ice cold saline and centrifuged in buckets packed with ice. Alternatively, it may be possible to wash the cells inside a cold room or in a thermostatically controlled centrifuge. Similarly, if the absorption stage has taken place at 37°C, warm saline must be used for the washing and the centrifuge buckets preheated and lagged (failing a hot room or thermostatically controlled centrifuge).

After the red cells are thoroughly washed, 1 ml. of saline is added to them and they are placed in a water bath at 56°C for 10 minutes. During this time the suspension is continuously agitated. The tube is then centrifuged maintaining the temperature at 56°C and the supernatant saline which contains the eluted antibody is removed as quickly as possible. The activity of some eluates deteriorates rapidly so they should be tested for antibody as soon as possible after being prepared.* The key to success in the preparation of eluates lies in the meticulous washing of the cells after the absorption stage and in the maintenance of the various temperatures necessary to keep the antibody in the attached or free state according to whichever is appropriate at the time.

* If it is desired to store an eluate, the antibody can be recovered into AB serum or human albumin instead of saline.

Technique No. 21.4. Detection of antibody by indirect anti-human globulin on trypsin treated cells

The chosen standard red cells are first trypsin treated as in technique No. 10.4. They are then used to test the serum by the indirect anti-human globulin technique (technique No. 10.3b).

Technique No. 21.5. Detection of antibodies by indirect anti-human globulin plus complement

The source of complement for this technique can be fresh human or guinea-pig serum. If human serum is chosen it must not contain antibodies which would agglutinate the test cells. It should be used undiluted. Guinea-pig complement is diluted 1 in 5 or 1 in 10 at which dilutions it will not usually agglutinate red cells. It is however advisable to check this on each batch before use.

The anti-human globulin should be one of wide specificity reacting with IgG as well as complement IgA and IgM globulin. The test is set up as for indirect test (technique No. 10.3b) but before incubation one unit volume of complement-containing serum is added to each tube. Control tubes are also set up, one for each of the standard cells used, containing equal volumes of complement, saline and standard cells. After this the procedure is as for indirect anti-human globulin.

Chapter 22

THE CHOICE OF BLOOD FOR TRANSFUSION AND DIRECT MATCHING METHODS

Blood transfusion has developed so rapidly in the last twenty years that it comes as something of a shock to realise that its history goes back into the remote past. In ancient thinking the words "blood" and "life" were almost interchangeable and many endeavours were made to transfer the healthy life blood of a young man to the aged and infirm. In most cases this was done by the recipient drinking the blood; the results were, of course, rather disappointing!

As early as the sixteenth century it was realised that the transference should be from blood vessel to blood vessel, but it is not known whether such an exchange was in fact performed. Harvey's discovery of the circulation of the blood in the early seventeenth century gave a new impetus to the interest in transfusion and Lower actually kept alive dogs, which had been exsanguinated, with blood from other dogs, transferred by connecting the carotid artery of the one to the jugular vein of the other by means of quills. The success of this venture led to attempts to transfuse Man. Animals (sheep and lambs) were used as donors, but the experiments were discontinued when the fourth recipient died. It is interesting to note that this patient had three transfusions in all, the first symptomless, the second showing typical symptoms of a hæmolytic transfusion reaction and the third resulting in the patient's death.

During the latter half of the nineteenth century experiments started again, sometimes using animal blood, sometimes human, but the results were so often serious or even fatal that transfusion was abandoned. Then in 1901 Landsteiner discovered the ABO blood group system and realised immediately the importance of his discovery. It was not until some fifteen years later, however, that it was universally accepted that blood grouping and direct compatibility tests were a necessary prelude to transfusion. It was then realised that if the recipient had agglutinins active at 37°C in his serum and the transfused blood had the corresponding agglutinogen, the blood would be destroyed *in vivo* and a hæmolytic transfusion reaction would result.

The possibility of the destruction of the recipient's red cells by transfused antibody was not considered to be a real danger because of the dilution factor. For this reason, up to about 1940, group O blood was considered safe for transfusion to all groups and was called Universal Donor Blood. Nowadays it is realised that transfusion with homologous blood, *i.e.* blood of the same type as the recipient, is to be preferred, not only because the transfusion of antibodies may be dangerous, but also because the number of potential donors is doubled; an important point when the demand for blood is steadily increasing. The titre of anti-A and anti-B antibodies in most donor blood is not dangerous so that in emergency, one pint of group O can be given with little risk, but in massive transfusions of group O blood to patients of other groups the quantity of antibody transfused becomes considerable* and may even result in the destruction of almost all the recipient's own red cells. In particular, it has been shown that exchange transfusion of infants suffering from hæmolytic disease should be performed with blood of the infant's own ABO group.

The discovery of the ABO blood groups was, however, merely the beginning. Today many blood group systems are known, by means of which some hundreds of types of blood can be differentiated. Should they all be taken into consideration in choosing blood for transfusion? It is obvious that they cannot be and except in special cases only two systems are in fact considered, ABO and Rh.

When blood is transfused there are many dangers present, two of which are directly concerned with the antigen content of the transfused blood, the first being that of sensitisation, the second that of incompatibility.

In the first case the recipient does not possess the antigen found in the transfused blood nor the corresponding antibody, but the transfusion acts as a sensitising dose so that antibodies are produced in response to the transfusion or to a subsequent stimulus by the same antigen. Blood for transfusion cannot be chosen to exclude every possibility of sensitisation but fortunately most of the blood group systems are not strongly antigenic in Man and can usually be disregarded. The main exception is the Rh system, and here the problems of sensitisation must be faced. In the ABO system (where antibodies occur naturally) and in other systems whenever atypical antibodies active at 37°C have been formed the problem is not that of sensitisation but of incompatibility.

* This is true even if donors with high titre antibodies, in particular hæmolysins, are excluded.

A consideration of the two systems, ABO and Rh, gives an idea of the factors involved and how best to arrive at the objective, the safe transfusion of blood.

The ABO blood group system is still the most dangerous. This is because the antibodies are naturally occurring and over 95 per cent of all recipients will have anti-A and/or anti-B in their serum. On the other hand ABO blood grouping is a straightforward procedure and the simplest of direct matching techniques will detect any incompatibility. Most of the mistakes which occur are clerical rather than technical. Too much trouble cannot be taken to ensure that samples are correctly labelled and that compatibility labels with the patient's full name, etc., are attached to the bottles to be transfused (*see* below). On the technical side, the grouping of both recipient and donor blood should be performed on red cells and serum independently by either tube technique (No. 3.2) or moist chamber slide technique (No. 3.1). The controls must never be omitted; this simple precaution would have prevented many mistakes which resulted in incompatible blood being transfused.

The final test which is performed after the careful grouping of both donor and recipient is the direct match. This test involves incubating the patient's serum with the red cells of the prospective donors at room temperature and 37°C by techniques appropriate to the detection of antibodies which might be present in the patient's serum and which might cause an incompatible transfusion.

However meticulously the grouping of donor and patient has been carried out prior to transfusion, and however thorough the search has been for atypical antibodies in the patient's serum, *the direct match* (*or cross match*) *should never be omitted.* The red cells that are in actual fact going to be given to the patient are the most important ones to include in any antibody detection test.

The ideal direct matching technique for detecting any ABO incompatibility is the incubation of equal parts of the recipient's serum with a 5 per cent suspension of donor red cells in saline at room temperature, either in a precipitin tube for 2 hours, or on a slide in a moist chamber for 30 minutes. The practice of direct matching merely in bovine albumin is dangerous, for ABO agglutination is depressed in this medium and a false negative reaction may be obtained. When the time available for direct matching is less than that recommended it is worth mixing recipient's serum and donor red cells for even as little as 5 minutes—a negative reading will not mean that the blood is necessarily compatible but if the reaction is positive, a tragedy can be averted.

In considering the Rh blood group system it must be remembered that the most antigenic of the Rh agglutinogens is D and it is almost always anti-D which is meant when people speak of "Rh antibodies". It will be remembered that anti-D antibodies (and similarly all antibodies related to the Rh system) rarely, if ever, occur naturally, they are immune antibodies produced in response to stimulation by the corresponding antigen. This can occur either by transfusion, injection of blood or during pregnancy. The antibodies are active at 37°C and are, therefore, capable of causing severe and even fatal transfusion reactions.

It had long been realised that pregnant and post-partum women were a greater transfusion risk than other types of patient, but until the discovery of the Rh factor it was not known why this was so. Of all Rh negative women (approximately 17 per cent of the total English population) 5 per cent or 1 in 20 will produce Rh antibodies during pregnancy. It usually takes more than one stimulus by an Rh positive fœtus before antibodies develop in maternal serum. The percentage of Rh negative women with antibodies ranges from 0·5 per cent (primipara) to 20 per cent (parities 5 and over). These antibodies increase after delivery reaching a peak titre 10–20 days post-partum and thereafter diminish with varying degrees of rapidity and may even be detectable years later. Ideally Rh negative patients should never be transfused with Rh positive blood. Indeed, this is only done either by accident or when Rh negative blood is in short supply when the claims of: (*a*) persons who already have an Rh antibody; (*b*) Rh negative women who are not past the child-bearing age, and (*c*) infants suffering from hæmolytic disease of the fœtus have to be given priority. It is exceedingly important that girls and young women who are Rh negative should only receive Rh negative blood, as their sensitisation may not only expose them to a possible incompatible transfusion reaction in the future, but also their Rh positive children, even the first, might suffer from hæmolytic disease of the newborn.

If it is necessary to give Rh positive blood to an Rh negative person a search for even a trace of Rh antibody in the recipient's serum should be made. We would suggest that the serum is tested against a panel of Rh positive and Rh negative cells by anti-human globulin and by papain techniques. A papain technique should be included in the direct match, as there may be Rh antibodies present which are not detectable by the anti-human globulin technique.

While the problem of sensitisation and antibody formation is seen most clearly in the immunisation of Rh negative individuals to the D antigen it must be remembered that the other factors are also antigens. The transfusion of Rh positive blood to Rh positive recipients may result in the production of anti-C, anti-E, anti-c, anti-e—the production of anti-c and anti-e can also be stimulated by the transfusion of Rh positive persons with Rh negative blood, a reminder that it is not always safe to use Rh negative blood even in emergency.

Testing of Recipients

It is preferable to test the recipient at least one day before the transfusion is given. In the case of patients known to be for major surgery this preliminary testing can be done on a sample taken at the out-patient clinic.

Taking of Sample and Documentation

The sample should consist of 10 ml. of venous blood taken aseptically into a dry sterile container and allowed to clot. It should be labelled with the patient's full name, date of birth (a much better aid than age to the establishment of identity), serial number, the ward and the date on which the sample was taken. Such a label, completed in every detail, should be attached to the sample at the patient's bedside before there is any chance of confusion with blood from another patient. Hospitals will work out their own error proof system of identifying patients and samples. The identity disc attached to the patient's wrist is almost certainly the best source of accurate information. Patients themselves may be too ill or too nervous to answer even simple questions of identity accurately. When a patient is required to confirm his identity he should not be asked whether he is John Smith but the questioner should ask "What is your name?" "Your date of birth?" etc.

Case notes attached to the patient's bed are not necessarily a reliable source of information without prior checking; patients are sometimes put into a different bed and their case notes left behind to be changed over later. More than one transfusion tragedy has occurred because a sample was incorrectly labelled.

Tests on Patients Requiring a Single Transfusion (no previous transfusions or abnormal obstetric history)

The ABO group and Rh type (using anti-D only) of the patient is determined. If found to be D negative, confirmatory tests with anti-CD and anti-DE sera can be done (techniques 12.2–4) but whatever the results of these a D negative patient should receive

Rh negative (cde.cde) blood. Blood of the same ABO group and Rh(D) type as the patient is selected and direct matched (technique No. 22.4). In the rare event of incompatibility with blood of any of the prospective donors being found, the antibody causing this should be identified before a further direct match is attempted. If there is little time available it may be necessary to find compatible blood without identifying the causative antibody—a large pretransfusion sample should be taken so that the antibody may be identified later.

Tests on Patients Requiring a Further Transfusion

The ABO group and Rh(D) type will almost certainly be known at this stage. Since a previous transfusion has been given which may have sensitised the patient, a test for antibodies is often helpful. It is suggested that this should consist of an indirect antihuman globulin and papain test either against red cell samples from the previous bottles of blood given (if available) or against a small panel of selected red cells. The chosen cells should be group O of Rh sub-types R_1R_1 (CDe.CDe), R_2R_2 (cDE.cDE) (or R_2r) and rr (cde.cde) and should also be capable of detecting the "warm" antibodies of other blood group systems, *viz.* anti-K, anti-Fy^a, anti-S, etc. If no atypical antibodies are found blood (of the same ABO group and Rh type as the patient) is direct-matched. In the event of atypical antibodies being found, these should if possible be identified before the blood is selected.

Tests on Patients for Multiple Transfusions*

In addition to the tests already cited above, it is often rewarding to perform a full Rh sub-typing on patients likely to need many transfusions. Even if it is not possible to give them blood of their own Rh sub-type a knowledge of the Rh antigens possessed by the patient will form a guide to the Rh antibodies that might be formed as a result of repeated transfusion.

Ideally this sub-typing is carried out on blood taken from the patient before any transfusions are given but sometimes this is not possible and the patient will already have donor red cells mixed with his own. In order that these donor red cells may interfere as little as possible with the sub-typing results the sample for this determination is taken as long after the previous transfusion as is practicable. Even with this precaution the typing may prove difficult (but *see* technique No. 22.1).

Here again any atypical antibodies found either as a result of

* Hæmolytic anæmias form a special case and are dealt with in Chapter 26.

the antibody tests or during direct matching, should be identified before blood is transfused.

Tests on Patients with Transfusion or Obstetric History Suggestive of Antibody Formation

The ABO grouping, full Rh sub-typing and antibody tests recommended above are the first step in the investigation of these cases. Any atypical antibody which may be present will in most instances be revealed at this stage and can then be identified. If no atypical antibody is found, an additional search against a larger panel of standard cells according to technique No. 21.1 will be necessary.

Tests on Patients whose Serum Protein Balance is Disturbed, *e.g.* those with Multiple Myelomatosis

In these cases an abnormality in plasma protein balance develops which results in a strong tendency for the patient's serum to cause pseudo-agglutination of all red cells including his own.

ABO grouping and Rh typing of such patients can only be carried out on well washed red cells. Serum ABO grouping is usually not possible by normal agglutination techniques, it can however be done by the anti-human globulin technique using patient's serum and standard A_1, A_2, B and O red cells.

The pseudo-agglutination has a characteristic appearance (*see* Plate 5*a*) and with experience becomes readily recognisable. The clumps of red cells seem to glow, there being less refraction of the light than with true agglutination where the clumps are almost opaque. However, pseudo-agglutination may mask true agglutination and, therefore, no opinion should be pronounced on the result of any test in which it appears. The indirect anti-human globulin test for antibodies can be used, as interference from pseudo-agglutination will not be encountered.

Tests on Patients who Have Received Dextran

These patients are in a similar category to those described above. The presence of dextran in the plasma results in heavy pseudo-agglutination which may mask the presence of true agglutination. The testing can usually be done on a pre-dextran sample but where this has not been taken the procedure is the same as for patients with an altered protein balance.

Tests on Patients with Atypical Antibodies

The methods employed for the identification of atypical antibodies have already been described in some detail (*see* Chapters

13 and 21). The identification should be completed before blood is chosen for the transfusion. It is because this may take some time that it is recommended that wherever possible testing should take place at least 24 hours pre-transfusion. It is often the practice to transfuse a patient whose serum contains an atypical antibody, before that antibody has been identified. It is argued that from the practical point of view the identity does not matter if a careful direct match is carried out. This is in fact only true if the atypical antibody is a fairly strong one. To rely entirely upon a direct match to detect a weak atypical antibody is to court danger, however carefully the tests are done. This is particularly true if the atypical antibody in the patient's serum is one that shows dosage. Anti-c, for instance, is characterised by showing marked dosage, therefore a weak anti-c might react with all cde.cde cells with two doses of "c", whereas some CDe.cde red cells with one dose of "c" might be negative. A weak unidentified anti-c, therefore, might appear compatible with blood of genotype CDe.cde but would in fact be incompatible *in vivo*. If an atypical antibody is properly identified the blood selected for transfusion can be typed with a stronger example of the same antibody from the laboratory's collection of typing sera and this danger eliminated. When the antibody is too weak to identify no such check is possible; in which case it must be realised that if the antibody shows any activity at 37°C, although the blood appears to be compatible *in vitro* on the results of the direct match, it may in fact be incompatible *in vivo*. The clinician must be warned of this possibility so that he can take the necessary steps, *i.e.* giving the transfusion slowly, watching for clinical symptoms and also, if desired, withdrawing a sample after about 50 ml. of blood has been given to be examined for hæmoglobin pigments (*see* Chapter 24).

Tests on Patients Undergoing Hypothermia

When patients are operated upon for heart defects under profound hypothermia, they also receive massive transfusions of blood, using a heart-lung machine.

This means that for a period of time of about 1 hour, recipient and donor bloods are in contact at about 10°C. At this temperature the vast majority of patients have cold antibodies, auto-antibodies, anti-H, anti-I, anti-P_1, and anti-A_1, etc. If the normal saline direct matching technique is performed at 10°C strong positive reactions are encountered in many cases, often with all bloods tested including the recipient's own blood. This suggests that the normal technique is not paralleling the position *in vivo* as cooling the patient to 10°C does not produce an auto-hæmolytic reaction in cases where an auto-antibody is present. Moreover transfusion in spite of a positive cross-match at 10°C is followed by no adverse sequelæ. A new cross-matching technique (No. 22.5) has been devised for these cases using mixtures of whole blood. This gives results which are closely correlated with the degree of agglutination that is found on the pump and shows that in almost all cases these cold antibodies are not causing agglutination in the conditions found in the actual transfusion. If this cross-matching technique gives strong positive results attempts must be made to find more compatible blood or the patient must not be cooled to 10°C but to a temperature at which the cross-match is compatible. Batchelor *et al.*, 1966.

Changes in Blood Group Systems in Malignancy

Changes in blood group antigens or antibody content may occur in cases of malignancy so that grouping of such patients occasionally presents particular problems. Sometimes there is a lack of the iso-antibodies (anti-A and/or anti-B); this is usually because the patient has little or no gammaglobulin in his serum. Electrophoresis of his serum will confirm that the gammaglobulin is absent. On the other hand occasionally more antibody is formed, *e.g.* anti-B has been found in A_1B, etc. Sometimes an excess of blood group substances occurs in the serum. This leads to neutralisation of the anti-A and anti-B grouping sera unless the patient's cells are carefully washed several times. Anti-I antibodies are common especially in cases of leukæmia.

The commonest change in red cells is that they become poly-agglutinable due to the exposure of the T antigen on the cells, anti-T occurring in all adult human sera. Other changes which may occur are reduction in strength of the A agglutinogen, the acquiring of a pseudo-B antigen by A cells and alteration in strengths of the Rh antigens.

If anomalies occur during the testing of the cells or serum of patients with malignancy, if at all possible, the blood groups should be fully investigated by a specialist laboratory before transfusion is undertaken.

Choice of Blood

The blood of choice is that of the patient's own ABO blood group and Rh(D) type and only when this cannot be obtained in time for the transfusion should an alternative be considered (*see* Chapter 23 for emergency procedure). This simple rule suffices for all patients whose sera do not contain any atypical antibodies. In the occasional case where atypical antibodies occur, the additional essential is that the blood does not react with the particular antibody or antibodies possessed by the patient. Table 22.1 gives the

Table 22.1

The Type of Blood to Choose for Transfusion to Patients whose Sera Contain Rh Antibodies

Atypical antibody present	Type of blood to give
Anti-D Anti-CD Anti-DE	rr (cde.cde)
Anti-C in D-positive patient	R_2r (cDE.cde) *or* R_2R_2 (cDE.cDE)
Anti-C in D-negative patient	rr (cde.cde)
Anti-E in R_1R_1 (CDe.CDe) patient (also anti-Ec)	R_1R_1 (CDe.CDe)
Anti-E in R_1r (CDe.cde) patient	R_1R_1 (CDe.CDe) *or* R_1r (CDe.cde)
Anti-E in D-negative patient	rr (cde.cde)
Anti-c	R_1R_1 (CDe.CDe)
Anti-e (also anti-Ce)	R_2R_2 (cDE.cDE)

most readily available type of blood for patients whose sera contain any of the various Rh antibodies. Note that in the case of anti-E occurring in a patient of R_1R_1 (CDe.CDe) it is safer to assume the presence of a mixture of anti-E and anti-c, although anti-c may not be apparent. If atypical antibodies active at 37°C belonging to other blood group systems are involved the selection of blood is straightforward, *e.g.* K negative blood for patients with anti-K, Fy^a negative blood for those with anti-Fy^a, S negative for those with anti-S. To obtain such blood of the patient's own ABO group it will almost certainly be necessary to consult the Transfusion Service.

Atypical antibodies which are completely inactive at 37°C can be ignored when selecting blood for transfusion. Before it is concluded that a cold antibody detectable by saline technique at room temperature is inactive at 37°C, the indirect anti-human globulin test with the addition of complement (technique No. 22.2) should be performed as 37°C activity demonstrable by this technique is accompanied by a diminished survival *in vivo* of red cells containing the corresponding antigen. The transfusion reactions due to such antibodies are usually mild, the main effect of the incompatibility being a failure to achieve full benefit from the transfused blood.

Direct-matching (or Cross-matching) of Blood for Transfusion

Non-emergency Transfusions

Serum from the recipient should be tested against the cells of the donor by technique No. 22.4 which includes:

(1) Saline tube technique at R.T.
(2) Saline tube technique at 37°C.
(3) Albumin Addition technique at 37°C.
(4) Indirect anti-human globulin technique at 37°C.
(5) Papain technique at 37°C (in special cases and especially where Rh positive blood is being given to an Rh negative recipient).

In cases where an atypical antibody has been detected by another technique this must also be included as part of the direct match.

Moreover, the indirect anti-human globulin plus complement method (technique No. 22.2) should be included wherever cold agglutinins are present in the recipient's serum. The testing of the recipient's serum with his own red cells by each of the techniques employed should be included as a negative control. The reasons for selecting each particular method are given below so that the dangers that may arise from omitting any of the tests may be appreciated.

(1) *Saline Tube Technique at Room Temperature.* This is the optimum temperature and medium for the detection of ABO incompatibility and potent cold agglutinins.

(2) *Saline Tube Technique at 37°C.* This is the optimum temperature and medium for the detection of "warm" agglutinins (complete antibodies).

(3) *Albumin Addition Technique at 37°C.* This is a good technique for the detection of most Rh incomplete antibodies although a few of them may show a prozone. Incomplete antibodies of other blood group systems may not show up well by this method. It is an easier technique at which to become proficient than the indirect

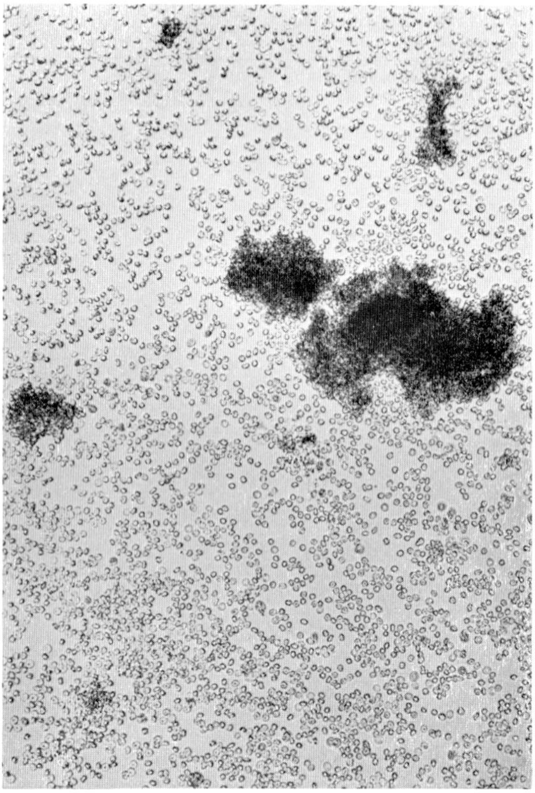

PLATE 9. "Mixed blood" appearance.

p. 225

anti-human globulin but may be omitted in a laboratory experienced in the latter technique.

(4) *Indirect anti-human globulin at* 37°*C*. This technique should never be omitted. It is highly efficient in the detection of all kinds of incomplete antibodies.

(5) *Papain Technique at* 37°*C*. This is the most sensitive antibody detection technique. It is not included in all direct matching because there is a tendency to give positives due to auto-antibodies and it is extremely sensitive so that weak cold antibodies are detected, for example anti-P_1 or anti-Lewis, whose presence does not constitute a transfusion hazard.

Techniques

Technique No. 22.1. Typing of patients with transfused blood in their circulation

For these cases the typing sera used should be the most potent available. The setting up of the tests with the appropriate anti-sera in no way differs from the methods already described. A negative reaction can be interpreted as applying to both recipient and donor, as can a strong positive reaction with practically no free cells. When, however, the red cells of one react with a particular anti-serum, while those of the other do not, a "mixed blood" picture is obtained (*see* Plate 9). The full interpretation of a "mixed blood" picture can only be made with a knowledge of the history of the case. For instance where Rh negative blood has been given in an emergency to a patient of Rh type unknown a "mixed blood" picture with anti-D serum on a post-transfusion sample clearly indicates that the recipient is Rh positive as the unagglutinated cells must be those of the Rh negative donor. In a more involved case, where it is desired to ascertain the full Rh sub-type of a patient for multiple transfusion who has already received Rh positive blood—the position is complicated in that the Rh sub-type of the donor also is unknown. The proportion of agglutinated to free cells is the only guide as to which cells belong to the recipient and which to the donor and where large amounts of blood have been transfused even this fails. If difficulty is experienced in judging the proportion of agglutinated to free cells, mixtures of known constitution should be made and used as a standard for comparison.

In cases where the proportions are almost equal, the problem can only be resolved by waiting until the circulation is relatively free from donor cells. If in the interim period it is essential to give further transfusions, the blood used must all be of the same sub-type. How this clarifies the position can be seen from the following protocol:

Sample	Date	Anti-A	Anti-B	Anti-C	Anti-D	Anti-E	Anti-c	Conclusion
Recipient	12/2/68	—	—	C	C	MB*	C	Mixture of O. R_1r and OR_1R_2
1st donor	14/2/68	—	—	C	C	—	C	OR_1r
2nd donor	15/3/68	—	—	C	C	—	C	OR_1r
3rd donor	20/4/68	—	—	C	C	—	C	OR r
Recipient	8/5/68	—	—	C	C	MB*	C	Mixture of O, R_1r, and OR_1R_2

* Mixed blood.

The O R_1r blood in sample (2) has come from the February, March, and April transfusions—blood transfused before 12th February, 1968, would no longer be in the recipient's circulation on 8th May, 1968. The reaction with anti-E is, therefore, due to the recipient's own red cells being E positive and the recipient has been typed as O R_1R_2.

Technique No. 22.2. The investigation of a cold agglutinin for 37°C activity by the indirect anti-human globulin plus complement technique

Apart from the following modifications this technique is identical with technique No. 21.5, to which reference should be made for all practical details.

The serum containing the cold agglutinin is tested against cells which: (*a*) give a positive, and (*b*) give a negative reaction by saline technique at room temperature. The separate reagents including the complement are warmed to 37°C before being mixed. The tests are maintained at 37°C during the washing stage but the actual reading can be done at room temperature.

Technique No. 22.3. Obtaining sample of donor from bottle

If blood is obtained from a Transfusion Centre which issues pilot bottles,* which are expressly designed for cross-matching purposes, the red cells of the donor are obtained from this. If, however, no pilot bottle is issued with the blood, a sample must be obtained directly from the bottle itself. The technique of removing a sample whether from the main or pilot bottle is the same. The perforation in the cap is exposed and swabbed with a suitable antiseptic. The surface is then flamed and a specimen of blood removed by means of a sterile syringe with fine gauge needle after treatment with glycerine-phenol (*see* Appendix I). The citrated blood is then washed and used for the direct-match.

* Where pilot bottles are issued these should remain attached to the main bottle.

Technique No. 22.4. Direct-matching

First the necessary arrangement of tubes in blocks is made to cover the whole direct-matching procedure, allowing for the testing of the patient's serum against red cells from each proposed donor and his own cells by the following techniques:

(*a*) Saline tube technique incubating at room temperature.
(*b*) Saline tube technique incubating at 37°C.
(*c*) Albumin addition technique incubating at 37°C.
(*d*) Indirect anti-human globulin technique incubating at 37°C.
(*e*) Papain technique incubating at 37°C for selected cases only.

Occasionally an additional technique, *e.g.* trypsin or papain will be required. The patient's serum is then run into all appropriate tubes and its presence in them checked.

The patient's red cells and those from each bottle (withdrawn by technique No. 22.3) are washed three times in saline, and are then diluted to make 2 per cent suspensions. An aliquot of cells from the patient and from each bottle is papain treated for use in the papain technique. The usual control for albumin and anti-human globulin tests of a weak incomplete anti-D with known D positive and D negative red cells is included. After the red cells have been added to the tubes, the saline tests are incubated for 2 hours, the albumin tests for 1 to 1½ hours after which one drop of albumin is added to each tube and they are allowed to stand for a further 30 minutes, and the indirect anti-human globulin tests for 1 hour. At the end of 1 hour the latter can be completed and read while the remainder of the tests are undergoing the further incubation. The tubes containing papain treated cells are centrifuged and read after 1 hour's incubation. Alternatively the Löw's papain technique (10.5a) can be used.

Results should be recorded in detail giving strengths of agglutination by means of the usual symbols. Incompatibility detected between the patient's serum and the red cells of any of the donors necessitates the identification of the causative antibody. For this investigation technique No. 21.1 may be required. A positive reaction between the patient's serum and his own cells due to auto-agglutination is likely to be reflected in the results obtained against donor red cells also, since auto-agglutinins are almost invariably pan-agglutinins. A positive reaction between the patient's serum and his own red cells must be followed up by a direct anti-human globulin test (technique 10.3b) since this is likely to be positive indicating that the patient's red cells are sensitised by antibody *in vivo*. In such cases a further investigation must be undertaken (*see* Chapter 26).

Technique No. 22.5. Direct-matching of blood for hypothermia patients

The Whole Blood Test. Whole blood for the patient is made up using equal volumes of the patient's serum and packed washed cells. Citrated blood in the proportions of 4 parts of blood to one of A.C.D. as in a bottle of stored blood of the appropriate group is used as the donor whole blood.

The patient's whole blood and the donor whole blood are then run into 9 × 50 mm. tubes in the following proportions:

Patient's whole blood	9	8	7	6	5
Donor whole blood	1	2	3	4	5

A tube containing patient's whole blood and a tube containing donor whole blood are included in the test as controls.

The blood is left at the appropriate temperature (usually 10°C) for 2 hours. Saline is cooled to the temperature of the test and is used to dilute the whole bloods on a microscope slide before reading microscopically.

This test is used in addition to the normal direct matching technique (No. 22.4).

Blood By-products and Substitutes

Packed Cells

These are used in cases where it is desired to give red cells without unduly increasing the blood volume. They are prepared from well sedimented whole blood, not more than seven days old, by removal of the supernatant plasma. The packed cells should be used as soon as possible after being prepared, never being stored for more than a few hours. This means that if more than two pints of packed cells are required for one patient they should be prepared in two batches.

Plasma

The supernatant plasma from bottles of blood not used for transfusion, either time-expired or bled specially for plasma preparation, can be removed and freeze dried. It can then be stored for up to eight years. (This is the official expiry limit although it is probable that freeze dried plasma is stable for much longer periods.) When it is needed it is reconstituted by the addition of sterile pyrogen-free distilled water. Plasma is used for transfusion in cases where a blood expander is needed but not red cells. For preparation of dried plasma the M.R.C. booklet by R. I. N. Greaves (No. 258, 1946) should be consulted.

Fresh Frozen Plasma—plasma separated within 24 hours of the blood having been taken is frozen at −20°C. This is used for transfusion of patients whose own plasma lacks clotting factors, in the main, hæmophiliacs.

Anti-Haemophilic Globulin-Rich Cryoprecipitates

It is possible by freezing in ethanol and dry ice and subsequent thawing at 4°C to prepare a cryoprecipitate from plasma which is very rich in A-H-G. (Pool and Hershgold, 1964.) This precipitate redissolved in 10–15 ml. of saline is much more satisfactory than fresh frozen plasma in the control of bleeding in hæmophiliacs.

The preparation can be done conveniently by means of double bag plastic packs. The blood is centrifuged in a precooled refrigerated centrifuge at top speed as soon as possible after taking. The plasma is expressed into the attached transfer pack and frozen by immersing in an insulated container containing dry ice in ethanol to which more dry ice is added during the 15 minutes which is adequate to freeze the contents.

The packs are then hung up in a 4°C refrigerator for 24 hours to thaw. They are then re-centrifuged to concentrate the precipitate and the plasma carefully returned to the primary bag. The cryoprecipitate adheres to the walls of the transfer pack. This is separated from the primary bag and stored frozen at −30°C. When needed it is reconstituted by the addition of 10–15 ml. of saline, a syringe can be used to inject the saline, and then to transfer the solution direct from the bag to the patient.

Technique 22.6. Assay of factor VIII in cryoprecipitate

Cryoprecipitate contains many of the clotting factors in small amounts but it is rich in factor VIII, possessing up to 80 per cent of the anti-hæmolytic activity of the original plasma (in 5 ml. instead of in 250 ml.). Some batches may contain less (sometimes as low as 26 per cent) so that periodic assays of the cryoprecipitate are useful, although it is, of course, not practicable to test every bag.

The cryoprecipitate is redissolved either in 5 ml. of residual plasma or in saline; 0·1 ml. of this fluid is diluted 50-fold—this gives an approximation to the original volume and is suitable for estimation against normal plasma.

Reagents

(1) *Buffered isotonic saline*: (Prepared by adding 2·20 g. NaCl per litre to tris buffer. Tris buffer is prepared by dissolving 24·30 g. $NH_2C(CH_2OH)_3$ in a litre of distilled water, taking 250 ml. of this solution, adding 42 ml. of N.HCl, and making up almost to a litre, and then adjusting the ph to 7·4 at room temperature.)

(2) *Light Kaolin*: 0·5 g. of Light Kaolin (B.D.H.) is suspended in 100 ml. of tris buffer.

(3) *Inosithin*: 1 gm. is dissolved in 100 ml. of tris buffer, shaking until completely dissolved (this takes some time). This preparation is stored deep frozen in 1 ml. aliquots. When needed it is further diluted 1 in 50 in the tris buffer.

(4) Citrated plasma from a severely affected hæmophiliac.

(5) Control normal plasma (pool of at least 3 normal plasmas).

(6) Calcium Chloride, 0·035 Molar.

(7) Solution of cryoprecipitate.

The control plasma and the cryoprecipitate plasma are diluted 1 in 10 and then serial dilutions up to 1 in 320 prepared and kept in an ice-bath. Into each of a series of clotting tubes is pipetted 0·1 ml. of undiluted hæmophilic plasma. The dilutions of control plasma, cryoprecipitate and a blank of buffered saline are added to the appropriate tubes. It is often sufficient to test the first four dilutions of the control, five of the cryoprecipitate solution, and one blank, making a convenient number of tubes, namely ten.

The tubes are placed in the 37°C water bath at one minute intervals (timed by stop-watch). 0·1 ml. of well-mixed kaolin suspension being added to each tube after it has been at 37°C for exactly one minute; all the tubes being shaken from time to time. After 10 minutes exactly, 0·1 ml. of inosithin and 0·1 ml. of $CaCl_2$ are added at one minute intervals as before, a stop-watch being started for each tube as the $CaCl_2$ is added. As the clotting times will be between 1 to 4 minutes a number of stop-watches will be needed. The whole procedure is then repeated and the mean of the clotting times for each duplicate pair plotted on a linear scale against the corresponding concentrations on a logarithmic scale taking 1 in 10 plasma as 100 per cent and 1 in 20 as 50 per cent and so on. The two sets of reading should fall on roughly parallel straight lines, and the factor VIII concentration of the cryoprecipitate determined as a percentage of that of the control plasma from the horizontal distance between the lines.

Protein fractions from Plasma

Plasma can also be used to prepare various protein fractions which are of great use for therapeutic purposes. Crude fibrinogen (50 per cent) is used for the making of fibrin foam or a purified fibrinogen (80 per cent), this purified product is rich in anti-hæmophilic globulin. Prothrombin and thrombin are prepared from the supernatant after the precipitation of fibrinogen. They are particularly useful in skin and nerve grafting. Gamma globulin is prepared and used as an effective prophylactic for measles. A final product which is 94 per cent human albumin is used as an intra-venous fluid taking the place of plasma particularly in the treatment of diseases associated with a low circulating albumin.

Dextran

This is not a blood by-product but a substitute for plasma. It is a non-toxic fluid containing a number of closely related polysaccharides composed of long chains of glucose units. It has a colloid osmotic pressure slightly greater than that of plasma. It has been used with success for patients suffering from burns and in other circumstances in which plasma would otherwise be given.

Care of a Hospital Blood Bank

It is not inappropriate as an addendum to this chapter to consider the workings of a hospital blood bank since this is the source of the donor blood that is used for direct-matching.

Keeping of Records

The documentation for such a bank is relatively straightforward. Blood is received weekly or fortnightly from the Transfusion Service and should be booked into a ledger keeping the various groups separate and also the Rh positive and Rh negative supplies within these groups. The fate of the blood should also be recorded here, *i.e.* to whom transfused and the outcome of the transfusion or, if unused, the date of return to the Transfusion Centre.

Refrigeration

The blood must be stored at a temperature of 4°–6°C. It is important that this temperature should not vary by more than plus or minus 2°C so that some kind of temperature recorder, such as the Cambridge recorder, must be employed to keep a running check on the temperature inside the refrigerator. If blood should happen to be over-cooled and thereby partially frozen, it must be discarded as dangerous for transfusion. Care should be taken to ensure that the temperature within the refrigerator is even and that there are no areas in which the blood might become frozen; in particular it must always be protected from coming in contact with the freezing compartment. It is convenient, where possible, particularly in hospitals running a large bank, to have alternative refrigerator accommodation in case one refrigerator breaks down or becomes inefficient.

Ageing of Blood

It is generally agreed that the effective life of a bottle of blood is three weeks from the day of bleeding the donor, although blood stored for longer periods can be used with safety but with slightly less good results. Blood should be used in strict date order, the oldest being issued first unless there are special indications for the use of fresh blood.

Fitness for Use

A bottle of blood is totally unfit for use if hæmolysed and/or infected. This so rarely occurs that the routine which would prevent a transfusion death from these causes is often omitted. Examination of both a smear for gross bacterial contamination and a spun sample for hæmolysis just prior to use eliminates this transfusion hazard.

Transfusion Apparatus

The old type glass-rubber transfusion apparatus is fast becoming obsolete as the supply of satisfactory plastic disposable sets increases. These sets have many advantages one of the most important of which is the reduction in the number of pyrogenic reactions. We have however included a note on the preparation and care of glass-rubber apparatus as this is still in use in some countries (*see* Appendix V).

Direct-matched Blood

A label must be attached to any bottle which has been direct, matched giving full details of the patient—name, date of birth, ward, and most important of all, the serial number from the patient's identity disc.* This will have been obtained from the label of the blood sample from the patient, used for direct match (*see* page 218). This number, on the label of the direct matched

* If as we suggest above the method of having a wrist identity disc is used.

blood, must be *checked again with the patient's wrist identity disc* before the transfusion is begun.

It cannot be emphasised too often that careful and meticulous direct matching procedure in the laboratory has sometimes been of no avail on account of mistaken identity in the wards.

BIBLIOGRAPHY

POOL, J., and HERSHGOLD, E. (1964), "High Potency Antihaemophilic Factor Concentrate prepared from Cryolglobulin Precipitate." *Nature, Lond.*, **203,** 312.

BATCHELOR, EUNICE M, BOORMAN, KATHLEEN E., LINCOLN, P. J., ZEITLIN, R. A. (1966). "Technique for the evaluation of cold antibodies in cases for operation under hypothermia." *J. Clin. Path.*, **19**, 348.

CHAPTER 23

EMERGENCY TRANSFUSIONS

AN emergency transfusion is a matter for close co-operation between the pathologist and the clinician who has requested and will give the blood. The degree of the emergency has to be weighed against the risks involved if there is insufficient time for the normal direct-match (technique No. 22.4) to be performed. There is no emergency so great that some sort of direct matching cannot be carried out even if it is done in the theatre while the transfusion apparatus is being set up or while plasma or blood substitutes are being given.

Sometimes a state of emergency is created unnecessarily as when the laboratory is requested at the last minute to provide blood for a patient whose time of operation was booked days beforehand. Once a laboratory allows itself to be persuaded to enact such requirements these will become a habit which may dangerously reduce the efficiency of the direct-matching service.

The wisdom of appointing experienced workers for emergency serological procedures cannot be over-emphasised; particularly is this essential for night emergencies when even a specialist may find the conditions a strain and the inexperienced find themselves without an authority to whom to refer in difficulty.

Equipment for Emergency Work

A laboratory which normally undertakes a fair amount of routine serological testing will probably find it unnecessary to make special preparations for emergencies which may occur during the day. They can be dealt with using the materials which are readily available but for night work a special rack of reagents should be set aside. This rack should contain the following:

(1) Anti-A, anti-B, anti-D, anti-sera all well tried for the emergency technique selected.
(2) Positive and negative control cells on these anti-sera.
(3) Anti-human globulin reagent diluted ready for use.
(4) Controls for the anti-human globulin test ready washed.

Choice of Rapid Typing Techniques for Emergency Work

Choice of method for emergency tests will be influenced by the availability of potent anti-sera. Rapid ABO grouping presents little difficulty providing both cells and serum are tested and a control of the patient's cells suspended in saline is examined under the conditions of the method chosen. Anti-D sera sufficiently potent for Rh typing on a slide may not always be available and therefore a reliable rapid method by which anti-sera of average potency can be used, will have to be selected.

There is considerable variation in preferred methods between different laboratories. The following points should be noted when selecting a method for emergency work. Several hundred tests by the chosen technique should be compared with tests done by standard tube method before it is put into general use. Choice should be made in favour of a method which will give false negative rather than false positive results. Rh negative blood can almost always be safely given to an apparently Rh negative recipient who is in fact Rh positive but the reverse procedure may be disastrous. It is an advantage to select a method by which the result may be confirmed microscopically if necessary.

The authors cannot claim detailed knowledge of every rapid Rh typing technique. Table 23.1 gives a representative selection; methods considered most reliable are described at the end of the chapter.

The methods are broadly divided into 3 classes:

(*a*) capillary,
(*b*) slide,
(*c*) tube with use of centrifuge.

Each class has both its advantages and drawbacks. Capillary methods are extremely sensitive and a wide range of anti-sera are suitable. The chosen technique either with or without the addition of papain can become very reliable in experienced hands particularly if a control of patient's red cells put up with AB serum in place of the typing serum, is included. The chief disadvantage is that the results cannot be easily confirmed under a microscope. It is possible to blow gently the contents of a capillary on to a slide but it is not easy to do without breaking up the fragile clumps of cells.

It is easier to acquire proficiency at slide tests and they are very reliable provided controls are never omitted. We have a personal preference for the moist chamber slide technique using the convenient perspex box holding strips of perspex, already described. In practice it will be found that most saline and many albumin

Table 23.1
Rapid Methods for Rh Typing

Type of method	Designation	Principle	Advantages	Disadvantages	Time taken: (*a*) For incubation	Time taken: (*b*) Complete test*	Reference
A. Capillary	1. Chown	Angled capillary. Positives show beaded appearance	Sensitive. Economical	Macroscopic only. Occasional false positive which should show up in control	20″	35″	Technique No. 23.1
	2. Chown with papain	As above	As above. Range of suitable sera increased because of papain	As above	15″	30″	Technique No. 23.2
B. Slide	3. Moist chamber	Saline or albumin type anti-D incubated in moist atmosphere	Wide range of anti-sera suitable. Rapid. Microscopic	Fewer false negatives than 3. Easy to prepare	15″	20″	Technique No. 9.1
	4. Papain slide	Incomplete anti-D + papain + cells on slide	Rapid. Microscopic	Only certain anti-sera suitable. Some false negatives. Papain control essential	15″	20″	Hekkir *et al.*, *Vox Sanguinis*, **2** (No. 2), 128, 1957
C. Tube	5. Papain tube	Incomplete anti-D + papain + cells in tube centrifuged	Rapid. Wide range of anti-sera. Microscopic	Papain control essential	10″	20″	Technique No. 23.3
	6. Centrifuge tube	Saline or albumin type anti-D incubated in tube and centrifuged	Rapid. Microscopic	Only certain anti-sera suitable. May give false positives with albumin anti-sera	15″	20″	Technique No. 23.4
	7. Polyvidone	Incomplete anti-D + polyvidone	Rapid	Macroscopic only. Tendency to false positives if read microscopically	15″	20″	McNeil *et al.*, *Amer. J. clin. Path.*, **22**, 1216

* Includes time for washing cells.

routine Rh typing sera are suitable so that supplies of anti-sera for this method is not a problem.

The papain slide test has been used by the originators for an impressively large number of tests. Our impression however was that only certain anti-D sera were suitable; we prefer the papain centrifuge tube test which is very good indeed and does not require the selection of particularly potent anti-sera as does the centrifuge technique No. 23.4.

The tube tests using a centrifuge are very easy to set up and centrifugation after approximately ten minutes' incubation hastens the development of the agglutination. Nevertheless, there is always the possibility with centrifuge methods of obtaining both false positives and false negatives when re-suspending the cell sediment after centrifugation. This tendency is reduced to a minimum when the anti-serum selected gives good macroscopic agglutination after the tube is tapped gently with the finger.

The polyvidone method is mentioned as being representative of a class of technique employing substances to develop rapidly the agglutination of the incomplete anti-D. There is a high tendency to rouleaux formation which makes the test unreliable unless read only macroscopically. It is not recommended.

In Table 23.2 can be seen the procedures that are recommended for varying lengths of time available for direct matching. The times quoted do not allow for the collection of the patient's blood or the assembly of the necessary apparatus and reagents. The ABO group and Rh type will often be known (arising from the practice of testing at the ante-natal or outpatients clinics); the procedure when this is so is given in section (*a*) while section (*b*) deals with completely untested cases (Table 23.2).

Procedure No. 1 in this table is the full-scale non-emergency technique which is recommended as being the safest procedure and is included for comparison. A reduction in the time allowed, to 2 hours (2) means a reduction in the incubation period with the attendant hazard of missing agglutination that may not be very strong by saline and albumin techniques. The indirect anti-human globulin technique with its normal incubation period of 1 hour will be unaffected. Procedure No. 3 relies upon the moist chamber slide technique (a slight modification of technique No. 3.1) to detect an ABO incompatibility and the rapid indirect anti-human globulin for warm atypical antibodies. In procedure No. 4 the emergency slide test (technique No. 23.6) is by no means infallible but is preferable to no direct-match at all. Procedures No. 5 and 6 recommend moist chamber slide grouping of patient (technique

No. 3.1) with a rapid method of determining whether the patient is D positive or D negative (*see* Table 23.1).

Table 23.2

Direct-matching Procedure

(*a*) ABO Group and Rh type of Patient Known

Time	Direct-match techniques	Remarks
(1) 2½–3 hr.	Saline R.T. Saline, albumin, and indirect anti-human globulin at 37°C. Papain, trypsin, trypsin anti-human globulin or indirect anti-human globulin + complement where indicated. Incubation of tests 2 hr.	The procedure for all but emergencies.
(2) 2 hr.	As (1), but incubation period reduced to 1 hr.	Cell sediments should be handled with extreme care as agglutination may not be complete.
(3) ¾hr.	Moist chamber slide technique at R.T. Indirect anti-human globulin at 37°C incubating for 20 min. in water bath.	Will detect ABO incompatibilities and strong atypical antibodies. May miss antibodies of low titre.
(4) Less than ½ hr.	Emergency slide test 23.6 followed by procedure (3).	Allow blood to go to ward on result of slide test.

(*b*) ABO Group and Rh type of Patient Unknown

Time	Testing of recipient	Direct-match techniques	Remarks
(5) 3 hr.	ABO moist chamber. Rh sandwich or moist chamber.	As for (1).	The typing of the recipient is checked by standard tube techniques at the same time as the direct-match.
(6) 1½ hr.	ABO moist chamber. Rh sandwich or moist chamber.	As for (3).	(as above)
(7) ¾ hr. or less	ABO slide.	As for (3) or (4).	Direct-match one bottle of Rh negative blood of appropriate ABO group. For any further blood required proceed as (6).

Procedure No. 7 allows no time for Rh typing. ABO grouping by slide method is done and Rh negative blood of the appropriate ABO group used pending Rh typing.

Many people use Eldon cards for emergency typing. We prefer using liquid serum and including controls with each test. On the other hand an Eldon card will give a rapid ABO group and could be used in emergency. We would prefer to give Rh negative blood rather than rely on an Eldon card Rh typing, nor could we recommend an Eldon card direct matching technique.

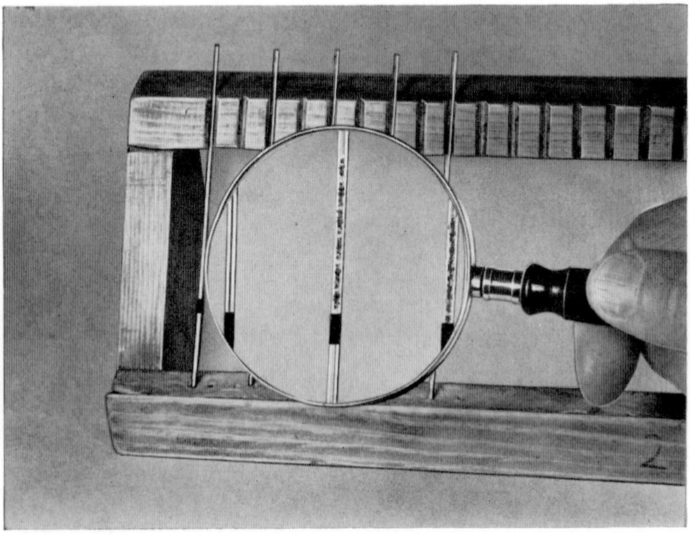

PLATE 10. The Chown capillary test.

p. 239

By now it will be appreciated that the authors do not favour the maxim: "In an emergency use O Rh negative". An adherence to this dictum can lead to anomalies. We well remember a particular case in which when asked why group O Rh negative blood had been given to a patient known by all concerned to be group A Rh positive the reply was: "Oh, it was an emergency".

Technique No. 23.1. Chown capillary technique (Plate 10)

The apparatus for this technique consists of capillary tubes, internal diameter 0·5 mm. (the diameter is important and must be between 0·4 mm. and 0·6 mm.) and length 10–15 cm., and a rack with notches to hold the tubes at an angle of 45°. This angle is critical. For reading purposes the tubes are illuminated from behind and a hand magnifying lens is used.

The anti-serum should be saline agglutinating and of such potency that it can be diluted at least 1 in 4 with saline. It is essential that the red cells should be thrice washed and made up to a 50 per cent suspension in saline. One end of a capillary tube is dipped into the anti-serum and a column of fluid approximately 2 cm. in height is permitted to run in. The capillary is next dipped into the washed cells and a column of red cell suspension equal in length to the column of serum is drawn up. Care must be taken to ensure that there is no air bubble between serum and cells. The capillary tube is then inverted so that the red cells are above the serum and the lower end quickly dipped into petroleum jelly to seal it. It is then placed in the special rack. Controls of known D positive and D negative red cells are included and also the patient's cells with AB serum.

The tests are incubated for 20 minutes at 37°C and then read against a white illuminated background with, if necessary, the assistance of a hand lens. A beaded appearance of cells formed along the lower side of the capillary indicates a positive reaction whereas a thin smooth line of red cells indicates a negative.

Comment. This method, when performed with suitable sera, washed cells and adequate controls, can, in the hands of the experienced worker, become very reliable. Unfortunately, it is quite often performed with unwashed or insufficiently washed cells, with undiluted sera, without discrimination between saline and albumin anti-sera and even sometimes with serum diluted in albumin. In these circumstances it is a very unreliable technique. The supplies of sera suitable for this technique are not adequate for all the Rh testing that has to be done; moreover it is very risky to assume that Rh sera issued for use by the tube technique will give satisfactory results by the Chown test.

Technique No. 23.2. Chown capillary technique (modified Gilbey) using papain

This is essentially the same as the previous technique. The anti-serum used is incomplete anti-D and need not be of particularly high titre. It is mixed in a tube with an equal part of Löw's papain before being drawn up into the capillary. With the papain present, the reactions develop a little more quickly than in the first Chown method described.

Technique No. 23.3. Papain tube technique

One volume of incomplete anti-D is pipetted into each of the requisite number of precipitin tubes followed by an equal volume of Löw's papain. Then a 2 per cent suspension of once washed red cells from the patient and from Rh positive and Rh negative controls are added. The tubes are incubated in a water bath at 37°C for 5–10 minutes and then slowly centrifuged.

Reading is effected by tapping each tube gently with the finger; positives give strong macroscopic agglutination. Tests appearing negative are examined under the microscope.

Technique No. 23.4. Centrifuge tube technique

This is essentially the same as the papain tube technique but omitting the use of papain. It is most satisfactory when a potent saline anti-D is used. Incubation is for 15 minutes in a water bath. The tubes are tapped gently but great care must be exercised to avoid the false positives which may be obtained when handling gently to avoid false negatives!

Technique No. 23.5. Emergency direct-match ($\frac{1}{2}$ to 1 hr)

When an emergency arises which will not allow time for the full direct-matching technique (technique No. 22.4) we recommend a modification (*see* Table 23.2) which will detect an ABO incompatibility and most atypical antibodies. It consists of two tests only:

(1) Moist chamber slide at R.T.

One drop of the patient's serum is mixed with one drop of 2 per cent suspension of washed red cells on a carefully labelled "long" slide (*see* technique No. 3.1) or on equally carefully labelled microscope slides, using one slide for each test. The tests are allowed to stand in the moist chamber for 10–15 minutes, and the results read, all negative reactions being checked microscopically.

(2) Indirect anti-human globulin at 37°C. As in technique No. 22.4, the tests should be made with the patient's serum against red cells from each proposed donor and his own cells. This control of own cells should never be omitted.

The indirect anti-human globulin test is set up in the usual way except that as the incubation time is cut to a minimum of 20 minutes, it is advisable to warm the tubes, saline, etc., to 37°C so that no time is lost. Moreover, a water bath is preferable to a hot air incubator. After 20 minutes' incubation the technique progresses normally (*see* technique No. 10.3a).

It is possible that this technique may fail to reveal an incompatibility due to a weakly reacting antibody. For this reason the clinician should always be informed that only an "emergency" direct match has been done.

Technique No. 23.6. Emergency direct-match (less than $\frac{1}{2}$ hr)

It should be emphasised that this method will not detect every incompatibility and it must never be used when the transfusion of blood can be delayed for as much as 30 minutes. In fact its use is restricted to those grave emergencies in which the only alternative would be to transfuse without a direct-match. It will detect most ABO incompatibilities, a few Rh incompatibilities, *e.g.* those caused by potent saline agglutinins, some very potent cold agglutinins but very little else.

The sample from the patient should be taken into heparin or sequestrine and centrifuged, or if no centrifuge is available allowed to sediment. Two drops of the supernatant cell-free plasma are mixed on an opalescent tile with one drop of blood direct from the bottle (*i.e.* whole blood diluted with ACD). The use of recipient plasma rather than serum allows blood from the bottle to be used without washing—serum would cause a clot. The sensitivity of the test is slightly reduced by using unwashed cells but there would be no time available for washing. The tile is gently rocked and read, preferably over a light, after 2 and 5 minutes. If there is any agglutination the blood should not be used. If the blood appears compatible it may be given, the results being confirmed while the transfusion is in progress.

Chapter 24

THE INVESTIGATION OF HÆMOLYTIC TRANSFUSION REACTIONS

A hæmolytic transfusion reaction may be defined as the occurrence of abnormal destruction of red cells of either the donor or the recipient following a transfusion.

After a normal compatible transfusion of fresh blood the donor's red cells are destroyed at a slow rate, approximately $\frac{1}{120}$th of the total being eliminated per day. When incompatible blood is given the donor's erythrocytes are usually rapidly destroyed, often within a few hours of transfusion, and clinical signs of the rapid red cell destruction may develop. Destruction of some of the recipient's own cells may follow transfusion of blood, the plasma of which contains high titre incompatible agglutinins.

Although the clinical diagnosis of incompatible transfusion is outside the province of the serologist, it is useful for him to be able to interpret the findings in a given case because the clinical picture will often influence the serological testing. Where the clinical diagnosis is in doubt the search for an antibody which could have caused the reaction need not be so extensive.

The clinical features any of which may accompany an incompatible transfusion reaction are as follows: rigor, generalised tinglings, bursting headaches, constricting chest pains, feelings of heat and severe lumbar pains. In addition, signs of collapse, cold clammy skin, cyanosis, feeble pulse and hypotension may be noted. Later, jaundice, hæmoglobinuria, oliguria may develop. Alternatively, there may be no clinical symptoms at the time of transfusion. This, of course, constitutes a grave danger since in these circumstances a large amount of blood can be transfused without the incompatibility being suspected.

When it is thought from the clinical findings that a hæmolytic transfusion reaction has occurred, the first point to establish is that hæmolysis of red cells has taken place. Some of the clinical features mentioned above, particularly severe rigors can accompany compatible transfusions and, therefore, cannot be used for differential diagnosis.

Hæmatological and Biochemical Investigations to Establish Hæmolysis

For these at least 10 ml. of blood taken as soon as possible after the incompatible transfusion has occurred together with later samples at intervals are required. It is useful to have available a good pre-transfusion specimen of serum from the patient.

A sample of blood removed from the patient by venepuncture within an hour of a hæmolytic reaction occurring will usually have plasma stained pink with free hæmoglobin. Providing it is certain that this staining cannot be due to mechanical red cell damage during the taking of the sample, this forms good evidence for intra-vascular hæmolysis having taken place.

If hæmoglobin is present in too small a concentration to be apparent to the naked eye, a spectroscopic examination of the plasma may reveal its presence. Usually hæmoglobin is rapidly broken down and hæmatin is formed which combines with the plasma albumin to form methæmalbumin, which also may be detected spectroscopically by Schumm's test (technique No. 24.1).

Evidence of red cell destruction is very often afforded by a raised concentration of bilirubin in the plasma which stains it a deep yellow. The bilirubin should be measured quantitatively by an appropriate technique. In many laboratories this will be done using an Auto-analyser. Alternatively, technique No. 24.2 (using the Van den Bergh reaction), technique No. 24.5 (a spectrophotometric method) or technique No. 24.6 (an ultramicro spectrophotometric method) all give satisfactory results; the last method is especially valuable when only very small amounts of serum are available. The increase in bilirubin is usually obvious to the naked eye, particularly if the colour of the post-transfusion plasma is compared with that of the pre-transfusion sample.

When rapid hæmolysis has taken place the increase in plasma bilirubin is a constant feature but it should be realised that bilirubin levels are controlled to a large extent by liver function, the capacity of the liver for dealing with the excretion of bilirubin affecting both the degree of clinical jaundice and the plasma bilirubin level. Additional evidence of hæmolysis may be deduced from a comparison between pre- and post-transfusion figures for hæmoglobin and red cell count. The red cells from each bottle of blood transfused, if no hæmolysis has taken place, will normally raise the hæmoglobin by about 6–8 per cent and the count by about 500,000 cells per cubic millimetre approximately. However, following transfusion there are blood volume changes which alter the hæmoglobin level and the red cell count so that no comparisons should be made on results obtained within 24 hours.

After incompatible transfusion hæmoglobinuria may occur. Other sequelæ may be oliguria or even anuria. Persistent anuria results in death usually at about 10–14 days after the transfusion. Hæmoglobin in the urine may be detected spectroscopically or biochemical tests may be made for the break-down products urobilinogen and urobilin. (Technique No. 24.3.)

A microscopical examination of the sediment from a centrifuged sample of urine will occasionally reveal red cell casts; an indication of severe renal impairment.

Having confirmed that hæmolysis of red cells has taken place, the next step is to establish the cause. Hæmolytic transfusion reactions commonly have a serological basis, but it should be noted that they may also occur when hæmolysed donor blood is given. This hæmolysis may be due to: (*a*) overheating; (*b*) freezing; (*c*) overlong storage; (*d*) contamination of the blood by hæmolytic bacteria. If the above possibilities have been satisfactorily excluded, a serological investigation should be planned.

Serological Investigations

In spite of (or perhaps because of!) the discovery of numerous blood group systems in the past ten years, an ABO incompatibility is still the commonest cause of a hæmolytic transfusion reaction. Less often the Rh factor is involved and from time to time most of the other blood group systems have been implicated.

It is proposed here to describe first of all a general routine which should be carried out whenever an incompatible transfusion reaction is suspected, after which incompatibilities due to the various systems will be considered separately. Occasionally the circumstances are such that an inkling of the cause of the reaction is known before a serological investigation is commenced. An example of such is the finding of a clerical or labelling error. In this case the serological tests will be appropriately modified. In all instances the specimens of blood required for a full investigation are the following:

(1) Pre-transfusion sample.
(2) Post-transfusion sample taken as soon as possible after the reaction has taken place.
(3) A later post-transfusion sample taken 5–10 days after the transfusion (specimens at other intervals may also be required).
(4) Samples from each bottle, wholly or partly transfused.

At the outset it is helpful to examine microscopically a 2 per cent red cell suspension in saline from sample (2) as it sometimes contains agglutinates. These are composed of donor cells which have been agglutinated by an antibody contained in the serum of the recipient. Eventually the agglutinated cells are broken down and removed from the circulation. In fact often their destruction is effected so rapidly that there are no agglutinated cells apparent when a suspension is examined. The absence of agglutinates is therefore no contra-indication to a diagnosis of hæmolytic transfusion reaction. An alternative reason for their absence is that no agglutination *in vivo* but merely sensitisation and subsequent hæmolysis of the transfused cells has taken place. Evidence for this can sometimes be obtained if a direct anti-human globulin test (technique No. 10.3b) is performed on sample (2) in cases in which no agglutination is apparent. A "mixed blood" appearance may develop through the agglutination of sensitised donor cells by the anti-human globulin serum which confirms their sensitisation *in vivo*. It is often worthwhile doing the direct anti-human globulin test even when there is some evidence of agglutination without it, since the anti-human globulin often increases the size and number of the clumps.

The next step is the retyping of the red cells of both donor and recipient and the re-direct-matching of blood from each bottle transfused using serum from both pre- and post-transfusion specimens (1) and (2) from the patient (technique No. 22.4).

The conduct of the case after this point will vary according to the results of the re-typing and re-direct-matching tests. It is probable that they will reveal which blood group system is involved or at least indicate the most profitable further line for investigation. If a particular blood group system is implicated by the above tests, details for further investigation can be found in the appropriate section of this chapter. When an incompatibility is detected without it being clear to which blood group system the causative antibody belongs an attempt should be made to identify the antibody (technique No. 21.1). Negative results (*i.e.* the blood appearing compatible) probably indicates either that a hæmolytic reaction has not taken place or that it has no serological basis. However, such a conclusion must be reached with caution, due consideration being given to the clinical, hæmatological and biochemical findings. Moreover, there are three circumstances in which the serological findings may be negative in spite of a hæmolytic reaction due to blood group antibodies. The first of these is caused by the absence of the causative antibody in both pre- and post-transfusion samples. The absence of the antibody in the pre-transfusion specimen is most unusual but occasionally occurs either because it has become inert as a result of storage or because the antibody causing the reaction only appeared in the bloodstream in response to stimulation by an antigen present in the blood given. In the latter case the transfusion reaction is usually delayed and relatively mild. The absence of the antibody in the post-transfusion sample (2) is unlikely to be due to a badly preserved sample since this will have been tested almost immediately after taking. The most usual reason for not being able to detect an antibody at this stage is that it has been absorbed by the transfused blood.

A second reason for negative findings, in spite of a genuine hæmolytic reaction having occurred, is that antibodies of high titre in the donor's blood have caused destruction of the recipient's own red cells. This possibility must always be borne in mind if group O blood has been given to patients of groups A, B, or AB.

A third reason for the apparent compatibility of the blood given may be that the techniques employed will not detect the particular antibody which may be present. The direct match should be repeated using additional methods such as the trypsin, trypsin anti-human globulin, and anti-human globulin plus complement. All the above reasons for an incompatibility remaining undetected must be considered before concluding that the blood given was compatible.

Hæmolytic Transfusion Reactions Due to ABO Incompatibility

Since anti-A and anti-B are naturally occurring antibodies, the hæmolytic process resulting from an ABO incompatibility is usually rapid.

The serological findings in a case of ABO incompatibility wherein the group O patient received a transfusion of 120 ml. of group A blood will be described as being typical of this class. (Table 24.1.) The "mixed blood" appearance shown by the post-transfusion sample with anti-A serum is due to the presence of transfused group A cells in the recipient's circulation. Its development is, of course, due to the reaction between the anti-A grouping serum and some of the transfused group A cells which have not yet been destroyed by the recipient's own anti-A. It can be seen that the anti-A has not been completely neutralised, in spite of the presence of circulating transfused group A red cells. This is by no means an uncommon phenomenon. The anti-A and anti-B titres before and at intervals following the transfusion are shown in Fig. 5.1. From the immune response of the anti-A it could have been deduced that group A blood had been given even if a sample from the donor had not been available. Thus in cases where no

Table 24.1

Incompatible Transfusion—A–O

	Cell grouping			Serum grouping	
	Anti-A	Anti-B	O serum Anti-A + Anti-B	A cells	B cells
Pre-transfusion sample of patient . . .	–	–	–	C	C
Post-transfusion sample of patient . . .	Mixed blood appearance	–	Mixed blood appearance	+	C
Bottle given . . .	C	–	C	–	C

	Donor's red cells			
	Saline		Albumin	Anti-human globulin
Repeated cross match	R.T.	37°C	37°C	
Pre-transfusion serum .	C	+ +	(+)	Not done*
Post-transfusion serum .	+	(+)	w	Not done*

* Anti-human globulin tests not carried out because saline tests were positive.

sample of donor blood has been kept, the immune response is a valuable guide to the group of the blood given.

When selecting blood for transfusion it is not usually necessary to take the sub-groups of A into account. Atypical anti-A_1 antibodies are normally only active at low temperature. It is only in the rare cases when they are active at body temperature that they will cause destruction of transfused A_1 red cells. Nevertheless in any suspected transfusion reaction where a group A or group AB patient has been given homologous blood, the red cells of patient and donors should be typed with anti-A_1 (technique No. 6.2). The pre- and post-transfusion samples of serum should be tested with known A_1 and A_2 red cells both at room temperature and at 37°C.

Destruction of Recipient's Red Cells by Incompatible ABO Antibodies of High Titre in Donor Plasma

If homologous blood is always used for transfusion this problem does not arise. However, should group O blood with high titre antibodies be given to patients of groups A, B, or AB, a hæmolytic transfusion reaction may result. The range of severity of the reaction is wide, occasionally resulting in the death of the patient, sometimes in less severe clinical symptoms, but more often merely in a failure to obtain the expected post-transfusion increase in red cell count and hæmoglobin level.

In cases where no incompatibility can be demonstrated between the recipient's serum and the donor erythrocytes but it is known

Table 24.2

Incompatible Transfusion—O–A

	Cell grouping			Serum grouping		Titre of Anti-A	Titre of Anti-B
	Anti-A	Anti-B	Group O serum Anti-A + Anti-B	A cells	B cells		
Pre-transfusion sample of patient . . .	C	–	C	–	C		
Post-transfusion sample of patient . . .	Mixed blood appearance	–	Mixed blood appearance	(+)	C		
Bottle given . . .	–	–	–	C	C	2,000	256

	Donor's red cells			
	Saline		Albumin	Coombs
Repeated cross match	R.T.	37°C	37°C	37°C
Pre-transfusion serum	–	–	–	–
Post-transfusion serum	–	–	–	–

that incompatible agglutinins have been transfused, these should be titrated. At the same time the sera should be titrated for anti-A or anti-B hæmolysins (technique No. 5.1), as it is considered that these hæmolysins play the major role in such transfusion reactions. Anti-A or anti-B agglutinin titres of less than 1,000 will not cause appreciable destruction of the recipient's blood unless associated with potent hæmolysins, except when the recipient is particularly anæmic or several bottles containing incompatible agglutinins are given.

Typical findings of a case of high titre antibodies in group O blood given to a group A patient are shown in Table 24.2. In the recipient's post-transfusion sample we have the anomaly of free anti-A agglutinins in the serum of a group A patient, evidenced by the serum reacting with group A cells. The persistence of free anti-A in the recipient's plasma renders group A blood (*i.e.* blood of the recipient's own group) temporarily incompatible. Therefore, if a further transfusion is contemplated, it is advisable to wait until the anti-A has been eliminated; or if this is not possible, to transfuse washed group O red cells resuspended in group AB plasma to avoid giving the patient more incompatible antibody.

That a hæmolytic transfusion reaction is due to transfused antibody is difficult to prove conclusively except by the demonstration of a normal survival of donor cells, by the inagglutinable cell count technique (the Ashby method), technique No. 24.4. If the donor cells are eliminated at the normal rate for compatible blood, then the hæmolysed red cells must be the recipient's own.

Hæmolytic Transfusion Reactions Due to Rh Antibodies

In the consideration of Rh antibodies as causative factors of transfusion reactions some attention must be given to the fact that they are atypical antibodies which normally only appear in the serum in response to stimulation by the corresponding antigen. If an Rh antibody is present in the patient's serum before the transfusion is given, the sequelæ are similar to those already described for hæmolytic reactions due to anti-A or anti-B. In the sample taken immediately after the transfusion agglutinates are not usually seen but they may develop if a direct anti-human globulin test is carried out. There is a greater possibility of this happening than with ABO incompatibilities because of the common occurrence of incomplete Rh antibodies.

Rh antibodies also show the typical immune response curve such as that shown in Fig. 5.1. A protocol of the findings in a case of a D negative patient whose serum contained anti-D antibodies, transfused with one bottle of D positive blood, is shown in Table 24.3.

A patient who has been sensitised either by previous transfusions of Rh positive blood or by an Rh positive fœtus *in utero*, but in whom antibodies have not yet developed, may be stimulated to produce them by a transfusion of Rh positive blood. In these cases the elimination of the transfused red cells is comparatively

Table 24.3

Incompatible Transfusion due to Rh Antibodies

	Cell grouping					Serum grouping	
	Anti-A	Anti-B	Group O serum Anti-A + Anti-B	Anti-D	Anti-D	A cells	B cells
Pre-transfusion sample of patient . . .	–	–	–	–	–	C	C
Post-transfusion sample of patient . . .	–	–	–	Mixed blood appearance +	+	C	C
Bottle given . . .	–	–	–	V	V	C	C

	Donor's red cells			
	Saline		Albumin	Indirect a.h.g.
Repeated cross match	R.T.	37°C		
Pre-transfusion serum	–	–	+	+
Post-transfusion serum	–	–	w	+

slow and the clinical symptoms are usually confined to the appearance of a fairly transitory jaundice which may easily be overlooked. If the appropriate tests are made the survival time of the transfused cells will be found to be greatly decreased (technique No. 24.4) and when they have all been eliminated from the circulation the atypical antibody will be detectable in the serum (techniques Nos. 10.1–5). This type of hæmolytic transfusion reaction in which the causative antibody is not present in the recipient's serum pre-transfusion but appears in response to the transfused blood is often called a "delayed reaction". The extreme case of a "delayed reaction" is one which shows "intermediate cell survival". The atypical antibody develops so slowly that the donor red cells remain in the circulation for a long time although they do not survive as long as normal compatible red cells.

All the Rh antibodies are potential causes of hæmolytic transfusion reactions. At one time anti-D was most commonly implicated but with the increasing consciousness of the undesirability of giving D negative patients D positive blood, transfusion reactions due to this antibody are becoming more rare. The Rh sub-typing of Rh positive patients is not routine practice, so that the possibility of other Rh antibodies being the causative factors, must be borne in mind when investigating hæmolytic reactions wherein both patient and donor are D positive. In these cases a full Rh sub-typing of patient and donors may give a clue to the identity of the antibody responsible. The general principles of antibody identification already discussed in Chapter 21 should be adhered to when investigating transfusion reactions due to atypical antibodies whether of the Rh or other blood group systems.

Hæmolytic Transfusion Reactions Due to Other Blood Group Systems

Little need be said regarding hæmolytic reactions due to other blood group systems, as these follow the same general pattern. Moreover they seldom occur although most of the known blood group antibodies (*see* Tables 15.1 and 15.2) have been incriminated in transfusion reactions from time to time. The antibody responsible can usually be identified if the procedure outlined in Chapter 21 is followed.

Demonstration of Transfused Red Cells *in vivo*

There are three ways of demonstrating the survival of transfused red cells *in vivo*. The basic principle is that there must be some method of distinguishing between the two red cell populations, that of the recipient and that of the donor. Two methods depend upon the fact that if the populations contain different blood group antigens, using an appropriate anti-serum one population can be agglutinated and the other left free. The third method makes use of isotope-labelled red cells, whose presence is, of course, detected by the radioactivity emitted.

The first method is simply a qualitative detection of transfused cells involving the selection of an anti-serum by which they are agglutinated leaving the recipient's own cells free; the finding of a "mixed blood" picture demonstrates that donor cells are still present in the circulation (cf. technique No. 22.1). It is obvious that the sensitivity of the test will depend upon the amount of blood transfused. Cells from a compatible transfusion of 500 ml. of blood can be detected up to about ninety days after transfusion.

The second method, the Ashby inagglutinable cell count technique (technique No. 24.4) is the most commonly used procedure for following the rate of survival of transfused red cells. Here it is the recipient's red cells which are agglutinated leaving those of the donor free for counting. The success of this method depends mainly upon the choice of a powerful and avid anti-serum. This high standard of avidity restricts the method in practice to cases where anti-A, anti-B, anti-M or very potent anti-D can be used. It will be found that for fresh compatible blood a sample taken 24 hours later contains more free cells than one taken at the end of the transfusion. This is because the recipient's blood volume is increased by the transfusion but will have returned to normal by this time. Whenever, therefore, the 24 hour count is the greater, it, and not that obtained immediately post-transfusion, is taken as denoting 100 per cent survival. From this point blood will normally be eliminated at the rate of approximately 1 per cent per day. When stored blood is used there may be an initial drop in count but thereafter the rate of elimination will normally be of the same order as for fresh blood. Incompatible blood will be eliminated much faster; in cases where a strong antibody, *e.g.* anti-A or potent anti-D, is present in the serum at the time of the transfusion all the transfused cells may be eliminated in a few hours. As has already been remarked intermediate survival may occur when an antibody which was absent at the time the transfusion was given is being produced in the recipient in response to an antigen contained in the transfused red cells.

The labelling of red cells with radioactive isotopes makes it possible to measure the survival of less than 1 ml. of cells. With such small quantities there is no risk of a hæmolytic transfusion reaction. This makes the test one of great value in determining whether an antibody detected *in vitro*, especially one which appears to have little or no 37°C activity, will in fact destroy transfused red cells *in vivo*. It thus forms a very sensitive and reliable biological test for compatibility. Another application is where it is thought that the patient's own cells may have an abnormal life-span, as his tagged red cells can be re-injected and studied in his own circulation. The method does not usually lend itself to the investigation of a hæmolytic transfusion reaction, although the injection of isotope labelled red cells from the same donors or from others having red cells of known antigenic constitution may be of value in certain cases.

Various isotopes have been used for these studies, *e.g.* ^{15}N, ^{59}Fe, ^{32}P, ^{51}Cr.

In particular, the method using ^{51}Cr has become an established routine in specialised laboratories. It seems unlikely, however, that the method will be adopted in general laboratories, at any rate for some years. It is not proposed, therefore, to give any description of the technique here, especially as the authors cannot speak from personal experience. For an authoritative account of the method and its applications *Blood Transfusion in Clinical Medicine* (Mollison) should be consulted.

Treatment

The treatment of an incompatible transfusion reaction will, of course, depend upon its severity. If the reaction is mild with a slightly raised serum bilirubin and no renal impairment, probably no treatment is necessary, nor indeed advisable. More severe cases may need to be treated with compatible packed red cells to maintain a hæmoglobin concentration above 10 gm. per cent. Hæmodialysis using the artificial kidney machine is indicated in any of the following situations:

(*a*) The blood potassium is more than 7·5 milli-equivalents per litre.
(*b*) A high blood urea over 400 mg./100 ml., with low urea clearance.
(*c*) If the sodium, chlorides and calcium blood levels are low. General deterioration of clinical condition, *e.g.* severe vomiting or coma, etc.

It is important that fluid balance is maintained (intake limited to 500 ml. if the patient is completely anuric) as over-hydration and œdema makes successful hæmodialysis less likely. In fact the immediate treatment when it is known that there has been intravascular hæmolysis is to give 100 ml. or 20 per cent mannitol followed by an infusion of 45 m.E.q. of sodium bicarbonate in an attempt to provoke a diuresis.

Techniques

Details of some of the more important biochemical techniques which have to be used when investigating hæmolytic transfusion reactions are described below as are the serological methods for demonstrating survival of red cells *in vivo*. The other serological methods have all been described in previous chapters and the technique reference numbers have been included in the text. A plan for the investigation of a transfusion reaction is given in Appendix II. (Procedure No. 7.)

Technique No. 24.1. Schumm's test

This is a sensitive test for small amounts of methæmalbumin, which it will be unnecessary to use if spectroscopic examination of the plasma has shown the typical absorption band in the red part of the spectrum at 624 mμ.

A convenient volume (about 0·5 ml.) of plasma is covered with a layer of ether. Then $\frac{1}{10}$th volume of concentrated ammonium sulphide (Analar) is added and the contents of the tube are mixed by shaking. The fluid is then examined spectroscopically. If methæmalbumin was present in the original sample a sharp band at 558 mμ will be seen. This is due to the formation of an ammonium hæmachromogen.

Technique No. 24.2. Estimation of serum bilirubin (van den Bergh reaction)

The reagents required are as follows:

(1) Absolute alcohol.
(2) Ammonium sulphate (saturated).
(3) Methyl red (2·9 mg. per litre at pH 4·63) = 0·04 mg. bilirubin in 10 ml. fluid. Stock standard solution is 290 mg. pure methyl red dissolved in 100 ml. glacial acetic acid. In a litre graduated flask 1 ml. of the standard and 5 ml. glacial acetic acid are placed; to this is added a little water and then 14·4 g. of crystallised sodium citrate are gradually washed in. When solution is complete the fluid is made up to 1 litre.
(4) Diazo reagent made by mixing two solutions A and B. A = 1 g. sulphanilic acid in 250 ml. N. Hydrochloric acid made up to 1 litre with water. B = 0·5 g. sodium nitrate in 100 ml. distilled water. Ten ml. of solution A is mixed with 0·3 ml. of solution B immediately prior to use.
(5) Buffer 3·6 g. disodium phosphate (Na_2HPO_4 $12H_2O$) in 100 ml. distilled water.

One ml. of well centrifuged serum is mixed with 0·5 ml. of diazo reagent and left for 2 minutes; 0·5 ml. of saturated ammonium sulphate and 8 ml. of absolute alcohol are added. The mixture is stoppered and shaken well to mix; it is then centrifuged and the colour of the supernatant fluid is compared colorimetrically with the methyl red standard.

If the concentration of azo-bilirubin in the test seems to be more than twice that in the standard, a suitable dilution of the original serum with the phosphate buffer is made. It is important to remember that this involves multiplying the final reading by the dilution factor. Calculation:

$$\text{Bilirubin (mg. per 100 ml.)} = \frac{\text{Reading of test}}{\text{Reading of standard}} \times 0{\cdot}04 \times 100$$

Technique No. 24.3. Qualitative test for urobilinogen and urobilin in urine

Two drops of N/10 iodine solution is added to 5 ml. of urine to oxidise any urobilinogen present to urobilin. Five ml. of a 10 per cent suspension of zinc acetate in alcohol is then added. The mixture is left to settle and the supernatant fluid examined for the appearance of a green fluorescence which indicates the presence of urobilin (which may have been present in the original urine either as urobilinogen or urobilin). Spectroscopic examination of the fluid reveals a broad absorption band (due to urobilin) at the green-blue junction.

Technique No. 24.4. Quantitative test for the survival of transfused red cells (Ashby technique)

From a well mixed sample of patient's blood taken into Wintrobe mixture, an accurate 1 in 50 dilution in 3 per cent sodium citrate is made. To a convenient volume (0·3 ml.) of the diluted blood an equal quantity of the appropriate anti-serum is added. The mixture is left at room temperature for 2 hours (or at 37°C if anti-D is being used) and then centrifuged at 1,500 r.p.m. for 1 minute. The tube is vigorously shaken to break up the agglutinates. The largest clumps are then allowed to sink to the bottom of the tube while the upper three-quarters of the suspension is transferred by means of a Pasteur pipette into a second tube which is centrifuged as before. The sediment is then re-suspended by a standard technique consisting of fifty inversions through an angle of 90°–120° at the approximate rate of one inversion per second. A counting chamber is filled from the top of the fluid; this minimises the number of agglutinates withdrawn. Most of the agglutinated cells will appear as tight clumps but any cells that are free but distorted in shape should be regarded as agglutinated and, therefore, not included in the count. Two spreads are made and a total of about a thousand free cells counted.

In calculating the number of transfused cells per cubic millimetre of whole blood, the figure for the inagglutinable cell count must be subtracted. Where no pre-transfusion sample is available an approximation to this figure may be obtained by a count made on blood of the same type as the recipient. It should be remembered that the dilution factor in this method is 1 in 100 whereas for total red cell count as normally performed it is 1 in 200.

When using this technique to follow the survival of transfused red cells, counts are performed at intervals and the results recorded graphically, so that the curve obtained can be compared with that given by fresh, compatible normal blood.

Technique No. 24.5. Serum bilirubin spectrophotometric procedure

Reagents

(1) *Phosphate buffer, pH* 7·4: 4·05 gm. of disodium hydrogen phosphate, Na_2HPO_4 and 1·74 gm. of monobasic potassium phosphate, KH_2PO_4, are dissolved in ion-free water and made up to 1,000 ml. The pH is checked.

(2) *Phosphate buffer pH* 5·0: 27·6 gm. of sodium dehydrogen phosphate, $NaH_2PO_4.H_2O$, is dissolved in about 700 ml, ion-free water and the ph adjusted to 5·0 with 5N NaOH, and made up to 1,000 ml. with water.

(3) Ethyl acetate, $CH_3COOC_2H_5$.

(4) n-Butanol, $CH_3(CH_2)_2CH_2OH$.

Procedure

(1) *Total Bilirubin.* Into 5 ml. of pH 7·4 phosphate buffer 0·1 ml. of serum is pipetted (or 0·02 ml. serum into 1·0 ml.). The test is well mixed and read against phosphate buffer at 455 mμ and 575 mμ in Beckman DU using micro cells for smaller amounts.

$$(\text{O.D.}_{455} - \text{O.D.}_{575})\ F_T = \text{mg./100 ml. Bilirubin}$$

F_T is calculated from the specific absorption of a known standard of sodium bilirubinate in 5 per cent human albumin. It must be calculated for each instrument and standard.

(2) *Unconjugated Bilirubin.* 0·8 ml. of ph 5·0 phosphate buffer is pipetted into a 15-ml. ground glass-stoppered tube; 0·1 ml. of serum and 2·5 ml. of ethyl acetate are added

and the mixture shaken very vigorously for three 30-second periods. The ethyl acetate layer is read in the Beckman DU or in the ultramicro spectrophotometer at 455 mμ and 575 mμ using ethyl acetate as the blank.

$$(O.D._{455} - O.D._{575}) \times F_U = \text{mg./100 ml. bilirubin}$$

F_U is calculated using a known standard.

By substituting butanol for ethyl acetate, bilirubin and its "monoglucosiduronide" are extracted. From this value and the values for total and unconjugated bilirubin, actual values for "mono-" and di-glucosiduronide can be calculated.

Technique No. 24.6. Serum bilirubin ultramicro-spectrophotometric procedure

Total Bilirubin. The test is performed in a 400 ml. polyethylene tube. 10 ml. of serum are diluted with 250 ml. pH 7·4 buffer. The test is well mixed and read in No. 151 spectrocolorimeter at 455 mμ and 575 mμ using buffer as blank.

Calculation

$$(O.D._{455} - O.D._{575})\, F_T = \text{mg./100 ml. Bilirubin}$$

Conjugated and Unconjugated Bilirubin. Again using a 400-ml. polyethylene tube, 10 ml. serum are mixed with 80 ml. pH 5·0 buffer and 250 ml. ethyl acetate. The top of the tube is covered with a 1-cm. square of parafilm and a stopper inserted. The tube is shaken well to ensure complete extraction. The ethyl acetate layer is read at 455 mμ and at 575 mμ in the No. 151 spectrocolorimeter using ethyl acetate as blank.

Calculation

$(O.D._{455} - O.D._{575})\, F_U$ = mg./100 ml. unconjugated bilirubin. By substituting n-butanol for ethyl acetate, unconjugated bilirubin and the monoglucosiduronide are extracted. From these results, the values for the mono- and diglucosiduronides can be calculated.

As in technique No. 24.5 F_T and F_U must be calculated for each instrument and standard.

CHAPTER 25

HÆMOLYTIC DISEASE OF THE FŒTUS

Ætiology, Ante-natal Care, Serological Testing of Mother, Baby and Father

Hæmolytic disease of the fœtus is caused by maternal antibodies which are incompatible with fœtal erythrocytes. These antibodies cross the placenta and attack the infant's erythrocytes and may also damage the fœtal tissues. The antibody causing the disease in the majority (about 95 per cent) of cases is anti-D. In about 5 per cent of cases other blood group antibodies have been found to be responsible, the less common antibodies of the Rh system and the ABO antibodies being the next in order of importance to anti-D.

Clinical Picture

A detailed account of the clinical features and of the treatment of hæmolytic disease of the fœtus is beyond the scope of this book. However, laboratory work and the clinical assessment of the case must, of course, go hand in hand. When the clinical picture is typical but no antibodies are detected by the standard routine, a more extensive investigation has to be made.

The most common clinical features of the disease are anæmia and jaundice. Usually they occur together but it is possible for an infant to have a low hæmoglobin without any jaundice and occasionally a high degree of jaundice is associated with hæmoglobin values of over 110 per cent. The anæmia is usually accompanied by an increase in reticulocytes and nucleated red cells. Infants with severe anæmia may have up to 50–60 per cent of reticulocytes and as many as 200,000 nucleated red cells per cubic millimetre of the peripheral blood. A proportion of infants die *in utero*, most of them with hydrops and showing some degree of maceration at delivery. It should be noted, however, that cases of hydrops fœtalis have been described in which no materno-fœtal incompatibility has been demonstrated.

The degree of jaundice in the infant can be measured by performing a bilirubin test on the cord serum. The time of onset of the jaundice in suspected cases of hæmolytic disease is important. In most genuine cases the infant is either born jaundiced or the jaundice appears within 24 hours of birth. If an infant becomes jaundiced at a later period of its neonatal life then the jaundice is usually "physiological" and is not due to hæmolytic disease of the newborn.

It might be expected that once an infant with hæmolytic disease had been born alive it ought to recover, as after birth the infant is cut off from a further intake of Rh antibody. However, some infants born alive with the disease die despite treatment. Some die within 24 hours from cardiac failure, some die of cardiac failure during or soon after exchange transfusion; some die of progressive anæmia (this should be prevented by "top-up" transfusions if the hæmoglobin level drops significantly 3–14 days after exchange transfusion) and others develop signs of damage to the central nervous system at about the third day and may die later on. Examination of the brain may show a yellow staining of many of the nuclei particularly in the basal ganglia. This pigmentation is known as kernicterus.

Nowadays the practice of keeping the serum bilirubin low by means of exchange transfusion, repeated if necessary, has virtually eliminated kernicterus in treated infants.

Serological Picture

The serological picture associated with hæmolytic disease of the newborn is of an infant having inherited an antigen from the father which is absent in the mother and which has caused her to form the corresponding antibodies. These antibodies traverse the placenta and cause damage to the fœtal red cells. In the majority of cases, a positive direct anti-human globulin test on the infant's red cells can be obtained thus demonstrating that they are sensitised by the antibody.

The knowledge that hæmolytic disease of the newborn has an antigen-antibody basis and the introduction of serological tests has greatly facilitated the differential diagnosis of the disease from other causes of stillbirth, neonatal death, neonatal jaundice, etc. It can now be rapidly diagnosed and often prognosed with some degree of accuracy before the baby is born.

When the clinical picture is typical or suggestive of hæmolytic disease serological tests should be done as soon as possible, especially if the mother is known to be Rh positive, as the confirmation of the diagnosis, the identification of the causative antibody and the provision of compatible blood may take the laboratory some time.

The result of the serological tests, however, must not be viewed out of perspective. Although positive serological findings may be used as a basis for the diagnosis of hæmolytic disease in cases when it is not certain clinically from what disease an infant is suffering, the mere finding of an atypical antibody in the mother which has sensitised the infant's red cells does not necessarily mean that the infant is a clinical case of hæmolytic disease and in need of treatment. In some cases where the serological findings are typical of the disease, the infant may be only very lightly affected or even apparently quite normal. Obviously in these instances treatment is undesirable.

An assessment of the value of the serological findings during pregnancy for prognosis is attempted below.

Ideally the first serological steps are taken in early pregnancy, so that when the baby is born it is a matter of only a few simple tests and the treatment can be begun in the first 12 hours of life.

Each Rh positive fœtus must be regarded as a potential "dose" of antigen for the Rh negative mother. The first one or two "doses" of antigen usually do not produce antibodies so that the first and often the second Rh positive child in a family will not suffer from hæmolytic disease. As might be anticipated, the number of Rh positive children in a family who escape the disease will largely depend upon the ease with which the mother becomes stimulated to form antibodies. The number of stimuli required for antibody formation varies from individual to individual; it is markedly affected by a transfusion of Rh positive blood.

The initial antibody production is liable to occur at any time from early pregnancy onwards. The non-appearance of antibodies by about the thirty-fourth week reduces the likelihood of their being produced in that particular pregnancy. However, it sometimes happens that the first appearance of antibodies is at about ten days post-partum or even occassionally much later; being found up to three to six months after delivery. This is almost certainly because fœtal red cells enter the maternal circulation at delivery and cause an immune response. Hence the importance of testing a post-delivery sample for the benefit of a future pregnancy.

Antibodies arising after the thirty-fourth week tend to be of low titre and associated with a mildly affected or clinically normal infant. The peak of the immune response is reached from 10–20 days following delivery and may, as just mentioned, be caused largely by entry of fœtal red cells into the mother at birth; thereafter the titre falls, but by sensitive techniques it can be detected months, and often years, after stimulation.

Surprisingly, in 97 per cent of cases where her Rh positive fœtus has stimulated a woman to produce Rh antibodies there is no materno-fœtal ABO incompatibility in contrast to normal pregnancies, for which the corresponding figure is 81 per cent. This is because when fœtal cells which are incompatible with the mother's ABO antibodies come into her circulation they are usually destroyed before they can act as an antigenic stimulus.

Most antibodies of the Rh and other blood group systems have been the causative factors in hæmolytic disease of the newborn. Nevertheless, the anti-D antibody is responsible for about 95 per cent of all cases which are sufficiently severely affected to need transfusion. It is, therefore, the D negative woman who is at greatest risk and for whom the most careful serological routine during and after pregnancy will have to be planned.

Ante-natal and Post-natal Serological Testing of Mother

It is usual at the present time for all pregnant women to have routine serological tests performed.

It is recommended that all women at their first attendance at a clinic should have ABO grouping, Rh typing with anti-D, and an antibody screening test with R_1R_2 cells by albumin and papain or trypsin techniques. If the papain technique is not included in the routine screening some Rh antibodies will go undetected. Many of these, later in pregnancy, will be detectable by other methods. A few will remain "papain type" antibodies throughout the whole of the pregnancy.

The women can be divided into six classes as shown below (*see also* Procedure No. 8).

D positive

D positive with normal history and no atypical antibody. No further tests.	D positive with history suggestive of hæmolytic disease. No atypical antibody. Tests as (4).	D positive with atypical antibodies, whatever the previous history. Tests as (6).
(1)	(2)	(3)

D negative

D negative with normal history and no atypical antibodies. Antibody test repeated at 32nd week, delivery, and 10th day. Baby is tested.	D negative with history suggestive of hæmolytic disease. No atypical antibody. Antibody test monthly from 28th week. Baby is tested.	D negative with antibodies, Titration at varying intervals (depending on the case) including delivery and 10th day. Husband and baby tested.
(4)	(5)	(6)

When an antibody is found at any time during pregnancy, it must be investigated for specificity and for strength. If the antibody is of the Rh system Chapter 13 will be helpful in determining the exact specificity. An anti-human globulin test with Rh negative K positive and Fy^a positive cells should also be included. In an appreciable proportion of cases where Rh antibodies have been produced and the husband is K+, anti-K antibodies are formed also. If the antibody is not Rh it can usually be identified by technique No. 21.1. If the antibody is so weak that identification is difficult, repeat samples should be requested monthly as the strength may well increase as the result of stimulation.

Once the antibody has been detected and identified no further tests are necessary or indeed helpful until about the 28th week of pregnancy. It is then that the changes in titration values may be of importance in the prognosis for the present pregnancy.

Prognosis and Handling of Case Based on Antibody Titration

Whether antibody titration during pregnancy will be any guide as to the prognosis for the infant *in utero* is still regarded as doubtful by some authorities. The best correlation seems to be with the anti-human globulin titre.

We find a strong positive correlation between the anti-human globulin titre of the maternal serum and the clinical condition of the baby. This is shown clearly in the accompanying Table 25.1 which shows the proportion of stillbirths, neonatal deaths and

Table 25.1

Proportion of Stillbirths, Neonatal Deaths and Severely Affected Infants at Different Levels of Maternal Titre

Maternal anti-human globulin titre at delivery	<32	32	64	>64
Percentage of infants stillborn	0·8	6	14	25
Percentage of infants dying in the neonatal period	2	2	7	12
Percentage of infants severely affected but recovering after transfusion (usually repeated)	4	12	26	40
TOTAL	6·8	20	47	77

severely affected infants at different levels of maternal antibody titre. The titres given are anti-human globulin titres performed by technique No. 25.4 without the addition of hæmolysed red cells, *i.e.* they are the anti-human globulin titre with which the partial absorption titre is strictly comparable. It can be seen that for titres below 32 only about 3 per cent of infants will die. In fact a large number of the babies (about 50 per cent) will require no treatment and the rest will recover after one exchange transfusion. In the 0·8 per cent of cases where the infant is stillborn there will almost invariably have been a previous stillbirth or neonatal death in the family; as mentioned below this would in itself be a reason for premature delivery and some of these 0·8 per cent could be saved in this way. Thus if during pregnancy the maternal antibody is below 32 the pregnancy should, in the absence of any other indications for induction, be allowed to go to term. The 2 per cent of neonatal deaths, shown in Table 25.1 were of heart failure during or following exchange transfusion, and research into methods of preventing this are needed.

Titres of below 32* by our techniques constitute 50 per cent approximately of all cases.

If the titre is 32 (a further 20 per cent of all cases) the same remarks apply except that as the percentage of deaths is higher (8 per cent) some clinicians may be inclined to induce early at this titre.

For titres of 64 and over premature induction should be considered. Other factors such as previous history, homo- or heterozygosity of the father, etc., will also influence this decision. The partial absorption titre is worth doing when the anti-human globulin titre is 64 or over, especially when the husband is heterozygous as if it is low there is a greater chance of the infant *in utero* being Rh negative and therefore unaffected.

The partial absorption (P.A.) (technique No. 25.4) titre is the anti-human globulin titre of the maternal serum after partial absorption with standard hæmolysed Rh positive cell suspension, by the method of Vos. There is evidence to show that these titres closely parallel the titres of free Rh antibody in the fœtal circulation; it is well known that anti-human globulin titres in cord sera tend to be high when the baby is severely affected with hæmolytic disease. In the assessment of any particular case, it is usually necessary to compare the results of a series of titrations before deciding whether the serological tests indicate that a stillbirth is likely to occur unless there is early induction. It has been recommended that weekly samples should be titrated, but probably fortnightly samples from the 28th week are adequate. If on any sample, however, there is a marked increase in anti-human globulin and P.A. titre to the significant level a further

* The actual numerical value may vary slightly if the anti-human globulin titre is done by a different method, especially if the proportion of serum dilution to red cells is varied.

sample should be taken one week later and if the rise is maintained the question of early induction will arise.

It will be appreciated that unless there is a history of stillbirth and/or neonatal death, it is solely when the anti-human globulin and P.A. titres are high (64 or over) and especially if they are rising that premature induction should be considered.

The titration of maternal antibodies at delivery and ten days post-partum also makes possible the selection of high titre donors of Rh typing serum. This is not of immediate benefit to the mother and baby concerned but without such sera, freely given by mothers who have seen the effects of hæmolytic disease on their own children, none of the ante-natal Rh testing, nor the treatment of infants with hæmolytic disease, nor even the provision of Rh negative blood would be possible.

Prognosis and Handling of Case Based on Previous History

If there is no previous history of antibody formation or hæmolytic disease at a previous pregnancy the present infant may be mildly or severely affected, even stillborn. When there is a previous mildly affected baby needing no treatment, the present infant is less likely to be severely affected. When there is a previous severely affected or stillborn infant the prognosis is bad and induction as soon as the infant is viable, usually between 34–36 weeks, gives the best hope of survival.

Intra-uterine Transfusion

The latest mode of treatment for hæmolytic disease of the new-born is by intra-uterine transfusion. This is normally only attempted when the prognosis is bad. The assessment is based on previous obstetric history, *i.e.* a stillbirth or neonatal death, on anti-human globulin titre, *i.e.* a titre of 64 or over at 28th week of pregnancy or beforehand and on the results of examination of liquor amnii obtained by amniocentesis. The basic principle of the spectrophotometric method (*see* technique 25.8) is to measure the quantity of bilirubinoid pigments present, making adjustment for hæmoglobin and background opacity. If the height of the spectral absorption curve at 450 mμ is measured above a line drawn to the curve from 365 mμ and 550 mμ this gives a direct measure of bilirubin as this "tangent" corresponds to the absorption expected if no bilirubin were present. This height is known as the optical density deviation. Typical curves are shown in Fig. 25.1(a)–(d). The pigment peaks shrink with increasing maturity due to a fall in protein and therefore in bilirubin levels. It is important therefore to have an exact knowledge of maturity to assess the significance of any optical density deviation.

Figure 25.1(e) is Liley's diagram for the interpretation of the significance of optical density deviation in relation to weeks of gestation.

Figure 25.1(a) shows an optical density deviation of 0·32 at 22½ weeks. On Liley's diagram this suggests a severely affected infant. Figure 25.1(b) shows no optical density deviation and was associated with a normal infant. Figure 25.1(c) and (d) are from the same case, in (c) the amniotic fluid was coloured with hæmoglobin pigments giving a peak at 400—this makes the "tangential" line difficult to draw and the optical density deviation not so reliable—for what it is worth it suggests a normal or mildly affected infant (dev. 0·035 at 34 weeks), the sample taken one week later was uncontaminated and gave a deviation of 0·08 this plotted onto Liley's diagram prognosed a mildly affected infant, which was in fact the case.

When the deviation prior to 32 weeks is sufficient to bring it into the shaded portion of Fig. 25.1(e) it is an indication for intra-uterine transfusion, after 32 weeks a high deviation suggests the advisability of immediate induction.

Specimens of amniotic fluid should be protected from light because bilirubin is photosensitive. The yellow colour of amniotic fluid results from the presence of closely related bilirubinoid pigments which makes biochemical estimation inferior to spectrophotometric assay. A modification was suggested by Alvey (1964); he measured the absorption at 454 and 574 mμ as the extinction coefficient of oxyhæmoglobin is identical at these wavelengths. The difference in the two readings he called the "Bilirubin Index." Using this method he claims to be able to subdivide his cases into three categories according to the levels obtained and to prognosticate an unaffected, mildly affected or severely affected infant accordingly.

The tests on the amniotic fluid are the most informative especially when the husband is heterozygous. The past history may be bad and the titre high and even rising but if there is no peak at 450 mμ and no bilirubin in the amniotic fluid this indicates that the child is Rh negative and not in need of treatment (*see* Liley, 1963a). The technique of intra-uterine transfusion was evolved by Liley (1963b). There are several modifications, one in fairly general use is that of Holman and Karnicki (1964). A needle is inserted into the fœtal abdominal cavity, the position being checked by X-ray.

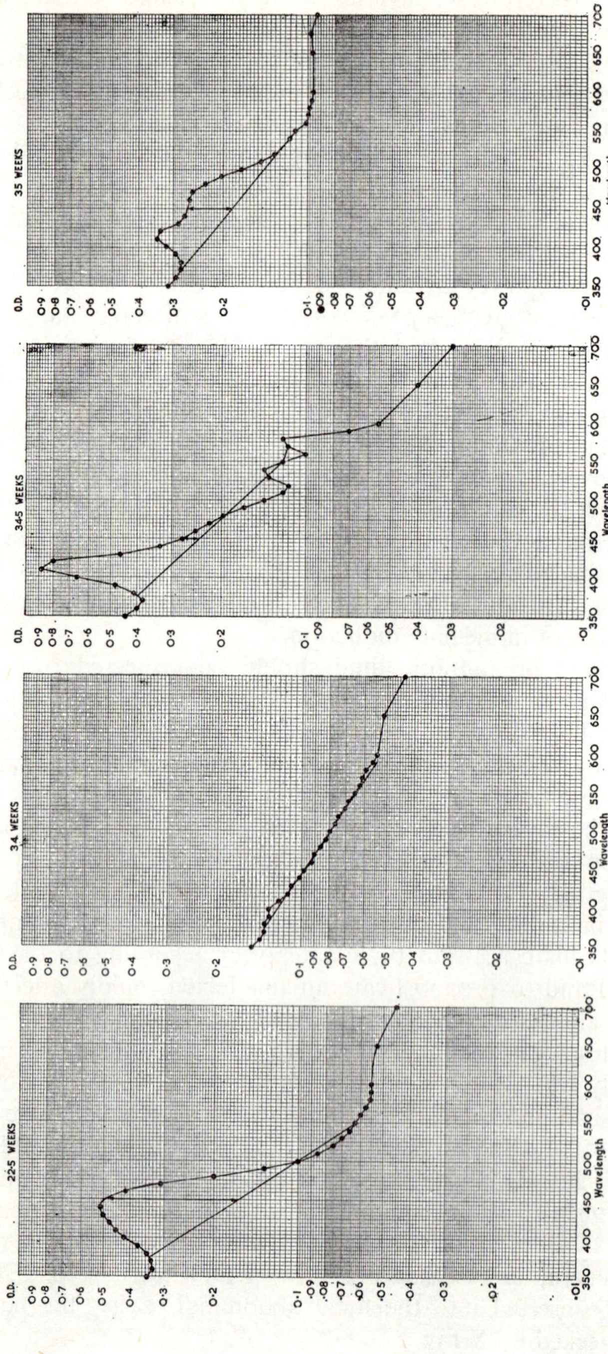
22·5 WEEKS
34 WEEKS
34·5 WEEKS
35 WEEKS
O.D.
Wavelength
350
400
450
500
550
600
650
700
(a)
(b)
(c)
(d)

(*a*) Curve showing optical density deviation of amniotic fluid where the infant was severely affected with hæmolytic disease.

(*b*) Normal curve of optical density (infant Rh negative).

(*c*) Curve showing difficulty in finding optical density deviation due to hæmoglobin pigments.

(*d*) Curve showing optical density deviation of amniotic fluid where the infant was mildly affected with hæmolytic disease (same case as (*c*)).

(*e*) Significance of optical density deviation at various periods of gestation (after Liley).

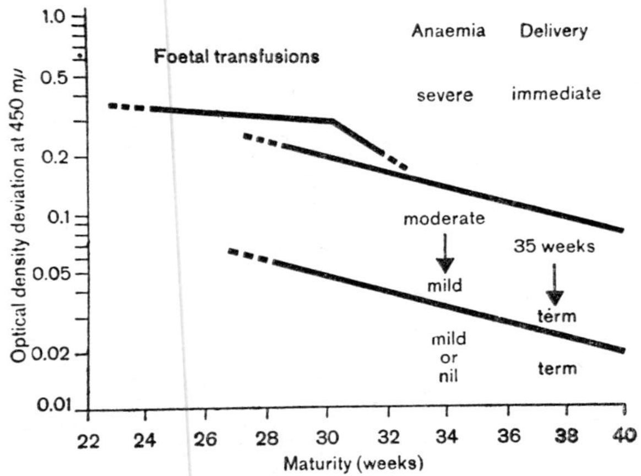

(*e*)

FIG. 25.1.

About 100 ml. of fresh blood is transfused. Most workers use group O Rh negative blood for the intra-uterine transfusion, but others use Rh negative blood of the same ABO group as the mother. In either case the blood is direct matched with the maternal serum. Possibly group O Rh negative cells suspended in AB plasma are the ideal as these avoid giving A or B blood to an O baby on the one hand, or anti-A and anti-B to an A or B baby on the other. When a sample of amniotic fluid is available the ABO group of the infant can be determined by inhibition technique on the spun down tissue cells in the fluid and the blood given can be of the same ABO group as the infant.

Intra-uterine transfusion is usually performed not later than the 32nd week of pregnancy. The procedure is often repeated two weeks later. Delivery is usually at about 36th week of pregnancy often by lower segment Cæsarean section.

When the cord blood is tested it may well be found to be almost entirely adult blood and type as Rh negative with a negative or only weakly positive direct anti-human globulin reaction. In spite of this the infant may need exchange transfusion, the criteria being falling hæmoglobin and/or rising serum bilirubin.

The infant should be tested at about the age of 6 months to determine its true group and Rh phenotype.

Prevention of Iso-immunisation by Injection of Anti-D Antibodies

To prevent an Rh negative woman from ever producing Rh antibodies is, of course, the ideal way of preventing hæmolytic disease of the fœtus. It has been found from experiments using male volunteers that immunisation can be prevented if injected Rh positive cells are destroyed by Rh antibody injected within 72 hours (Finn *et al.*, 1961) (Gorman *et al.*, 1964). The next step was to see whether injection of anti-D prevented antibody formation in Rh negative women following pregnancy with a Rh positive infant.

Clarke (1968) in a review article on the results of several years work showed that a high degree of protection was obtained using concentrated purified IgG anti-D antibodies. It is now standard practice to protect Rh negative women in this way. At delivery an estimate is made of the number of fœtal cells in the maternal circulation. This is done by an elution technique based on the method devised by Betke and Kleihauer (1958) the modification we find most satisfactory is used by Shepherd from the variation proposed by Nierhaus and Betke (1968), it is given in technique

No. 25.7. If any fœtal cells are seen IgG is given to the mother; at present the recommended dosage is 2 ml. containing 200 μg. for 1–5 cells per 50 low power fields, and this dose can be doubled or even trebled if larger numbers of fœtal cells are detected. If the infant is ABO incompatible with the maternal serum any fœtal cells entering the maternal circulation are usually promptly destroyed therefore it is not necessary to give anti-D. It is however advisable to look for fœtal cells as if there is a large spill into the maternal circulation it may be a wise precaution to give anti-D to speed the destruction of the fœtal cells. At present in England Rh negative women are only receiving anti-D after their first and second Rh positive infant but as more anti-D becomes available it is probable that they can be protected whatever their parity.

The anti-D used for injection comes from the following sources, (*a*) from women who have produced it as the result of pregnancies, some of them giving donations of satisfactory titre for many years after the causative pregnancy, (*b*) from older women, and (*c*) men who already have a weak Rh antibody—which can be stimulated by injection of Rh positive cells, and (*d*) from male volunteers immunised to produce an antibody *de novo*.

The titre in the original serum must be at least 64 by albumin technique (in many cases it is of course much higher). The sera are pooled and the concentrated IgG prepared by a Swiss variation of the Cohn fractionation technique.

It seems likely that hæmolytic disease due to anti-D will within the foreseeable future become extremely rare. For the next twenty years or so, of course, cases will continue to occur in families where the mother already has Rh antibodies. A few cases will also occur where the spillage of fœtal cells and the immunisation of the mother has occurred some weeks prior to delivery or where the number of fœtal cells in the maternal serum at delivery has been too large for the dose of anti-D given. There may be other factors which would prevent treatment.

Some fascinating new work on a natural inhibitor of Rh antibodies deserves mention (Guimbretiere and Guimbretiere, 1969).

Of 193 Rh negative women with anti-D, 31 showed a disappearance of Rh antibodies. In each case an inhibitory factor in Rh serum was found. When 155 Rh negative women who had given birth to Rh positive children without the development of antibodies were tested, 100 were shown to possess an Rh antibody inhibitor. Nine of these women had had more than five Rh positive children. When a search for an inhibitor was made among 100 male blood donors, none of them showed inhibitory power.

The Rh inhibitor was demonstrated experimentally by titrating selected anti-D sera (titres adjusted to about 1 in 15) using the serum to be tested for its inhibitory power as a diluent. When an inhibitor was present such titres were usually reduced to 0. The best results were obtained with trypsin treated red cells suspended in a veronal acetate buffer at pH 7·35. Surprisingly it was found during the course of the experiments that sera containing inhibitors did not inhibit all anti-D sera against which they were tested but displayed a constant pattern of inhibition—so constant that they could be divided into three types. In 1964 Freiesleben and Jensen described an anti-D which could be inhibited by a factor found in all human sera. This may be similar but is not identical with the three types described above.

Serological Testing of Father

The father should be tested for ABO group and for Rh sub-type. A knowledge of his ABO blood group (and that of the mother) will enable the laboratory to have suitable blood standing by for the infant. (*See* below.)

The so-called Rh "genotyping" of husbands is, of course, really phenotyping with the available sera. As explained in Chapter 12 laboratory tests cannot in many cases determine an individual's precise genotype; it can only determine the phenotype or as it is often called the probable genotype. This is why most laboratories when asked to perform an Rh genotyping test will report the actual reactions obtained followed by the comment "probable genotype" or phenotype.

When a woman has developed antibodies as the result of stimulation by a fœtal antigen inherited from the father, the question that needs to be answered is whether this man is homo- or heterozygous for the antigen concerned. When the antigen is, for example, C or E the question can be answered accurately by the use of anti-C and anti-c or anti-E and anti-e sera. In the vast majority of cases, however, the antigen in question is D and here no simple test is possible; it is, however, possible by testing with anti-C, anti-D, anti-E, and anti-c, with the addition in some cases of anti-e, to obtain an idea as to the chances that any given individual is homo- or heterozygous with regard to D. In Table 11.3 (Chapter 11) the Rh sub-groups are arranged in phenotype groupings determined by these sera and there it can be seen that some phenotypes comprise many genotypes and most phenotypes include homozygous DD and heterozygous Dd genotypes. In each phenotype, however, there is always one genotype that is

Table 25.2

Interpretation of the Rh D Positive Phenotypes in Terms of DD (Homozygous) and Dd (Heterozygous)

Reactions with anti-sera					Phenotype	Genotypes				Relative frequency of Heterozygous: Homozygous	Relative frequency of Heterozygous: Homozygous for whole phenotype
C	D	E	c	e		Most frequent	% of phenotype	Next most frequent	% of phenotype		
+	+	−	+		R_1r	R_1r(Dd)	93·7	R_1R_o(DD)	6·2	15 : 1	15 : 1
+	+	−	−		R_1R_1	R_1R_1(DD)	95·5	R_1R'(Dd)	4·5	1 : 21	1 : 21
+	+	+	+		R_1R_2	R_1R_2(DD)	88·4	R_1R''(Dd)	7·5	1 : 12	1 : 8
−	+	+	+	+	R_2r	R_2r(Dd)	93·3	R_2R_o(DD)	6·2	15 : 1	15 : 1
−	+	+	+	−	R_2R_2	R_2R_2(DD)	85·6	R_2R''(Dd)	14·4	1 : 6	1 : 6
−	+	−	+		R_or	R_or(Dd)	96·8	R_oR_o(DD)	3·2	30 : 1	30 : 1
+	+	+	−		R_1R_z	R_1R_z(DD)	97·1	$R'R_z$(Dd)	2·4	1 : 40	1 : 41

more common than the rest and, with one exception, among these common genotypes d is associated with c.

In Table 25.2 the probable genotype is given for each phenotype followed by the next most probable as well as the percentage occurrence of each of these and whether each one is homo- or heterozygous for D. The figures given for the relative frequencies in each phenotype apply to a random population and are of course applicable to husbands of Rh negative women who have not formed antibodies. The husbands of Rh negative women who have formed Rh antibodies are a selected rather than a random population. This means that there is a much higher probability of the husband being homozygous with regard to D than is suggested by the figures given here. In any individual case, however, if the most probable genotype is one heterozygous for D it is quite justifiable to consider that there is the chance of a D negative unaffected child resulting from the present or any subsequent pregnancy. Where the parents are very anxious to have another child but are hesitant because the husband appears to be homozygous for D it may help to test his parents and any surviving children he may have; the finding of a D negative parent or a D negative child would prove that he must be heterozygous for the D antigen.

Serological Testing of Baby

The tests on the baby's cord blood include: (*a*) ABO grouping; (*b*) Rh typing with anti-D sera; (*c*) direct anti-human globulin test; (*d*) full antibody test on cord serum; (*e*) red cells against maternal serum by saline, albumin and indirect anti-human globulin techniques. Before any tests are attempted, the cells must be carefully washed three times. Difficulty is sometimes experienced if the samples of blood are contaminated with Wharton's jelly which often causes aggregation of the red cells. When this occurs it may be necessary to obtain a fresh sample by heel prick. Contamination with Wharton's jelly can be avoided if the sample is obtained by vene-puncture from a placental vein.

ABO Grouping. Anti-A and anti-B agglutinins do not develop until a few months after birth; any such agglutinins that may be detected in the serum of the cord are of maternal origin having traversed the placenta, and are usually present in low titre only. Thus it is impossible to rely upon serum grouping to confirm the results obtained by testing the infant's red cells with anti-A and anti-B grouping sera. It is, therefore, recommended that the infant's red cells be grouped by two methods.

Rh Typing. The red cells of babies present a special problem in

Rh typing. Firstly, if the cells are not completely free of Wharton's jelly, any anti-serum containing bovine albumin may give false positive results. Secondly, both false positive and false negative reactions may be obtained when the red cells have been sensitised *in vivo* by a maternal antibody. An extra control when typing the red cells of babies is a tube containing equal volumes of the infant's washed cells suspended in AB serum and bovine albumin. If this shows clumping after being incubated for the same time as the D typing tests, it will be necessary either to obtain a fresh sample from the baby, or in cases where the direct anti-human globulin test is positive to attempt elution of antibody from the red cell surface (technique No. 25.2).

It is very rarely that any C or E determinants which the cells may possess will be blocked as well; typical findings in these cases are negative or indeterminate reactions with anti-D sera associated with strong positive reactions with anti-CD or anti-DE sera. In these circumstances also the antibodies should be eluted from the red cell surface.

Direct Anti-human Globulin Test. It is advisable to test with more than one anti-human globulin reagent or with a single reagent at more than one dilution. Occasionally a prozone is noted; with certain concentrations of antibody coating the red cells, a negative reaction or weak positive is obtained. The use of a different reagent or increasing the dilution of the same reagent will probably give a positive result.

Full Antibody Test on Cord Serum. In cases in which the maternal serum contains an atypical antibody, this may or may not be found free in the infant's serum. A high titre of incomplete antibodies in the cord serum is sometimes associated with slow recovery from hæmolytic disease. In spite of treatment by exchange transfusion, some remaining antibody carries on the destruction of the infant's own red cells.

Red Cells Against the Maternal Serum by Saline, Albumin, and Indirect Anti-human Globulin Techniques. Tests against the maternal serum are pertinent since the infant's red cells must contain the antigen responsible for the maternal stimulus and therefore if these tests are negative it is fairly safe to assume that the case is not one of hæmolytic disease. When a rare, or "private" antigen, not contained in any of the standard cells is the cause of the immunisation, the infant's and father's red cells will be the only ones capable of revealing the corresponding antibody. Obviously if there is an ABO incompatibility between the maternal serum and the infant's red cells these tests will not provide any information about possible maternal atypical antibodies. In such cases, if the clinical and hæmatological pictures strongly suggest hæmolytic disease, other antibody tests will have to be exhaustive.

Prognosis for Future Pregnancies

(*a*) *Mothers with Rh Antibodies.* Once a mother has formed antibodies and had one child with hæmolytic disease she tends to go on having affected children if her husband is homozygous, and the disease tends to show itself in its more severe forms with each successive affected child. However this is not always so; occasionally a D positive child who is only slightly affected is born after several children who suffered severely. Of course, if the husband is heterozygous there is always the chance of a normal D negative child following one with hæmolytic disease.

(*b*) *Mothers with no Rh Antibodies.* An Rh negative woman will almost always have one, if not several, Rh positive children before she produces antibodies which make her subsequent Rh positive children at risk. In this connexion it should be remembered, especially by those who come into contact with women who are worried by the fact that they are Rh negative, that almost all Rh negative women will have a normal first and second baby. In fact, only 1 in 30 will ever have a child affected with hæmolytic disease. Moreover, a third of the babies even of mothers who have Rh antibodies are either normal or so lightly affected that they do not require treatment; and of the remainder the majority recover uneventfully after treatment. As transfusion of Rh positive blood to an Rh negative individual acts as a more efficient stimulus to antibody production than an Rh positive fœtus, it is essential that all Rh negative women of child-bearing age, and all Rh negative girls from infancy upwards, requiring transfusion should receive only Rh negative blood. Otherwise it is most probable that they will form Rh antibodies at their first pregnancy with an Rh positive fœtus. Providing, however, the Rh negative woman is untransfused or transfused only with Rh negative blood it is extremely unlikely that Rh antibodies will be formed as the result of a first pregnancy, which will at the worst merely sensitise the mother to produce antibodies during a subsequent pregnancy.

As stated above, while it is yet too soon to be sure whether the prophylactic treatment with purified anti-D gamma globulin will be efficacious in every case, it is probable that the prognosis for the Rh negative woman has been improved so that of those without Rh antibodies less than 1 per cent will ever make them.

Hæmolytic Disease Due to Blood Group Antigens Other than D

The Other Antigens of the Rh System

Of the other antigens and antibodies of the Rh system c and anti-c have been most often incriminated as causing hæmolytic disease of the newborn, but as all the Rh antibodies are "warm" antibodies active at 37°C they must all, if found, be regarded as likely to cause the disease.

The routine antibody screening, as has been explained in Chapter 13, should detect and identify any of the Rh antibodies, although their specificity will need confirmation, *see* Tables 13.1 and 13.2. If the mother is Rh positive, her Rh sub-type should be determined as well as that of the father. Blood of suitable Rh sub-type can then be selected for the baby. In addition, at least two pints of compatible blood should be held in readiness for the mother, since, in the event of an A.P.H. or P.P.H., she will need at short notice blood of known Rh sub-type which is not normally available in the hospital.

If any of the Rh antibodies (*e.g.* anti-c) is detected at the first antibody testing (*i.e.* at about 12–15th week of pregnancy), the mother must be tested at regular intervals as if she was Rh negative with antibodies. If the antibody is only detectable by enzyme techniques throughout pregnancy, the baby will almost certainly be clinically normal. If it becomes detectable by anti-human globulin techniques it must be titrated and in the main the prognosis will be related to titre as for anti-D. There is however a tendency for the disease process to be less severe especially if the antibody is anti-E. Should the anti-human globulin titre reach 128 however, this is an indication for induction whatever the antibody specificity.

Sometimes the antibody is not detectable early in pregnancy and as the mother is Rh positive she may not be tested again. In any case where the infant is jaundiced and the mother is Rh positive, Rh sub-typing and tests for all Rh antibodies should be an essential part of the investigation especially if the direct anti-human globulin test on the baby's cells is positive.

ABO

Hæmolytic disease due to ABO incompatibility between maternal serum and fœtal red cells is not common although its frequency is next to that due to Rh.

It is not unusual for the first child in a family to be affected with the disease. This is not surprising when it is considered that anti-A and anti-B agglutinins are naturally occurring. In view of the constant and the high incidence of hetero-specific pregnancies it might be expected that hæmolytic disease due to ABO incompatibility would be of common occurrence. That it is not, is thought to be due to the presence of soluble A and B substances in the fœtal fluids which neutralise the anti-A and anti-B antibodies before they can attack the fœtal red cells. This, however, cannot be the whole story since there is no marked association of the disease with babies who are non-secretors.

The disease is often mild; but can be severe and may even include kernicterus.

The problem for the serologist is that of proving conclusively that a given case is one caused by ABO incompatibility. The mere presence of anti-A or anti-B antibodies in high titre in the maternal serum, even of the immune type, does not justify their incrimination as a cause of the disease for such high titre antibodies can be present in association with a normal baby. Moreover, the direct anti-human globulin test may be only weakly positive or even negative although the infant is showing definite symptoms. In any case it is well worth attempting an elution and identification of the sensitising antibody. (Technique No. 21.3.)

The finding of anti-A or anti-B in the eluate from an A or B baby respectively confirms the diagnosis of ABO hæmolytic disease. It should be pointed out however, that antibody can be eluated in some cases from the cells of a clinically normal infant. This parallels the finding of a Rh positive clinically normal infant with a positive direct Coombs when the maternal antibody is anti-D.

A full investigation of the serum by technique No. 21.1 to eliminate the possibility of there being an atypical antibody which might be causing the disease must be made before assuming that it is due to anti-A or anti-B. If these results are negative and the maternal serum can be shown to have the typical features of an immune serum it is safe to treat the case as one caused by ABO incompatibility, whether or not the direct anti-human globulin test is positive. This means that the infant if requiring a transfusion should receive washed group O red cells resuspended in AB plasma since it is undesirable to give the baby further anti-A or anti-B antibody incompatible with its own red cells. The direct-matching is performed in the usual manner (technique No. 22.4) using maternal and not infant's serum. Thus, even in the event of the disease not being due to ABO incompatibility but to some other maternal antibody, blood compatible with this and therefore suitable for transfusion to the infant will have been given.

It will be appreciated from the comparative rarity of ABO hæmolytic disease compared with the frequency of the group combinations in which it is likely to occur, notably O mother and A or B infant, that only a few maternal anti-A or anti-B antibodies are capable of causing the disease.

It has been shown that when the child suffers from ABO hæmolytic disease the maternal serum will show immune characteristics including lysis of A or B cells and in particular will have a high titre incomplete IgG component. This cannot be determined directly because of the presence of agglutinin which masks the incomplete antibody. Witebsky (1948) described a method by which the agglutinin was partially neutralised by A or B substance and the "immune" antibody estimated by titration in human AB serum. This test has been modified by testing the partially neutralised serum by the indirect anti-human globulin test. A further modification using pure anti-IgG reagent has been suggested recently (Polley *et al.*, 1965).

This latter test (technique No. 25.5a) is positive in almost all severe cases of ABO hæmolytic disease. On the other hand it is less satisfactory as a prognostic test—we use a modified version as a screening test (technique No. 25.5b)—but many cases where the baby does not need transfusion are giving values in the same range as is found in cases of hæmolytic disease.

Recently a new test has been introduced by Sherwood (1969) by which a solution containing the IgG anti-A and/or anti-B antibodies can be prepared free of IgM or IgA antibodies. This method absorbs out the IgM and IgA fractions with DEAE cellulose in a buffer of 0·02 molarity at pH 8 (technique 25.6).

Preliminary work using this test shows that it is the most satisfactory both for the prognosis and diagnosis of ABO hæmolytic disease (Boorman *et al.*, 1969).

Another test which attempted to prognose the clinical condition is based upon the remarkable fact that immune anti-A sera react with group AB pig cells (Winstanley *et al.* 1957). (All pigs have a B antigen but some have also an A antigen.) This antibody called anti-A_p has been studied by Tovey *et al.* (1962) who found it to occur as a lysin in 453 of 10,647 O sera but only 32 of the infants had hæmolytic disease, of which 14 suffered sufficiently severely to necessitate transfusion. A further absorption test (A/A test) was devised which was more satisfactory. The same team has recently suggested a further test (the N.A. test), which also relies on absorption, this time using secretor saliva; the method of Sherwood (1969) (technique 25.6) is therefore more reliable.

Immune anti-A antibodies are also characterised by a high titre with A_x cells. This certainly selects high titre immune sera but in over half of the cases this is not associated with hæmolytic disease. A high titre with A_x cells is however often found where the infant is affected.

Voak (1968) showed by elution experiments that ABO hæmolytic disease was associated with high titre of maternal IgG antibody regardless of whether the antibody was monospecific anti-A or anti-B, a mixture of monospecific and cross reacting antibodies (*see* Chapter 32) or entirely cross reacting. He thus differs from Wiener *et al.* (1955 and 1966) who thought that cross reacting antibodies (called by them anti-C) were almost entirely responsible for the disease. Our experience agrees with that of Voak and we find that it is the IgG titre of the serum whether of a group O or a group A or B mother which is of critical importance in predicting or diagnosing ABO hæmolytic disease.

To summarise, if an infant is jaundiced it is likely to be due to ABO hæmolytic disease if some or all of the following criteria are present (listed in inverse order of significance).

1. Mother and baby ABO incompatible.
2. Mother group O and baby A or B.
3. Mother's serum lyses standard A or B cells and infant's cells.
4. Mother's serum contains anti-A_p lysin.
5. Mother's serum has a titre of 8 or over with A_x cells.
6. Positive A/A test or N.A. test (Gold *et al.*, 1969).
7. Mother's anti-human globulin titre using anti-IgG reagent in range 64–1,000 after neutralisation with a standard amount of A substance.
8. Mother's anti-human globulin titre 800 or over for anti-A and 400 or over for anti-B on the IgG fraction of the serum.

Other indications are a weak positive direct anti-human globulin test on infant's cells, saline suspended or papain or bromelin treated and the finding of free incompatible anti-A (or anti-B) in the infant's serum by saline or anti-human globulin techniques at 37°C.

Other Blood Group Systems

Hæmolytic disease caused by the less common antibodies in no way differs in its manifestations and treatment from that caused by Rh. The crux of the investigation is the demonstration and identification of the causative antibody and if treatment is needed, the selection of compatible blood.

It is worth remarking—since at times serologists, however experienced, become obsessed with the consideration of one blood group system to the exclusion of others which may be relevant—that infants who are Rh negative must always receive Rh negative blood whatever rare and fascinating antibody the maternal serum may contain.

Treatment of Infants Suffering from Hæmolytic Disease

Not all infants suffering from hæmolytic disease will require treatment. In any assessment of a given case, clinical, hæmatological and serological findings must all be considered. The decision to transfuse cannot depend upon positive serological findings alone, since these bear little or no relation to the severity of the disease process. On the other hand, the finding of anæmia (cord hæmoglobin below 95 per cent) and/or raised serum bilirubin (above 5 mgm./100 ml. approximately) are strong indicators for treatment. It must be realised too, that some cases in which no treatment is necessary at birth, may deteriorate during the first few days of life.

Treatment is by transfusion of blood compatible with the maternal antibody causing the disease. This means that where the mother is D negative, the infant D positive and the atypical antibody in the mother is anti-D, D negative blood (*i.e.* Rh negative cde.cde) is chosen for the transfusion.

The direct-match should be performed, wherever possible, with the mother's serum. Full details as to the choice of blood and the mode of direct-matching are given below. (Technique No. 25.3.)

The type of transfusion given may be either "simple" or "exchange". In a simple transfusion about 200 ml. of blood is given through a suitable vein; the internal saphenous is often chosen. It is now common practice to treat the infant by exchange transfusion. This is usually done within 24 hours of birth through the umbilical vein by means of a polythene catheter and an apparatus (several adaptations are in use) which will allow of about 10–15 ml. of blood being withdrawn from the infant and then 10–15 ml. of blood from the bottle being introduced through the catheter. The process is repeated until at least 90 per cent replacement of the infant's blood for the transfused blood is obtained. An accurate "input and output" record must be kept so that the pitfalls of, on the one hand, a reduced blood volume (which would lead to hæmodilution) and, on the other hand, an over-loaded circulation can be avoided. In order to avoid giving too much diluent (540 ml. of stored blood contain 120 ml. of anticoagulant) about 150–180 ml. of the supernatant plasma is removed from the blood, so that it is slightly concentrated. Two bottles of blood will be needed to obtain at least a 90 per cent exchange.

After treatment, hæmoglobin and serum bilirubin estimations should be made at regular intervals. If these are unsatisfactory a further transfusion may be necessary.

Selection and Direct-matching of Blood for Transfusion of Babies Affected with Hæmolytic Disease

Choice of Blood. The blood chosen should be of the same ABO blood group as the baby and should not contain the antigen corresponding to the maternal antibody which has caused the disease. Where the disease is due to an ABO incompatibility it is obvious that the two sections of this rule are in conflict; the second being the most important takes precedence and the blood given

Table 25.3

Selection of Blood for Transfusion of Infant

ABO grouping of Rh negative blood to have ready cross matched against maternal serum for possible exchange transfusion of infant for the ABO mother-father combinations.

Blood group of father	Blood group of mother			
	O	A	B	AB
O	O	O and A	O and B	A and B
A	O (A)*	O and A	O and B (A)* (AB)*	A (B) (AB)
B	O (B)*	O and A (B)* (AB)*	O and B	B (A) (AB)
AB	A* and B*	A (B)* (AB)*	B (A)* (AB)*	A and AB (B)

( ) Indicates that blood of this group is only rarely needed.
* Indicates that blood of this group cannot be cross matched against maternal serum.

is group O which has been washed to prevent the transfusion of anti-A and anti-B antibodies.

The blood used should be as fresh as possible and certainly not more than 5 days old as this will give minimal initial destruction and maximal survival in the infant's circulation. If the baby needs a transfusion it is probable that this will be given in the first few hours of life, it is convenient therefore to have suitable blood standing by before the baby is born. If the causative antibody is identified it will be simple to choose blood which is compatible with it. In the majority of cases it will be anti-D and the type of the blood to be transfused will be Rh negative (cde.cde). The ABO blood group needed, however, is not quite so easy to prognose. Table 25.3 shows how a knowledge of the ABO blood groups of mother and father will enable a determination of the possible groups of the baby to be made. If a sample of amniotic fluid has been obtained for spectroscopic investigation it can also be tested for the infants ABO group using technique No. 8.2. Bearing in mind that there is rarely an ABO blood group incompatibility between the maternal serum and the infant's erythrocytes in cases of hæmolytic disease of the fœtus due to Rh incompatibility, it is possible to have Rh negative blood of one, or at most two, blood groups standing by, which will in all but 3 per cent of cases not only be of the suitable ABO blood group but also compatible with the maternal ABO antibodies, if any. This latter point is important as the direct-match wherever possible should be performed with maternal serum.

Techniques

Technique No. 25.1. Direct anti-human globulin test on infant's red cells

A few drops of the infant's red cells are washed four times in saline. One drop of packed washed cells is then mixed with one drop each of two different anti-human globulin reagents (or with two different dilutions of a single reagent) on an opalescent tile. The usual controls necessary for such tests, *i.e.* each reagent with: (*a*) D positive red cells weakly sensitised with incomplete anti-D (*b*) D negative red cells treated with the same anti-D (*c*) unsensitised cells of group AB, and (*d*) the infant's own red cells mixed with saline, are included.

The tests are set out and read as described in technique No. 10.3a.

Technique No. 25.2. Rh typing of infant's red cells blocked with incomplete antibodies

The first procedure is the elution of antibody from the infant's red cells. This is done by technique No. 21.3. A temperature of 45°C is normally adequate for the dissociation of sufficient antibody for the cells to give satisfactory positive reactions with anti-D typing serum.

The heat-treated red cells are used for Rh typing (technique No. 10.1) preferably using saline anti-D.

If it is desired to show that the antibody recovered from the infant's red cells is anti-D it may be necessary to heat the cells at 56°C to obtain in the eluate sufficient antibody for identification.

Technique No. 25.3. Direct-matching of blood for baby

Blood of the baby's ABO group is selected, two bottles for an exchange or a half bottle for a simple transfusion.

Immediately after delivery a sample will have been taken from the mother and it is the serum from this sample which is used for the direct-match. The blood is direct-matched against the maternal serum by technique No. 22.4.

As discussed above there will be 3 per cent of cases where it is not possible to direct-match the selected blood against the maternal sample because of an ABO incompatibility. The procedure here is to direct-match using a potent serum of the same specificity as the maternal serum. Alternatively group O cells suspended in AB plasma direct-matched against the maternal serum can be used for the transfusion.

Technique No. 25.4. Partial absorption technique

Preparation of Hæmolysed Red Cells

Heparinised or citrated blood is collected from group O Rh positive donors. The cells are carefully washed three times in a large volume of saline, pooled and packed. It is a good idea to include several common Rh genotypes, *e.g.* CDe.CDe and CDe.cDE donors. The cells are finally packed by centrifuging at 3,000 r.p.m. for 30 minutes. An accurate 25 per cent saline suspension is made which is divided into 2 ml. samples. These are frozen at —20°C and used as required.

The Test

Equal volumes of a 1 in 4 dilution of maternal serum and thawed hæmolysed red cells are mixed and left at room temperature for 15 minutes. The mixture is serially diluted, at the same time comparative dilutions of the maternal serum are prepared (remembering that the mixture corresponds to a $\frac{1}{8}$ dilution of the original maternal serum). A range of dilutions from $\frac{1}{8}$ to $\frac{1}{1,024}$ is normally sufficient.

An equal volume of a 5 per cent suspension of standard Rh positive red cells are added to each dilution and the tests incubated at 37°C for 1 hour. They are then washed (as in technique No. 10.3a). It is probably easier to obtain standard results if the final stage of the anti-human globulin reaction is performed in tubes rather than on slides or tiles. Two volumes of anti-human globulin (*i.e.* excess) are added to each cell button and either allowed to stand for ½ hour or immediately centrifuged. The reactions are then read macro-, and microscopically.

For interpretation of results see above and the original papers.

Technique No. 25.5a. Indirect anti-globulin test on partly neutralised anti-A (or anti-B) in maternal (usually Group O) sera

The neutralisation stage is devised so as to add an amount of A substance which just fails to reduce the titre of IgG antibody while greatly reducing the titre of IgM(19s) anti-A. For this purpose a 1 in 800 dilution of a 2 mg. per ml. preparation of purified human A substance is usually satisfactory. Alternatively the inhibition of the IgM antibodies can be effected with whole group A_1 blood. Equal volumes of blood in A.C.D. from four different A_1 donors are pooled.

Serial doubling dilutions of the serum are prepared and to four volumes of each dilution are added either one volume of a 1 in 800 dilution of human A substance (2 mg. per ml.) and one volume of a 20 per cent suspension of washed A_1 red cells or one volume of pooled A_1 whole blood.

The mixtures are then incubated at 37°C for 1½ hours, the cells washed three times and a 20 per cent suspension prepared in saline. One drop of the washed cells is mixed with one drop of saline on an opal tile and a second drop is mixed with a drop of anti-IgG globulin serum. The degree of agglutination is read and the test is regarded as significant if the titre using the anti-IgG is 64 or over and it shows a definite enhancement over the saline titre—the higher the titre the more likely the infant is to suffer from ABO hæmolytic disease. If the titres in saline and anti-IgG are both equally high it is not possible to assess the amount of anti-IgG type antibody present and the test is inconclusive.

Technique No. 25.5b. Anti-IgG globulin screening test for high titre anti-A or anti-B

The principles of the screening test are identical with those of technique 25.5a. Three dilutions are selected so that the sera can be divided into low, medium and high titres. For ante-natal testing this simple division is probably sufficient, low titre cases can be disregarded. Medium titres are checked at 34th week and delivery for any rise and high titres are regarded as prognostic of hæmolytic disease if the present infant proves to be ABO incompatible.

The dilutions chosen are 1 in 50, 1 in 100 and 1 in 200. Four volumes of each dilution are mixed with one volume of the 1 in 800 dilution of A substance (2 mg. per ml.) and one volume of a 20 per cent suspension of A_1 red cells added. The mixtures are incubated for 1½ hours at 37°C, the cells washed three times and a 20 per cent suspension made in saline. One drop of the washed cells is tested with saline and another with anti-IgG and the results compared as in technique No. 25.5a.

Technique No. 25.6. A short method for the preparation of a serum fraction containing the IgG antibodies

The technique is based on the well tried DEAE cellulose column chromatography technique (*see* Appendix IV), DEAE is equilibrated with the Sorensens phosphate buffer ph 8·0 and 0·02 M (*see* technique No. Appendix IV.1). This is conveniently done in a column by running about 2 litres of buffer down a 2 × 30 cm. column containing 5 gm. of DEAE cellulose (Whatman D.E.11), It is made up to 100 ml. with buffer, by blowing out into a measuring cylinder and adding buffer up to 100 ml.

0·1 ml. of serum is added to 2·2 ml. of the 5 per cent (w/v) DEAE cellulose solution (well mixed) in 1 × 5 cm. tubes. The tubes are stoppered and then slowly rotated (on for instance a matburn rotator) for 20 minutes at room temperature. After centrifugation, the supernatant is removed and made isotonic by the addition of 10 per cent saline (0·1 ml. to 1 ml. of supernatant).

The serum fraction is titrated by saline and anti-human globulin techniques at R.T. The doubling dilutions for the saline technique start with the neat fraction which represents approximately 1 in 25 dilution of the original serum.

The anti-human globulin technique consists of 4 volume doubling dilutions starting with saline in the first tube so that the initial dilution is 1 in 50. As titres less than 1 in 200 are not significant the first two tubes can be discarded. One volume of a 20 per cent suspension of packed cells is added to each tube. After 2 hours incubation at room temperature the tubes are washed twice (this is adequate as the first dilution is one in two hundred). The washed cells are tested with a broad spectrum anti-human globulin reagent at the optimum dilution for detection of IgG antibodies. It is not necessary (as it was in techniques No. 25.5(a) and (b)) to use a pure anti-IgG reagent). Titres of 800 and over almost invariably indicate that the infant, if ABO incompatible with the maternal serum, will be affected and suffer from hæmolytic disease of the newborn. Occasionally titres of 200 or 400 will be associated with an affected infant.

Technique No. 25.7

The demonstration of fœtal cells in the maternal circulation (modified from Nierhaus and Betke (1968)).

Reagents

80 per cent ethanol.

Stock solution A. 0·75 per cent hæmatoxylin in 96 per cent ethanol.

Stock solution B. 2·4 gm. $FeCl_3$ and 2·0 ml of 25 per cent HCl are made up to 100 ml. with double distilled water (our single distilled water appears to be satisfactory).

Elution solution. Two parts of A are mixed with one part of B and one part of 80 per cent ethanol to give a mixture of pH 1·5.

The solution can be used for up to six weeks, but after about 4–5 days it will require filtering as a precipitate of ferric chloride is formed. After filtration it is perfectly satisfactory for use.

Counterstain. Either 0·1 per cent erythrosin or 0·5 per cent aqueous eosin.

Method

Whole blood is diluted with an equal quantity of saline and used for making films. The slides are fixed in 80 per cent ethanol for 5 minutes at room temperature. They are thoroughly dried. They are then placed for 20 seconds in the elution solution, rinsed in distilled water and counter stained for 2 minutes. At least fifty fields are examined using a $\frac{1}{6}$ objective. The finding of any fœtal cells is an indication for treatment of the mother anti-D immuno-globulin.

Comment

This method produces good films with the fœtal cells easily distinguishable. The white cells, including lymphocytes, stain grey, the adult red cells appear as "ghost" cells while the fœtal cells stain bright red.

Technique No. 25.8. Examination of amniotic fluid for bilirubinoid pigments

The sample of amniotic fluid should be protected from light in transit to the laboratory *e.g.* kept in a dark bottle. If kept in the laboratory it should be placed in the refrigerator until it is tested. Usually undiluted fluid can be used but if there is a great deal of bilirubinoid pigments present it may be diluted with an equal part of distilled water. A glass cuvette of 1 cm. light path is filled and readings taken between 375 mμ and 700 mμ at 10 mμ intervals. These are plotted on two cycle logarithmic graph paper to give a curve similar to those shown in Fig. 25.1.

A line is drawn to touch the curve at 365 mμ and 500 mμ, this excludes bilirubin, and the height of the peak at 450 mμ above the line is measured. This gives the optical density deviation which is plotted on Liley's diagram (Fig. 25.1e) according to the week of gestation. The position of this point is an indication as to whether an intrauterine transfusion should be given, premature labour induced or the pregnancy allowed to proceed to term.

BIBLIOGRAPHY

ALVEY, J. P. (1964), "Obstetrical management of Rh incompatibility based on liquor amnii studies." *Amer. J. Obstet. Gynec.*, **90**, 769.

BETKE, K., and KLEIHAUER, E. (1958), "Fetaler und bleibender Blutfarbstoff in Erythrozyten und Erythroblasten von menschlichen Feten und Neugeborenen." *Blut*, **4**, 241.

BOORMAN, KATHLEEN E., SHERWOOD, F., and BATCHELOR, EUNICE (1970), "A preliminary report on the value of titrations of anti-A and anti-B IgG antibodies in serum fractions prepared by the short method using DEAE cellulose." (To be published.)

BOORMAN, KATHLEEN E., DODD, BARBARA E., and MOLLISON, P. L. (1942), "The clinical significance of the Rh factor." *Brit. med. J.*, **ii**, 535, 569.

BOORMAN, K. E. (1954), "The prognosis for the Rh negative woman." *Revue d'Hematologie*, **9**, 3, *bis* 475.

CLARKE, C. A. (1968), "Prevention of Rhesus iso-immunisation." *Lancet*, **2**, 1.

FINN, R., CLARKE, C. A., DONOHOE, W. T. A., MCCONNELL, R. B., SHEPPARD, P. M., LEHANE, D., and KULKE, W. (1961), "Experimental studies on the prevention of Rh hæmolytic disease." *Brit. Med. J.*, **i**, 1486–1490.

FREIESLEBEN, E., and JENSEN, K. G. (1964), "Inhibition of an anti-D by a normal serum factor." *Vox Sang.*, **9**, 65.

GOLD, E. R., FUDENBERG, H. H., and TOVEY, G. H. (1969), "Three stage screening test for ABO hæmolytic disease." *Int. Arch. Allergy*, **35**, 345.

GORMAN, J. G., FREDA, V. F., and POLLACK, W. (1964), "Prevention of iso-immunisation to the Rh factor using high titre anti-Rh gamma globulin." *Proc. Int. Soc. Blood Trans.*

GUIMBRETIERE, J., and GUIMBRETIERE, L. (1969), *Existence of a Natural Immunoprophylaxis in the Hæmolytic Disease of the Newborn.* Moscow: XII International Congress in Blood Transfusion.

HOLMAN, C. A., and KARNICKI, J. (1964), "Intra-Uterine Transfusion for Hæmolytic Disease of the Newborn." *Brit. Med. J.*, **ii**, 594.

LEVINE, P., BURNHAM, L., KATZIN, E. M., and VOGEL, P. (1941*c*), "The role of iso-immunisation in the pathogenesis of erythroblastosis fetalis." *Amer. J. Obstet. Gynec.*, **42**, 925.

LEVINE, P., KATZIN, E. M., and BURNHAM, L. (1941*a*), "Iso-immunisation in pregnancy, its possible bearing on the etiology of erythroblastosis fetalis." *J. Amer. med. Ass.*, **116**, 825.

LEVINE, P., and STETSON, R. E. (1939), "An unusual case of intra group agglutination." *J. Amer. med. Ass.*, **113,** 126.

LEVINE, P., VOGEL, P., KATZIN, E. M., and BURNHAM, L. (1941*b*), "Pathogenesis of erythroblastosis fetalis: statistical evidence." *Science*, **94,** 371.

LILEY, A. W. (1963a), "Errors in the assessment of hæmolytic disease from amniotic fluid." *Amer. J. Obstet. Gynec.*, **86,** 485.

LILEY, A. W. (1963b), "Intra-uterine Transfusion of Fœtus in Hæmolytic Disease." *Brit. Med. J.*, **ii,** 1107.

NIERHAUS, K., and BETKE, K. (1968), "Eine vereinfachte Modifikation der sauren Elution für die cytologische Darstellung von fetalem Hämoglobin." *Klin. Wschr.*, **46,** 47.

POLLEY, M., MOLLISON, P. L., ROSE, J., and WALKER, W. (1965), "A simple serological test for antibodies causing ABO-hæmolytic disease of the newborn." *Lancet*, **i,** 291.

POTTER, EDITH L. (1947), *Rh: Its Relation to Congenital Hæmolytic Disease and to Intra Group Transfusion Reactions.* Chicago: The Year Book Publishers.

SHERWOOD, F. (1970), "A short method for the estimation of IgG antibodies in serum." (To be published.)

TOVEY, G. H., LOCKYER, J. W., BLADES, A. N., and FLAVELL, M. C. G. (1962), "Antenatal prediction of ABO hæmolytic disease." *Brit. Jnl. Hæmatology*, 825.

VOAK, D. (1968), "The serological specificity of the sensitising Antibodies in ABO Heterospecific Pregnancy of the Group O mother." *Vox Sang.*, **14,** 271.

VOS, G. H. (1958), "The partial absorption test. A new technique for titrating Rh antibodies of pathological significance." *Aust. Ann. Med.*, **7,** 340.

WIENER, A. S., and UNGER, L. G. (1955), "Excess of group O mothers in ABO hæmolytic disease with special reference to the role of the blood factor C." *Exp. Med. Surg.*, **13,** 204.

WIENER, A. S., and WARD, F. A. (1966), "The serological specificity (blood factor) C of the ABO blood groups." *Amer. J. clin. Path.*, **46,** 1, 27.

WINSTANLEY, D. P., KONUGRES, A., and COOMBS, R. R. A. (1957), "Studies on human anti-A sera with special reference to so-called 'immune' anti-A. I The A^p antigen and the specificity of the hæmolysin in anti-A sera." *Brit. J. Hæmat.*, **3,** 341.

WITEBSKY, E. (1948), "Interrelation between the Rh system and the ABO system." *Blood*, **3,** *Suppl.*, 2, 66.

WOODROW, J. C., CLARKE, C. A., DONOHOE, W. T. A., FINN, R., MCCONNELL, R. B., SHEPPARD, P. M., LEHANE, D., RUSSELL, SHONA H., KULKE, W., and DURKIN, CATHERINE M. (1965), *Brit. Med. J.*, **i,** 279.

ZEITLIN, R. A., and BOORMAN, K. E. (1963), "The prognostic value of Coombs and partial absorption titration in hæmolytic disease of the newborn." *Jnl. of Obstetrics and Gynæcology of the Brit. Commonwealth*, Vol. LXX, **5,** 798.

ZEITLIN, R. A., and BOORMAN, K. E. (1965), "Premature induction, its advisability and limitations as a means of preventing intrauterine death, due to hæmolytic disease of the fœtus." *Proc. Int. Soc. Bld. Trans.*, p. 2087.

CHAPTER 26

HÆMOLYTIC ANÆMIAS

THE hæmolytic anæmias, *i.e.* anæmias consequent upon a reduced life-span of the patient's red cells, are by no means a simple subject capable of being dealt with in one short chapter; those interested are referred to one of the standard textbooks, especially Dacie and Worlledge, 1968. A brief account will be given here together with details of the serological techniques used.

The hæmolytic anæmias may be divided into two main classes: congenital and acquired.

The congenital hæmolytic anæmias include hereditary spherocytosis (congenital acholuric jaundice), hereditary elliptocytosis, Mediterranean anæmia, sickle-cell disease, etc. These are all the result of an inherited abnormality of the patient's red cells. This abnormality is intrinsic in the cells and is not associated with any antibody either attached to them or in the plasma. This means that the direct anti-human globulin test on the cells is negative and that no abnormal antibodies will be detected in the serum. Serological tests, therefore, do not give a positive diagnosis in these types of anæmia, but where a diagnosis of hæmolytic anæmia has been made on the hæmatological findings, the negative direct anti-human globulin test points to a congenital rather than an acquired type in which the test is positive. This can be confirmed by investigation of the patient's family and by the finding of an unimpaired survival of transfused normal red cells in the patient's circulation. Moreover, red cells from patients suffering from one of the congenital hæmolytic anæmias show a diminished survival rate in the normal recipient.

The second group, the acquired hæmolytic anæmias, may again be divided into two main sub-divisions, *viz.* hæmolytic anæmias associated with the formation of auto-immune antibodies and a very miscellaneous collection due to various other causes. Among the latter are included hæmolytic anæmia caused by drugs, infections, associated with leukæmia, etc. Also among the non auto-antibody types is hæmolytic disease of the newborn which is caused not by an auto-antibody but by a maternal immune antibody. This disease has been dealt with in some detail in Chapter 25.

The auto-immune antibody type of acquired hæmolytic anæmia presents a most interesting study—not the least because it is an exception to the fundamental law of immunity that immune antibodies are only produced in an individual to antigens which the individual himself lacks. The cause of such abnormal behaviour is by no means clearly understood but it is a fact that in these cases auto-antibodies are formed and can be detected both on the patient's red cells and in his plasma. Sometimes the auto-immune antibody is directed against a well known and easily identifiable antigen such as the Rh antigen e (anti-e was the first of the well known blood group antibodies to be detected as an auto-immune antibody). However, in almost all cases of auto-immune antibody type of acquired hæmolytic anæmia part, at least, of the auto-antibody is pan-reacting, so that the patient's serum is incompatible not only with his own red cells but also with those of all donors who could be chosen for him. Often I-negative blood is compatible, the apparently pan-reacting antibody being anti-I. These pan-reacting antibodies are normally only detectable by the indirect anti-human globulin, enzyme and hæmolysin techniques.

Auto-antibodies are associated with many forms of acquired hæmolytic anæmia and they undoubtedly play a part in the hæmolytic process. This does not mean, however, that the ætiology of the disease is understood nor indeed that it does not differ from case to case. Usually there is no known cause for the development of the antibody and the term "idiopathic" acquired hæmolytic anæmia is applied to such cases. This is in contrast to the cases which are "secondary" to other diseases or pathological processes such as virus pneumonia, chronic lymphatic leukæmia, disseminated lupus erythematosus, etc. An important disease of the latter class is paroxysmal cold hæmoglobinuria secondary to syphilis. Patients taking the drug α-methyldopa not infrequently give a positive direct anti-globulin test and although most of them show no evidence of increased red cell destruction the occasional patient develops auto-immune hæmolytic anæmia. The clinical and serological findings are the same as those of the warm antibody type of the disease (*see* below). The antibodies often have Rh specificities.

In spite of a wide variety in ætiology the auto-antibody types of hæmolytic anæmia have similar serological characteristics and there are a few well recognised serological techniques which are useful in their investigation.

Serological Investigation of a Patient Suspected of Suffering from Acquired Hæmolytic Anæmia

The samples required are patient's serum separated at 37°C and patient's red cells taken into A.C.D. (acid-citrate dextrose) solution or into sequestrene.

The direct anti-human globulin test is positive* in all cases of auto-immune hæmolytic anæmia; the auto-antibody is sensitising the patient's own cells. Although the positive anti-globulin test is strong presumptive evidence of auto-immune hæmolytic anæmia it is not absolutely diagnostic. Positive results may be due to antigen-antibody complexes adsorbed to the red cell surface or antibodies against drugs bound to the red cells. There is also the possibility of a positive direct anti-globulin test due to α-methyldopa administration as mentioned above.

The auto-immune antibodies, fall into two distinct types: (1) "warm" where the cold-agglutinin titre of the serum at 2°C is within normal limits in most cases but antibodies active at 37°C are present; (2) "cold" where there is a very high titre of cold agglutinins (often within the range 512–200,000 at 2°C) in the patient's serum. Although the direct anti-human globulin test is positive in both these two classes it can be used to confirm the differentiation between them (*see* Table 26.1). In cold antibody type, the positive direct anti-globulin test is due to complement on the red cells and not to specifically bound antibody. The antibody which is IgM globulin is usually active *in vitro* up to 30–32°C. The temperature in the blood vessels near the periphery may be within this range, in which case the antibody will bind complement to the red cells *in vivo* as well as causing agglutination. After rewarming to 37°C the antibody elutes off the cells but the complement components remain and these give the positive reaction with anti-non gamma (or anti-C_1) anti-globulin reagents.

Three types of anti-human globulin are used in the test: (1) a broad-spectrum reagent directed against human globulins reacting well with "warm" and "cold" type antibodies, (2) anti-IgG globulin directed specifically against the IgG fractions which gives a positive reaction with "warm" antibodies but negative with "cold" antibodies which are complement binding, and (3) anti-non IgG or anti-C^1 which reacts only with non IgG globulins and in particular with the C^1 (complement) which is bound onto the red cells by cold antibodies.

* Sometimes when a remission of symptoms occurs the direct anti-human globulin may be temporarily negative.

The anti-non IgG can be prepared by specific injection of suitable rabbits but is often prepared from a suitable broad spectrum reagent by neutralisation of the anti-IgG fraction with purified human IgG globulin.

Leddy (1966) has published the results of studying the direct anti-globulin test using rabbit anti-human globulin sera specific for the heavy chains of IgG, IgA and IgM and against complement (C^1) components. Three patterns of reaction were obtained, (*a*) agglutination with anti-IgG only, (*b*) with anti-C^1 only, (*c*) agglutination with both anti-IgG and anti-C^1 sera. Anti-IgA and anti-IgM sera were negative. Other workers have obtained an occassional positive test with anti-IgM sera. IgA antibodies do not appear to bind complement and have not yet been shown to be auto-antibodies.

Binding of complement without detectable antibodies on the red cell surface and in the absence of cold agglutinins in the serum is not uncommon in warm type hæmolytic anæmias. No antibody activity is found in the eluates made from the red cells in such cases.

The differentiation into "warm" or "cold" types of hæmolytic anæmia is of great value to the clinician in determining treatment.

Sometimes the antibodies appear to be mixtures of "cold" and "warm" types.

Wherever possible it is useful to identify the antibody present and to do this both an eluate from the red cells and the serum separated at 37°C are investigated.

The specificity of the antibody sensitising the red cells is best investigated on antibody eluted from the patient's cells, rather than on the serum, in which the amount of free antibody may be small and may also be contaminated with antibodies stimulated by previous transfusions.

Tests on Red Cells

(1) Direct Anti-human Globulin Test for IgG and Non IgG Differentiation

See technique No. 26.

(2) Elution of Antibody from Red Cells

This is done either by Landsteiner technique (which is given in technique No. 21.3 except that the first paragraph which describes the sensitising of the cells is irrelevant as the cells are already sensitised *in vivo*), or by the Weiner technique No. 26.4. The latter technique is particularly successful in eluting hæmolytic anæmia antibodies. The antibody will not normally elute from 'cold' sensitised cells but it can sometimes be eluted by the cæsium chloride technique (technique 26.10). In the case of "warm" sensitised cells the antibody may be pan-reacting or may have Rh specificity, or be a mixture of both.

(3) **ABO Grouping and Rh Typing**

These tests may present difficulties owing to auto-agglutinins and sensitised red cells.

If auto-agglutinins are present, the patient's serum against A, B and O cells may not give results consistent with his true ABO group and so the cell grouping may have to be relied upon entirely to give the right answer. If the patient's cells are collected into A.C.D. or sequestrene and washed three times at 37°C, there is little likelihood of interference by auto-agglutinins in the ABO grouping of the red cells but the Rh typing results may be falsified by the presence of the incomplete antibodies on the red cells accounting for the positive direct anti-human globulin result. This is because strongly sensitised red cells become agglutinated if suspended in a serum albumin mixture or even in serum alone. It is, therefore, strictly necessary to include controls of the patient's red cells suspended in AB serum or AB serum/albumin mixture where appropriate when Rh typing or sub-typing. The best approach to the problem is to use high titre saline sera which will withstand a certain amount of dilution with saline. In cases of extreme difficulty elution of antibody from the surface of the cells by technique No. 21.3 may have to be undertaken. Full Rh sub-typing should be done if possible, although for reasons given above it may not be possible to test for anti-c or anti-e for which high titre saline sera are not usually available.

It is as well to test for all known blood group systems (procedure No. 3) while the patient has no transfused red cells in his circulation. (For the standard techniques for each system see the appropriate chapters.) If the testing has to be done on a "mixed" sample, technique No. 22.1 may be found helpful. In view of the sensitisation of the patient's cells *in vivo* it is not possible to carry out typing tests which depend upon the indirect anti-human globulin technique. To obtain answers to these it may be necessary either first to elute the auto-antibody from the red cells (technique No. 21.3) or if opportunity arises to type the red cells when they are in a non-sensitised phase (which may occur when the patient is in remission).

Testing of Serum for Atypical Antibodies

In general the more severely the patient is afflicted by the disease the greater is the chance of demonstrating free antibody.

The procedure for this is similar to that described in Chapter 21 but it must be remembered that antibodies in cases of hæmolytic anæmia have rather special characteristics. Mixtures of specific antibodies may be present and some of these may be directed against antigens contained in the patient's own red cells (*e.g.* anti-e, *see* above) or anti-I.

These can often be sorted out only after absorption with specially selected red cells, *e.g.* homozygotes, such as EE, KK and II. Eluates of antibody from the patient's cells either by technique No. 21.3 or 26.3 should be examined in the same way as the serum. Antibody tests on both serum and eluate should be done by several techniques in parallel, always including anti-human globulin and papain.

Even in cases where there appears to be no free antibody in the serum of the patient as judged by the anti-globulin technique, papain will often reveal the presence of an antibody.

The type of direct anti-globulin test gives a clue to the type of reaction that may be expected when the patient's serum is tested with enzyme treated cells. For example when the direct anti-globulin test is positive only with anti-IgG reagent, the free antibody agglutinates but does not usually hæmolyse enzyme treated cells and is likely to be IgG; when the direct test is positive only with anti-C^1 reagent the free antibody agglutinates and hæmolyses enzyme treated cells and is likely to be of the IgM type. When both antiglobulin reagents give a positive reaction, the free antibody may be IgG or IgM.

Hæmolysins

Although *in vivo* hæmolysis is a feature of auto-antibody hæmolytic anæmia, "warm" hæmolysins are difficult to demonstrate. Rapid auto-hæmolysis may indeed take place *in vitro* but this is no proof that it is brought about by complement or antibody. Hæmolysis may take place for mechanical reasons owing to the presence of spherocytes. This kind of hæmolysis can be demonstrated even when complement is inactivated.

However, hæmolysins active at 37°C can sometimes be demonstrated at an acid pH (*see* technique No. 26.8) or by using trypsin treated red cells, or red cells from patients suffering from paroxysmal, nocturnal hæmoglobinuria.

Cold hæmolysins are more common and are usually readily demonstrated if the patient has a high titre of cold agglutinins at 2°C. This is particularly true if the pH is adjusted to between 6·5 and 6·8.

Trypsin treated normal cells or P.N.H. cells are readily hæmolysed even without the addition of acid but higher hæmolysin titres are observed with an adjusted pH. No correlation between titres of hæmolysins either "warm" or "cold" and severity of the disease has been noted.

A special feature of the paroxysmal cold hæmoglobinuria type of acquired hæmolytic anæmia is the Donath-Landsteiner hæmolysin. This antibody hæmolyses the red cells of the patient or a normal person but only if the sensitisation stage of the process takes place in the cold and the sensitised cells are subsequently raised to 37°C. If complement is withheld by heat inactivation, hæmolysis is prevented. The optimum pH for hæmolysis is in the region of pH 7·0 to 8·0. The Donath-Landsteiner antibody has the specificity anti-P, *i.e.* it is similar to the antibody made by p^K persons which agglutinates P_1 and P_2. There appears to be some correlation between the strength of the antibody and the severity of the disease.

Techniques

Technique No. 26.1. Quantitative antiglobulin test

This involves making serial fourfold dilutions of the anti-human globulin and then performing a direct anti-human globulin test using each dilution as the anti-human globulin reagent. Readings at 2, 5, and 10 minutes will probably be necessary, *see* protocol in Table 26.1. This technique is more satisfactory than the single dilution technique as cells sensitised with different types of antibody do react differently according to the dilution of the anti-human globulin; in particular the non-γ-globulin (cold) type of antibody gives a lower titre and does not show a prozone.

Technique No. 26.2. Screening technique for detecting antibodies present in serum from hæmolytic anæmia patients and determining their reactivity

It will have been realised that the full investigation of a serum for agglutinins, incomplete antibodies, papain reactive antibodies, and hæmolysins with a full panel of 5–10 red cell samples at several temperatures is a long and complicated procedure and very wasteful of serum (50 ml. of serum would not be too much for a detailed investigation). It is therefore helpful to screen the serum first to determine how the antibodies react. For this purpose the serum can be tested against a pool of red cells chosen to contain all the common antigens. In practice a pool of R_1R_1, R_2R_2 and rr cells, one at least of which is K+ and another Le^a+ will probably be satisfactory. Fresh human serum of the same group as the patient will be needed as a source of C^1. The tests should

Table 26.1

Differentiation of "Warm" and "Cold" Auto-immune Antibody Types of Hæmolytic Anæmia by Means of the Quantitative Direct Antiglobulin Test

	Dilutions of reagent							
	1/4	1/16	1/64	1/256	1/1,000	1/4,000	1/16,000	
Case (1) . . .	5+	2+	—	—	—	—	—	
Case (2) . . .	2+	4+	5+	5+	3+	—	—	
Cells sensitised with Rh antibody . . .	1+	3+	5+	5+	4+	3+	—	Read after 2 min.
O Rh negative control .	—	—	—	—	—	—	—	
Group AB Rh negative control . .	—	—	—	—	—	—	—	
Case (1) . . .	5+	4+	4+	+	—	—	—	
Case (2) . . .	3+	5+	5+	5+	5+	4+	2+	
Cells sensitised with Rh antibody . . .	2+	4+	5+	5+	5+	5+	4+	Read after 5 min.
O Rh negative control .	2+	—	—	—	—	—	—	
Group AB Rh negative control . . .	2+	+	—	—	—	—	—	
Case (1) . . .	5+	5+	4+	+	—	—	—	
Case (2) . . .	3+	5+	5+	5+	5+	4+	3+	
Cells sensitised with Rh antibody . . .	2+	4+	5+	5+	5+	5+	4+	Read after 10 min.
O Rh negative control .	2+	+	—	—	—	—	—	
Group AB Rh negative control . . .	3+	2+	+	—	—	—	—	

Conclusion. Case (1) is a "cold" auto-antibody type.
Case (2) is a "warm" auto-antibody type.

be done at 10°C, 18°C and 37°C. In every case the serum and cells must be brought to the chosen temperature before mixing and in the case of the anti-human globulin test maintained at the chosen temperature during washing. The experiment is duplicated, one set at pH8 and the other at pH7. The tests are put up as for the indirect anti-human globulin test (technique No. 10.3a) and examined after 1½ hours for agglutination and/or lysis. They are then washed and the anti-human globulin test completed using a broad spectrum reagent at the two dilutions, and a saline control. Similar tests are put up but with the addition of complement (*see* technique No. 26.5). If no antibody is detected in any of these tests, the serum is tested by papain technique at the three temperatures.

When free antibody is found the optimum technique is chosen and the antibody identified against a full panel of standard cells; more than one antibody may be present and absorption and elution experiments may be necessary to differentiate between them. Antibodies detected should also be classified as to whether they are auto- or iso-antibodies.

If there is a cold antibody present its thermal range should be estimated as should its titre at 4°C.

Technique No. 26.3. Direct anti-human globulin test for IgG and non IgG differentiation

As explained above three reagents are used in this test: (1) a broad spectrum reagent. This will be issued with instructions for use at two different dilutions, the stronger chosen to give a good positive with the C^1 (complement) so that cold complement binding antibodies are detected and the other the optimum dilution for the IgG globulin or warm type antibodies. Both dilutions should be used. (2) anti-IgG reagent. This is specially prepared reagent which reacts with IgG globulins only and should be used at the recommended dilution. (3) anti-C^1 reagent. Specially prepared anti-C^1 may not be available but it can be prepared from a good broad spectrum reagent. To do this the broad spectrum reagent is diluted 1 in 4 and to it is added an equal volume of a 1 per cent solution of pure human IgG globulin. The mixture is allowed to stand for at least 10 minutes before being used in the test. This neutralised reagent will store satisfactorily for 2–3 weeks frozen at −20°C but should be stored in small aliquots as continual freezing and thawing will reduce its efficiency.

The patient's red cells are washed 4 times in a large excess of saline and the direct anti-human globulin test (technique No. 10.3b) is performed using the three reagents (four tests to allow for the two dilutions with broad spectrum reagent) and with saline as a negative control. The reagents are controlled with known IgG and non IgG sensitised cells (the former are usually conveniently prepared by sensitising D-positive cells with a weak incomplete anti-D serum and the latter Le^a positive cells with an incomplete anti-Le^a) and with unsensitised cells. Table 26.2 shows typical results. Note that as in case (3) there may be a mixture of warm (IgG) and cold (non-IgG) antibodies sensitising the cells.

Table 26.2

Differentiation of "Warm" and "Cold" Auto-immune Antibody Types of Hæmolytic Anæmia by Means of the Direct Antiglobulin Test

	Reagents				
	Broad Spectrum		Anti	Anti-C^1	Saline
	$\frac{1}{10}$	$\frac{1}{80}$			
Case (1)	4+	5+	5+	—	—
Case (2)	5+	3+	—	5+	—
Case (3)	5+	5+	3+	5+	—
Warm-coated cells (IgG)	4+	5+	5+	—	—
Cold-coated cells (C^1)	5+	4+	—	5+	—
Unsensitised cells	—	—	—	—	—

Conclusion. Case 1 is a "warm" auto-antibody type.
Case 2 is a "cold" auto-antibody type.
In Case 3 there is a mixture of antibodies.

Technique No. 26.4. Weiner's technique for the elution of antibodies from the red cell surface

Sensitised red cells from a case of hæmolytic anæmia are washed three times with saline, tightly packed and all supernatant fluid removed. They are then placed in the deep freeze at about —20°C until the cells are completely hæmolysed. Alternate freezing and thawing will hasten this process. After finally thawing, ten times the original volume of 50 per cent (v/v) ethanol precooled to at least —6°C is added. The tube is rapidly inverted and the alcohol thoroughly mixed with the hæmolysed red cells and immediately returned to the deep freeze for 30–60 minutes. The tube is then centrifuged at 3,000 r.p.m. for at least 5 minutes. The supernatant is discarded and the tube filled with distilled water. The tube is then shaken thoroughly to mix and recentrifuged. The supernatant is again removed and a certain quantity of saline depending on the quantity of packed cells used (*e.g.* approximately equal volume) is added to the sediment which is thoroughly mixed with it. The tube is then incubated at 37°C for 30–60 minutes, centrifuged and the supernatant (eluate) collected.

Eluates can be prepared from as little as 0·1 ml. of cells but it is best to start with 1–2 ml. of packed cells. In our experience this is a good technique providing the cells are well coated with antibody at the outset. It can also of course be applied to cells sensitised with antibody *in vitro* as opposed to hæmolytic anæmias where the cells are sensitised *in vivo*.

Technique No. 26.5. Modification of indirect anti-human globulin test using acidified serum and complement

The pathological cold incomplete antibodies often sensitise cells more readily if the serum is acidified. The serum is acidified by adding 10 per cent by volume of N/4 HCl.

The indirect anti-human globulin test (10.4a) is then performed using acidified and unacidified patient's serum to sensitise normal cells. Moreover, these cold antibodies appear to need complement and therefore, inactivation of the serum will prevent the reaction. This is not true of the warm antibodies which react equally well even when the serum has been heat inactivated. If the patient's serum is old, fresh normal human serum (from which the incomplete cold antibody has been absorbed) or guinea-pig complement must be added.

Technique No. 26.6. Qualitative Donath-Landsteiner test

Direct. A 10 ml. sample of venous blood is taken and immediately divided between two dry tubes warmed to 37°C. One is kept at 37°C in a water bath while the other is first placed in crushed ice at 0°C for 30 minutes then, without disturbing the clot, transferred to the water bath at 37°C for an hour. If the test is positive the second tube will show gross hæmolysis, the serum will be coloured deep red, while the tube kept at 37°C throughout the test will show no trace of free hæmoglobin. This test is diagnostic of paroxysmal cold hæmoglobinuria.

Indirect. This test must be made on patient's serum which has been separated from the clot without cooling (*i.e.* at 37°C).

Nine parts of serum are mixed with one part of washed packed normal group O red cells (tube 1). The mixture is allowed to stand in crushed ice at 0°C for 30 minutes and then transferred to the 37°C water bath for 1 hour. A second tube (tube 2) is included using equal parts of the patient's serum and fresh normal serum to act as a source of complement (or guinea-pig complement). The negative controls are provided by keeping a duplicate (tubes 3 and 4) of tubes 1 and 2 at 37°C throughout.

A positive test shows hæmolysis in tubes 1 and 2 or in tube 2 alone (if the patient's serum is deficient in complement) with no hæmolysis in tubes 3 and 4.

Technique No. 26.7. Quantitative Donath-Landsteiner test

Serial doubling dilutions of the patient's serum are made in fresh normal serum. An equal volume of a 2 per cent suspension in saline of normal washed group O red cells is added to each tube. The test is immersed in crushed ice at 0°C for 30 minutes and then in a 37°C water bath for an hour. The tubes are centrifuged and the degree of hæmolysis read according to the following scale:

++++ or 4+ = complete hæmolysis
+++ or 3+ = deep red supernatant
++ or 2+ = red supernatant
+ = pale red supernatant
± or tr. = definite but weak hæmolysis compared with control

The hæmolytic titre is the reciprocal of the highest dilution giving a ± or tr. reaction.

Technique No. 26.8. Acid lysin technique

The antibodies which are associated with hæmolytic anæmias will sometimes hæmolyse normal cells *in vitro* provided that the serum containing them is acidified. A convenient way of ensuring the optimum condition for hæmolysis is to make the serial dilutions in fresh acidified normal serum. (The serum should be acidified by the addition of a tenth part by volume of N/4 HCl.) One volume of a 2 per cent suspension of normal group O red cells is added to each dilution, the tests allowed to stand for 2 hours, at 15°C if the antibody is of the cold type and at 37°C for "warm" antibodies, centrifuged and read for hæmolysis as above.

Technique No. 26.9. Hæmolysin technique using P.N.H. red cells

The red cells from patients with paroxysmal cold hæmoglobinuria are more readily lysed by hæmolysins than are normal cells. If an ordinary titration using normal unacidified serum as diluent is tested with group O P.N.H. cells a hæmolysin titre is obtained. This titre will often closely parallel the cold agglutinin titre of the serum.

Technique No. 26.10. Elution of antibodies using cæsium chloride

The cells which have been sensitised either *in vivo* or *in vitro*, are washed three times in a large excess of 0·85 per cent NaCl and packed hard by centrifugation. One quarter of their volume of 1·2 M cæsium chloride is added. The cells are resuspended and incubated at room temperature for 45 minutes. The suspension is then centrifuged at 600 g. for 20 minutes and the supernatant carefully removed. This is the eluate but it has to be made isotonic. This is done by dialysing at 0°C for 12–18 hours against four changes of large quantities of normal saline. If the eluate is not satisfactory a higher molarity of cæsium chloride can be tried. 1·2 M is the most satisfactory for the Rh antibodies, including auto-antibodies, 1·6 M even 2·0 M may give better results for cold antibodies and anti-B; anti-A shows improved elution at 2·4 M.

Technique No. 26.11. Rubin's method for elution of antibodies

This is an adaptation by Rubin (1963) of a method devised by Vos and Kelsall (1956).

The sensitised cells are washed three times in 0·85 per cent saline, packed and then an equal volume of 0·85 per cent saline added to the washed cells. To this mixture is added two volumes of diethyl ether. The container is stoppered and repeatedly inverted for one minute. The mixture is then centrifuged for 10 minutes at 3,000 r.p.m. After centrifugation three clearly defined layers are visible. The upper layer is ether, then comes a layer of denatured stromata and the bottom layer is the eluate. This will be found to be hæmoglobin stained. The two top layers are removed by vacuum suction and the eluate placed in a water bath at 37°C for 15 minutes to remove any traces of ether.

Comment

In spite of the slight disadvantage of producing an hæmoglobin stained eluate this is a most satisfactory method for elution of Rh antibodies, whether auto as in hæmolytic anæmias or from cells sensitised *in vitro.*

The Problem of Selection of Blood for Patients with Acquired Hæmolytic Anæmia

It is rarely possible to select blood for hæmolytic anæmias, which is entirely compatible by normal standards. The auto-antibody will usually agglutinate all red cells at least by indirect anti-human globulin and papain techniques if not by other methods also.

Moreover, the problem is intensified when the patient develops blood group antibodies not only to antigens which he lacks and by which he has been immunised by transfusion, but also to antigens which he himself possesses. In such cases it is very difficult to decide whether to transfuse blood of the patient's own sub-type or blood which is compatible with the sensitising antibody but which will inevitably contain antigens which the patient lacks. For example, an R_2r patient who has anti-e auto-antibodies would be given R_2R_2 blood but an rr patient with anti-e would be given rr blood because of the risk of producing anti-D; an R_1r patient with auto anti-e would be given R_2R_2 blood unless he then produced iso anti-E when R_1r blood (or rr blood) would have to be given.

Usually the best that can be done is to select blood that is compatible with any antibodies of blood group specificity that the patient may possess and then compare the reactions that are obtained with this blood against those obtained between the patient's serum and his own cells from which auto-antibody has been eluted. Blood is chosen for transfusion if its reactions are no stronger than the reactions obtained with the patient's serum against his own cells. Often blood can be found which seems more compatible than the patient's own.

BIBLIOGRAPHY

ANDERSON, R. E., and WALFORD, ROY (1963), "Elution of antibodies from sensitised red blood cells by means of caesium chloride." **33,** 8, 135.

DACIE, J. V. (1962), *The Hæmolytic Anæmias: Congenital and Acquired.* 2nd ed., J. & A. Churchill Ltd.

DACIE, J. V., and WORLLEDGE, SHEILA, M. *Auto-allergic blood diseases, in Clinical Aspects of Immunology.* Blackwell, Oxford.

LEDDY, J. P. (1966), "Immunological aspects of red cell injury in man." *Seminars in Hæmatology*, **3,** 48.

RUBIN, H. (1963), "Antibody elution from red cells." *J. clin. Path.*, **16,** 70.

TIPPET, P., NOADES, J., SANGER, R., RACE, R. R., SAUSAIS, L., HOLMAN, C. A., and BUTTIMER, R. J. (1960), "Further studies on the I antigen and antibody." *Vox Sang.*, **5,** 107.

VOS, G. H., and KELSALL, G. A. (1956), "A new elution technique for the preparation of specific immune anti-Rh serum." *Brit. J. Hæm.*, **2,** 342.

WEINER, W., BATTEY, D. A., CLEGHORN, T. E., MARSON, F. G. W., and MEYNELL, M. J. (1953), "Serological findings in a case of hæmolytic anæmia, with some general observations on the pathogenesis of this syndrome." *Brit. med. J.*, **ii,** 125.

WHITBY, L., and BRITTON, C. J. C. (1957), *Disorders of the Blood.* 8th ed., J. & A. Churchill Ltd.

CHAPTER 27

HUMAN BLOOD GROUPS IN RELATION TO GENETICS AND ANTHROPOLOGY

THIS chapter does not set out to do more than indicate the way in which the discovery of so many human blood groups is providing new tools for studying Mendelian inheritance and racial differences and development.

The study of the inheritance of the blood groups themselves is a fascinating one and many new discoveries have been made in the last twenty years. The geneticist has long felt that the blood groups are ideal material for the study of human genetics. Here are easily determinable inherited characteristics, unaffected by environment, so what more could a geneticist desire. This approach is to some extent justified as it is true that there are at least nine blood group systems for which anti-sera giving reliable results are fairly readily obtainable. On the other hand, as for example in Rh sub-typing or in testing with anti-Le^a and anti-Le^b, the results when obtained are capable of more than one interpretation.

There are two ways of using the human blood groups to study human genetics. The first and most obvious is to study each blood group system individually. There is still much to be learned for instance about the inheritance of even the ABO blood group system. In this study of the blood groups themselves we are finding not only examples of straightforward Mendelian inheritance but also of the effect of one gene on another, of "position" and "dosage" effects, of closely linked genes, etc. The second way is to use the blood groups as markers of chromosomes. So far out of the twenty-three autosomes there are blood group markers for at least nine and possibly several more; *see* the associations excluded column of Table 15.2. The full blood grouping of families, combined with the study of other inherited characteristics has already yielded some fruit. The largest contributor to this field is the sex-linked blood group Xg (*see* Chapters 19 and 34).

The work of the geneticist in demonstrating the mode of inheritance of blood groups has a practical application in questions of disputed identity, in particular of paternity (*see* Chapter 29).

The blood group systems are also of use to the anthropologist, because they are inherited characteristics which are determined by either a single set of allelomorphic genes or by a comparatively

Table 27.1

Blood Group Distributions in Various Populations

ABO

Population	Tested by	No. tested	Gene frequency		
			p(A)	q(B)	r(O)
English	Boorman (1950)	1,966	0·272	0·061	0·667
French	Moullec (1953)	1,458	0·264	0·045	0·691
Serbians	Simonovic (1953)	6,863	0·288	0·138	0·574
Sikhs	Bird *et al.* (1951)	600	0·180	0·230	0·590
Chippewa Indians (Full Blood)	Matson and Levine (1953)	161	0·064	0·000	0·936

Rh (D only)

Population	Tested by	No. tested	Gene frequency	
			D	d
English	Race *et al.* (1943)	4,618	0·6047	0·3953
Swedes	Grubb (1953)	10,222	0·5821	0·4179
Chinese (Peking)	Pan (1950)	2,324	0·9225	0·0775
Koreans	Blood Bank of Hawaii (1950)	156	1·0000	0·0000
Basques	Guash (1950)	649	0·5065	0·4935
Burmese	Mollison and Reddy (1946)	229	1·0000	0·0000

M and N

Population	Tested by	No. tested	Gene frequency	
			M	N
English	Ikin *et al.* (1952)	1,166	0·5373	0·4627
American Whites	Wiener *et al.* (1943)	6,129	0·5393	0·4607
North American Indians (Full Blood)	Landsteiner *et al.* (1942)	120	0·7625	0·2375
Fijians	Simmons *et al.* (1945)	200	0·3325	0·6675
Australian Aborigines	Wilson *et al.* (1944)	649	0·2974	0·7026
Latvians	Race *et al.* (1948)	172	0·6715	0·3285

simple set of gene complexes. Moreover, it is once again important that environmental factors do not play a large part in determining blood group frequencies. The classical anthropometric standards based on skin, hair and eye colour, stature and shape of the cranium all suffer from grave disadvantages as they are not in the main the result of a single simple system of genes, indeed often being controlled by a number of independent genes and the influence of environment is very marked.

It is useful, therefore, in studying the divisions of the human race to have not only the classic anthropometric observations but also the gene frequencies of as many blood group systems as possible. All the known blood group systems show variations in gene frequency in different populations. The details of such variations are much too complex to be considered here. *The Distribution of the Human Blood Groups* (Mourant, 1954) gives a very comprehensive account with several maps showing at a glance the distribution of the ABO, Rh, and M and N genes.

Table 27.1 gives a few comparisons of blood group gene frequencies in different populations. It is not intended as a comprehensive survey; Mourant in his textbook has some eighty pages of such tables, listing most of the published and unpublished data, giving the frequency of the blood groups—and even then he has omitted most of the published data for the ABO system. It will be seen that for the three systems selected in Table 27.1 there are wide variations; apart from the large racial distinctions small interrelated communities will naturally produce a different picture from those populations where there is a fair degree of movement and intermarriage. With the ABO system, unlike the Rh and MN there are many local variations—the finding of a relationship between a particular ABO blood group and susceptibility to certain diseases (*e.g.* carcinoma of the stomach, duodenal ulcer, etc.) makes it tempting to envisage the ABO blood groups as being liable to fluctuation due to selection.

These racial and geographical differences in distribution of the blood groups are not only of anthropological interest but also of practical importance to the serologist. A knowledge of the blood group gene frequencies of the population among which he works will influence his daily practice; for instance, in parts of the world where the D negative population is small the ante-natal and blood banking organisation can be modified accordingly.

Gene Frequencies

It is obvious that gene frequencies cannot always be directly determined, but must be calculated from the numbers of each phenotype observed. The phenotypes, *e.g.* the four ABO blood groups, can, of course, be counted. These will vary in different races and even in different geographical locations for the same race. It is important, therefore, when giving figures for blood group distributions or gene frequencies to state the source of the sample tested.

The mode of calculation of gene frequencies is similar whatever the genes may be. If the fundamental principles for the calculation of the A, B, and O gene frequencies are understood, it will be found that they are applicable to any human blood group system. It is worth while, therefore, considering them in some detail; those who are familiar with the subject can omit the step by step explanations.

The gene frequency is simply the number of times a particular gene occurs among all the genes belonging to a particular system and can be expressed as a percentage of the total number of genes in the system. The combined frequencies of any set of allelomorphic genes will obviously be 100 per cent. In actual fact for convenience the gene frequency is usually expressed as a decimal of 1·0 where 1·0 represents the whole system, so that the combined frequencies will add up to 1·0. The frequencies of the genes A, B, and O are denoted by the letters p, q, and r respectively, so that

$$p + q + r = 1 \quad \quad . \quad . \quad . \quad . \quad (1)$$

It is necessary to know the number in each phenotype in the whole population, for which the gene frequencies are being calculated. It is not, however, essential to group the whole population but merely a large sample and it is obvious that the larger the sample the more likely it is to be representative of the whole. N people therefore are tested where N is a very large number and of them there are (O) group O individuals, (A) group A individuals, (B) group B individuals, and (AB) group AB individuals, where (O), (A), (B), and (AB) are actual numbers counted. Therefore $(O) + (A) + (B) + (AB) = N$

The group frequency of O is therefore $\frac{(O)}{N}$

The group frequency of A is therefore $\frac{(A)}{N}$

The group frequency of B is therefore $\frac{(B)}{N}$

The group frequency of AB is therefore $\frac{(AB)}{N}$

These are actual numbers so that if the gene frequency can be expressed in terms of the group frequencies, expressions can be derived involving p, q, r and numbers from which p, q, and r can be calculated.

Group O consists entirely of the homozygous genotype OO and therefore its group frequency is $r \times r$ or r^2

$$i.e.\ \frac{(O)}{N} = r^2 \quad . \quad . \quad . \quad . \quad . \quad (2)^*$$

Group A consists of two genotypes, homozygous AA and heterozygous AO—the frequency of AA is $p \times p$ or p^2 and the frequency of AO is $2 \times p \times r$* (the 2 is because it is possible to have AO or OA), so that the group frequency of A is $p^2 + 2pr$

$$i.e.\ \frac{(A)}{N} = p^2 + 2pr \quad . \quad . \quad . \quad . \quad (3)$$

Similarly group B consists of two genotypes homozygous BB and heterozygous BO—the frequency of BB is $q \times q$ or q^2 and the frequency of BO is $2 \times q \times r$ so that the group frequency is $q^2 + 2qr$

$$i.e.\ \frac{(B)}{N} = q^2 + 2qr \quad . \quad . \quad . \quad . \quad (4)$$

Group AB consists of only one genotype AB and the group frequency is $2 \times p \times q$

$$i.e.\ \frac{(AB)}{N} = 2pq \quad . \quad . \quad . \quad . \quad . \quad (5)$$

Now take the five equations

$$p + q + r = 1 \quad . \quad . \quad . \quad . \quad . \quad (1)$$

$$\frac{(O)}{N} = r^2 \quad . \quad . \quad . \quad . \quad . \quad . \quad (2)$$

$$\frac{(A)}{N} = p^2 + 2pr \quad . \quad . \quad . \quad . \quad . \quad (3)$$

$$\frac{(B)}{N} = q^2 + 2qr \quad . \quad . \quad . \quad . \quad . \quad (4)$$

$$\frac{(AB)}{N} = 2pq \quad . \quad . \quad . \quad . \quad . \quad (5)$$

* If this point is not clear the reader is referred to the short account of the mathematical principles involved at the end of the chapter.

Add equations (2) and (3) together

$$\frac{(O)}{N} + \frac{(A)}{N} = r^2 + p^2 + 2pr$$

$$= (p + r)(p + r) \text{ (Factorising)}$$

$$= (p + r)^2$$

$$= (1 - q)^2 \; (\because p + r = 1 - q \text{ from (1)})$$

$$\sqrt{\frac{(O)}{N} + \frac{(A)}{N}} = 1 - q \text{ (taking square roots of each side)}$$

or

$$q = 1 - \sqrt{\frac{(O)}{N} + \frac{(A)}{N}}$$

This gives q in terms of actual numbers counted and so q can quite easily be calculated.

To obtain p add equations (2) and (4) and proceed as before.

$$\frac{(O)}{N} + \frac{(B)}{N} = r^2 + q^2 + 2qr$$

$$= (q + r)^2$$

$$= (1 - p)^2$$

$$\sqrt{\frac{(O)}{N} + \frac{(B)}{N}} = 1 - p$$

$$p = 1 - \sqrt{\frac{(O)}{N} + \frac{(B)}{N}}$$

Then from (1)

$$r = 1 - p - q$$

or from (2)

$$r = \sqrt{\frac{(O)}{N}}$$

The second value is not so accurate as it relies only on the number of group O bloods counted.

Example

In an actual count of the grouping of 500 individuals there were

214 of group O
234 of group A
32 of group B
20 of group AB

(*a*) Calculation from first principles

$$p + q + r = 1 \qquad (1)$$

$$\frac{(O)}{N} = \frac{214}{500} = 0{\cdot}428 = r^2 \qquad (2)$$

$$\frac{(A)}{N} = \frac{234}{500} = 0{\cdot}468 = p^2 + 2pr \qquad (3)$$

$$\frac{(B)}{N} = \frac{32}{500} = 0{\cdot}064 = q^2 + 2qr \qquad (4)$$

$$\therefore \quad \frac{(AB)}{N} = \frac{20}{500} = 0{\cdot}040 = 2pq \qquad (5)$$

$$\therefore \quad 0{\cdot}428 + 0{\cdot}468 = p^2 + 2pr + r^2$$

$$= (p + r)^2$$

$$= (1 - q)^2 \ (\because p + r = 1 - q \text{ from } (1))$$

$$\sqrt{0{\cdot}428 + 0{\cdot}468} = 1 - q$$

$$q = 1 - \sqrt{0{\cdot}896} = 1 - 0{\cdot}947 = 0{\cdot}053$$

Similarly $$p = 1 - \sqrt{0{\cdot}492} = 1 - 0{\cdot}701 = 0{\cdot}299$$

$$\therefore \quad r = 1 - 0{\cdot}053 - 0{\cdot}299 = 0{\cdot}648$$

or $$r = \sqrt{0{\cdot}428} = 0{\cdot}654$$

(*b*) Substitution in derived formulæ

$$q = 1 - \sqrt{0{\cdot}428 + 0{\cdot}468} = 0{\cdot}053$$

$$p = 1 - \sqrt{0{\cdot}428 + 0{\cdot}064} = 0{\cdot}299$$

$$r = 1 - 0{\cdot}053 - 0{\cdot}299 = 0{\cdot}648$$

or $$r = \sqrt{0{\cdot}428} = 0{\cdot}654$$

In actual practice the two values for r are never quite equal, no sample ever being absolutely representative of the population from which it is drawn. There are various ways of using the calculated figures to obtain improved estimates of the gene frequencies. Two useful methods are those given by Stevens (1938) and Hartmann and Lundevall (1944).

For those with little mathematical background a very short discussion of the equations used in the calculation of the gene frequencies and the frequency of any given genotype in a random population, is appended.

The easiest way of understanding how these frequencies are obtained is to study a concrete example. For a full mathematical proof of the formulæ obtained, the reader must turn to an elementary book on statistics.

Imagine a box of balls containing twice as many white balls as black. If picked at random from the box, the number of black balls to white picked out, if the sample is large enough, will be in the proportion of 1 : 2. That is, one out of every three articles will be a black ball—and from this sample it may be concluded that this is also true of the whole box and that the frequency of occurrence of black balls in the box is one in three, $\frac{1}{3}$ or 0·33.

The frequency of occurrence of ABO genes is of course more complicated than this because every individual has two ABO genes—in other words, the balls are picked out from two boxes each of which contains black and white balls in the same proportions. To take the simplest case, if each box has one black ball and two white balls, in how many different ways can one object be picked from each box and how often will each particular pair occur. There are obviously three different pairs, namely two black balls, one white and one black ball and two white balls. If from box I a black ball is chosen, then from box II (1) a black ball, (2) a white ball, (3) a white ball can be chosen to pair with the black ball so that from this first selection two black balls once and one black and one white ball twice result. If from box I a white ball is chosen, then from box II (1) a black ball, (2) a white ball, (3) a white ball can be chosen so that this time one black and one white ball once and two white balls twice result. Similarly, selecting the other white ball from box I, it can be paired with each of the objects in box II to give again one black and white ball once and two white balls twice. This makes nine possibilities (Fig. 27.1).

Box I	*Box II*	*Possible pairs*
	1 ●	Two black balls
1 ●	2 ○	One black and one white ball
	3 ○	One black and one white ball
	1 ●	One black and one white ball
2 ○	2 ○	Two white balls
	3 ○	Two white balls
	1 ●	One black and one white ball
3 ○	2 ○	Two white balls
	3 ○	Two white balls

FIG. 27.1. The pairing of balls chosen from two boxes.

The diagram clearly shows, for example, that two black balls will pair together on one occasion out of nine or to express it mathematically when the frequency of black balls is $\frac{1}{3}$ (or 0·33), the frequency of choosing two black balls is $\frac{1}{9}$ or $(\frac{1}{3})^2$. The frequency of white balls is $\frac{2}{3}$ (0·66) and the frequency of choosing two white balls is $\frac{4}{9}$ or $(\frac{2}{3})^2$. So there emerges the general rule that when objects (or genes) are the same (*e.g.* in homozygous individuals) the frequency of occurrence of a pair is the square of the frequency of the object or gene (*e.g.* if the frequency of the gene z is x the frequency of the genotype zz is x^2; similarly, the frequency of AA = p^2, of BB = q^2 and of OO = r^2). The frequency of choosing one black and one white ball is $\frac{4}{9}$ or $2 \times \frac{1}{3} \times \frac{2}{3}$. Here a general rule may be derived that the frequency of the mixed (*e.g.* heterozygous) pair is twice the product of the individual frequencies of each member of the pair. (This is provided that the order in which the articles are chosen does not matter—it will be seen in the example that there are two cases in which a white ball is chosen prior to a black and two in which a black ball is chosen prior to a white ball. So far there has been no reason to suppose in blood group inheritance that it is of any significance from which parent the gene originates.) It can now be seen why, if the frequency of the A gene is p and that of the O gene r the frequency of genotype AA is p^2, of genotype OO is r^2, and of genotype AO is 2pr.

BIBLIOGRAPHY

CHALMERS, J. N. M., and LAWLER, SYLVIA, D. (1953), "Data on linkage in man; elliptocytosis and blood groups. I. Families 1 and 2." *Ann. Eugen., Lond.*, **17**, 267.

HARTMANN, O., and LUNDEVALL, J. (1944), *Blood distribution in Norway with special regard to the* MN *and* O A_1 A_2 B *System.* Oslo: 1 Kommisjon Hos Jacob Dybwad.

MOURANT, A. E. (1954), *The Distribution of the Human Blood Groups.* Oxford: Blackwell Scientific Publications.

STEVENS, W. L. (1938), "Estimation of blood group gene frequencies." *Ann. Eugen., Lond.*, **8**, 362.

CHAPTER 28

THE COLLECTION AND TESTING OF DONOR BLOOD

WHILE much of the following applies to all the transfusion centres, the detail of the organisation is that of the South London Regional Transfusion Centre.

In this country all donors are volunteers. They are recruited by a number of methods, by direct contact with a patient, relatives or friends, by voluntary organisations, *e.g.* British Red Cross and W.V.S., by donors bringing along their friends and so on —and, in our experience the most effective method, by a local "campaign". These campaigns are conducted in the busy shopping areas by means of a loudspeaker van and a team of nurses who carry forms for the enrolment of volunteers. The volunteer is called to a blood collection session near to his home. This session is run by a mobile team equipped to set up a clinic in any large hall, hospital ward, etc. The team comprises a doctor, a team leader, some five or six donor attendants, a driver clerk, a driver technician, and a junior technician. The equipment carried, which enables the unit to be quite self-supporting, ranges from a large refrigerator capable of holding two to three hundred bottles of blood, donor couches, rest beds and blankets to local anæsthetic and injection "gun", donor cards, bottle labels, bottles, taking apparatus, crockery, tea and biscuits, tea towels, electric kettle, washing-up bowls, etc.!

On attendance at the session a medical history is taken; any donors who have ever had jaundice are rejected, as there is the possibility that their serum may contain the virus which gives rise to serum jaundice. This virus can be transmitted by blood transfusion and the resultant jaundice may be very severe, in some cases resulting in liver atrophy and the death of the patient. Malaria is another disease which can be transmitted from donor to recipient. Donors who have had malaria are accepted as their blood can be used for the preparation of serum. Some of them have a high iso-agglutinin titre and their serum is invaluable for anti-A and anti-B typing. Serum which is not suitable for this purpose is pooled and dried.

The new donor is tested for ABO group by an open tile method using undiluted grouping serum and whole blood from a finger or ear prick. This method has an appreciable error but it enables the donor bottle to be given a group label which will be correct in at least ninety-nine cases out of a hundred; only one bottle per hundred will have to be relabelled after the full testing has been done in the laboratory. It has been agreed that donors shall not be bled if their hæmoglobin level is less than 85 per cent. Only a screening test is done, as elaborate and time-consuming tests cannot be performed during a blood collecting session where about thirty to forty donors are bled per hour. The screening method makes use of the fact that a drop of blood let fall into copper sulphate solution of specific gravity 1·052 will sink to the bottom if the Hb is 85 per cent or over but will float if the Hb is below this figure. Those who fail this rapid screening test have a 5 ml. oxalated sample taken from which a more accurate estimation of the hæmoglobin level is made in the laboratory. Should it be 85 per cent or over the donor is recalled next time the mobile team is in his area but if not he is not recalled until passed by his own doctor as fit to donate blood.

The donor who has passed the hæmoglobin screening test has his name entered on to a serially numbered work-sheet from which his number is copied on to the back of his card; it is also printed on three small labels issued to him together with a larger coloured group label. The label for each group has a different colour: group O, blue, group A, yellow, group B, pink and group AB, white. In addition, on each label is printed either Rh negative for donors known to be of Rh sub-type cde.cde, or Rh positive for all others.

The donor is then bled (technique No. 28.1); a local anæsthetic being given before the insertion of the taking needle. Except for donors who are bled "dry", *i.e.* into a dry bottle for serum, 420 ml. of blood is collected from each donor into 120 ml. of A.C.D. solution.* When the needle is withdrawn from the arm, blood in the tubing is not allowed to flow into the bottle but is used to fill (*a*) a pilot tube attached to the bottle, for laboratory use, and (*b*) a bijou also attached containing A.C.D.; this sample is for direct matching tests. Each of these containers has one of the small labels attached to it, while the third together with the coloured groups label is attached to the main bottle.

The donor rests for about 10 minutes, and is given tea and biscuits before he leaves.

Immediately the blood is taken it is put into the refrigerator. The pilot tubes are placed in strict numerical order and transferred to the serological laboratory. Serological tests are normally done

* For A.C.D. solution, *see* Appendix I.

on the day following the actual blood-taking and the organisation is such that some 800 to 1,000 donor samples can be tested each day by a team of seven.

The tubes are arranged in numbered blocks each containing forty tubes in rows of ten so that one block corresponds to one work-sheet, the number of the block is entered on the sheet, and the strict numerical sequence of the tubes is checked. Red cell free serum is taken off into numbered racks, inactivated at 56°C for ½ hour and then used for the VDRL (technique No. 28.2) or the Price Precipitation Test (technique No. 28.3)* and for the serum check on the ABO grouping. It is more satisfactory to use inactivated serum for the latter test since fresh serum may cause hæmolysis of the standard A and B red cells. The red cells are tested for ABO group by technique No. 3.2, for Rh (D) type by technique No. 9.3 and the D negatives further investigated by techniques Nos. 12.1–4. All Rh (D) negative donors are screened by papain techniques (techniques No. 10.4 and 28.2b) for the presence of Rh antibodies. If these are found they may be sufficiently potent to be used for Rh typing and subsequent donations are also used for this purpose provided that the titre remains high. Blood with a low titre of Rh antibodies is issued for known Rh negative adults; it is not used for emergency transfusion or for babies.

All R′, R″ and D^u donors are used for the transfusion of Rh positive recipients, as all D negative recipients are transfused with Rh negative (cde.cde) blood.

The results of all the above tests are entered on the original work-sheet; where more complicated tests are necessary the results are entered on a "Repeat Sheet" and the conclusions entered back on to the original sheet. The original work-sheet has a perforated section where the group and Rh type of each bottle of blood is entered and at the same time the blood is inspected for fitness for use. Then the perforated portion of the work-sheet goes to the blood issue department together with the "passed" bottles of blood for issue to the hospital blood banks. In a few cases, *e.g.* where the donor's serum contains an atypical agglutinin, it is useful to have a bench work card which is filed under the donor's name and on which results can be entered whenever he is bled.

The donor holds a booklet giving his group and Rh type to which a certificate is added at each donation; in addition special cards are issued to the Rh negative, R′ and R″ donors for their own protection should they ever need to be transfused. The National Blood Transfusion Service also gives badges to their

* Or any other standard test for syphilis.

long-service donors, bronze for 10 donations, silver for 25 donations and silver-gilt for 50 donations.

Donors who have a sufficiently high titre of anti-A and/or anti-B iso-agglutinins are used as donors of grouping sera. Their donations are very valuable indeed as every one who donates a pint of blood for this purpose helps in the testing of several hundred bottles of blood and/or patients. Such donors are bled into dry sterile bottles and their blood allowed to clot. The serum is prepared and tested as described in Chapter 4.

Recent advances in the study of post-transfusion hepatitis have included the discovery of an antigen in the sera of patients with serum and infectious hepatitis, and in other diseases if therapy included multi-transfusions. The first example was found in an Australian aborigine—hence it is now known as Australia antigen. It is particulate and resembles a virus when examined under the electron microscope. It is thought that the antigen is responsible for both the infectious and serum hepatitis.

Antibody to the Australia antigen has been detected only in multi-transfused patients, particularly those with hæmophilia.

It has been found in some patients who did not develop clinical hepatitis; on the other hand the presence of the antibody even in high titre in some cases did not prevent the development of the disease (Holland *et al.*, 1969).

The Australia antigen and antibody is detected either by a micro-Ouchterlony technique of diffusion in agar gel or by a more sensitive complement-fixation technique.

The antibody is rare; if enough could be found it could be used for the screening of all donors for the presence of Australia antigen and thus at least a proportion of those who were potential sources of serum jaundice would be eliminated.

Techniques

Technique No. 28.1. Bleeding a donor

The blood is taken into an M.R.C. bottle containing 120 ml. of A.C.D. The bottle is gently shaken to wet the sides with the anti-coagulant, the cap is swabbed with 75 per cent alcohol containing 10 per cent Rockall before inserting the needles of the airlet and the taking apparatus. The airlet is inspected by eye to detect any which are non-patent. One drop of phenol-glycerine (glycerine plus 5 per cent phenol (Sherwin 1956))* is run down each

* When a bottle of blood cools from approx. 37°C to 4°C the contents contract and air is sucked in; the phenol-glycerine is very effective in preventing entry of organisms which might infect the blood.

needle to form a protective antiseptic layer over the puncture in the rubber wad—this can be done very conveniently by means of a plastic oil-can containing the phenol-glycerine.

Meanwhile the donor is prepared; the arm chosen is usually the left for right-handed persons and the right for left-handed but the veins at the bend of the elbow are palpated and if one arm has a larger and firmer vein than the other, this is chosen. The donor lies in a comfortable position, the arm supported at the elbow by a small pillow so that it is well extended. The cuff of a sphygmomanometer is adjusted round the upper arm. The skin over the selected area is cleansed by swabbing thoroughly with soap solution followed by the alcohol and Rockall mixture. The cuff of the sphygmomanometer is inflated to give a pressure of 100 mm. Hg which can be reduced to 40 mm. after the taking needle has been inserted in the vein. The medical officer gives an injection of local anæsthetic and inserts the taking needle into the vein. The donor holds a small pad in the palm of the hand which he squeezes gently to aid the flow of blood. The bottle is gently rotated to give good mixing of blood and anti-coagulant. The donor's name, address, serial number, etc., are checked and the bottle and pilot-tube labelled while actually at the bedside. If the flow lessens or stops a further airlet should be inserted immediately in case the one already in position while appearing patent is not really so. The pressure in the cuff of the sphygmomanometer should on no account be released before this has been done, as, if the stoppage is due to excess pressure in the bottle, air might be drawn into the donor's vein and an air embolism result. When the bottle is full to the 540 ml. marking the pressure is released and the tubing clamped. The needle is withdrawn from the donor's vein and placed in the pilot tube, the blood in the apparatus being allowed to run into the tube. A small pressure pad is placed over the puncture and strapped into position where it should remain for 24 hours.

The needles are removed first from the bottle and then from the pilot tube. The rubber wad exposed through the perforations in the cap is covered with adhesive tape and the bottle vis-capped.

Technique No. 28.2a. The VDRL reaction

Materials

VDRL antigen (we use "Wellcome" brand); Buffered saline. This is made up by dissolving 0·093 gm. $Na_2HPO_4.12H_2O$
0·170 gm. KH_2PO_4 and
10·0 gm. NaCl in one litre

of distilled water and adding 0·5 ml. of formaldehyde. The pH of this solution is 6·0 ± 0·1.

Normal saline *i.e.* 9 gm. NaCl to one litre of distilled water.

Preparation of antigen emulsion. The antigen is made up by dropping 0·5 ml. of the antigen into 0·4 ml. of buffered saline, rotating the solution while the antigen is being added and for a further 10 seconds to ensure a good mixing. Then 4·1 ml. of buffered saline is added, the bottle (a 30 ml. bottle is recommended) is stoppered and vigorously shaken for a further 10 seconds. The prepared antigen emulsion is stored in a 4°C refrigerator until needed. This emulsion is quite stable but a fresh supply should be made each week. Each batch should be tested with known negative and positive sera; if the results are not clear cut the preparation of the emulsion has not been satisfactory and a fresh batch should be prepared giving especial attention to the mixing.

The quantitative slide test. Using the VDRL as a screening test the quantitative slide test is the method of choice.

The sera to be tested are inactivated for 30 minutes at 56°C. The actual test is satisfactorily performed in welled tiles, and plastic tiles with eight rows each of ten wells are a convenient size.

Each serum is tested by placing 0·05 ml. of serum into a well of the slide and adding one drop ($\frac{1}{60}$th ml.) of antigen emulsion. The slides are rotated for 4 minutes on a mechanical rotator (a suitable one is supplied by Luckhams). The tests are read microscopically immediately after rotation at 100× magnification against a black spot background. The latter is not essential but we find it more satisfactory particularly when large numbers of tests have to be read. The positive reaction is a clumping of the emulsified particles. Large and medium clumps are read as a definite positive, an even distribution of small clumps as a weak positive—no clumping as negative. Occasionally irregular clumping or a loose formation of clumps is seen; this is a zonal reaction and the serum should be retested at 1 in 5 and 1 in 25 dilutions in normal saline.

Comment. A simple and reliable technique. A few false positive reactions are obtained but in a screening test this is a good fault.

Technique No. 28.2b. Blood group antibody screening using VDRL dilutions

Some time ago we wished to add a second antibody screening test to all our donor samples without greatly increasing the work. A method using the VDRL tests as a source of the donor's serum was devised by Leak and Walker. When the VDRL tests have been read one drop of papain treated OR_1R_2K positive red cells are added to each well. The tiles are stacked and the top one covered by an empty tile. They are then incubated for 30 minutes, gently rotated for about 4 seconds and examined for agglutination with the naked eye. Any serum giving a positive reaction is investigated by normal techniques to determine the specificity of the antibodies detected.

Comment. This has proved a very useful additional technique —we have not missed an Rh antibody (anti-D, anti-c, anti-e, etc.) detected by the more conventional techniques, anti-K has been detected, anti-Le^a and anti-Le^b and anti-P_1. Papain type auto antibodies are also detected.

Technique No. 28.3. Price precipitation test for syphilis

This is a modification of the Kahn test which has certain advantages:

(1) The results are more easily read than those of the Kahn test.
(2) The results given by different batches of antigen are identical.
(3) The antigen can be kept made up for use for long periods.
(4) The results are more specific than those of the Kahn.

Preparation of Antigen for Use in the Test. To make up 12 ml. of antigen (for 300–400 serum tests) 20 ml. of the alcoholic extract of ox heart muscle* is added to 12 ml. of normal saline. To do this, 20 ml. of alcoholic extract is measured into a large centrifuge tube or other suitable container, and 12 ml. of normal saline into another. The alcoholic extract is then poured on to the saline and the mixture poured back and forth six times. It is allowed to stand for 30 minutes. (It is important not to pour the saline on to the alcoholic extract.)

The mixture is centrifuged at 2,000 r.p.m. for 10 minutes after which the supernatant fluid is poured off and discarded. The precipitate is further drained of fluid by allowing the tube to stand in an inverted position on filter paper for 5 minutes. Any fluid still remaining on the side of the tube can be wiped off with filter paper or a cloth. Twelve ml. of normal saline is added to the precipitate. Mixture is effected with a pipette and the resulting suspension is transferred to a brown glass bottle with glass stopper or vulcanite screw cap. To avoid infection 0·022 ml. of 6·8 per cent sodium azide is added to each millilitre of suspension. When not in use the antigen is kept at 4°C.

* This can be prepared locally or obtained from the V.D.R.L. reference laboratory.

It is recommended that sufficient antigen for one week's work is made at a time.

The Test. Two tests are performed on each serum, so that a pair of tubes is required for each test, racks can be arranged as for the Kahn test.

Into the first tube is placed five volumes neat serum and into the second five volumes of serum and five volumes of saline, five volumes of the mixture being discarded. A known positive control is included with each batch of tests. One volume of antigen is now added to all tubes, and the tubes are shaken for 5 minutes. Subsequently 1 ml. of normal saline is added to each tube.

The results are read either with a ×6 lens and slit lamp or with the aid of a concave mirror as above.

The positive reactions appear as in the Kahn but the aggregates are usually larger.

The pipettes used for the technique are dropping pipettes, one giving a drop of five times the volume of the other. A convenient size is 0·11 ml. for the larger drop and 0·022 ml. for the smaller.

Standardisation

The precipitation titre is determined by making up four mixtures of 1 ml. heart extract with 0·4 ml., 0·6 ml., 0·8 ml., and 1 ml. respectively of normal saline. These are prepared as described above for use in the test, adding 0·6 ml. saline to each precipitate formed. Each antigen dilution is then tested against a known moderate positive serum, a normal serum and saline by the P.P.R. method.

Experience has shown that a suitable antigen is always obtained by mixing 0·6 ml. of normal saline to 1 ml. of alcoholic extract of heart muscle.

Comment

This technique may be selected in preference to 28.2a if desired. However, proficiency in reading takes longer to acquire.

BIBLIOGRAPHY

Cossart, Y., Taylor, P. E., Vahrman, J., and Zuckerman, A. J. (1969), "Australia-SH antigen in hepatitis patients in London." *Brit. med. J.*, **27**, 755.

Holland, P. V., Walsh, J. H., Morrow, A. G., and Purcell, R. H. (1969), "Failure of Australia antibody to prevent post-transfusion hepatitis." *Lancet*, **II**, Sept. 13, 553.

Leak, M., and Walker, G. Personal communication.

Okochi, D., and Murakami, S. (1968), "Observations on Australia antigen in Japanese." *Vox Sang.*, **15**, 374.

CHAPTER 29

THE FORENSIC APPLICATION OF BLOOD GROUPS

FORENSIC science deals often with problems of identity. Blood groups are excellent aids to these pursuits. They do not however show a positive identity, for example: "This man is the father of this child" or "This bloodstain originated from this person" but they do show a positive non-identity, for example: "This man is *not* the father of this particular child" or "This bloodstain *cannot* have originated from that person".

It is not our intention to write exhaustively on the subject of forensic blood grouping and immunology. Many of the techniques used are beyond the scope of this book. However, some of them are merely adaptations of those already described in other chapters and others can be readily mastered by workers who have become familiar with the practical application of blood grouping to clinical and transfusion problems. It must be stressed that although a good theoretical and practical grounding in blood grouping is essential for the forensic serologist, it does not by itself provide the necessary experience for forensic work. This must be gained in the laboratory while studying forensic problems which are very different from clinical ones.

The chapter is divided into two parts each dealing with the forensic aspect of (*a*) paternity tests and (*b*) blood grouping of stains.

(1) Blood Grouping applied to cases of Doubtful Paternity

Since blood group antigens are inherited according to Mendelian laws, they may be of value in problems of identity, for example in cases of doubtful paternity. The two relevant rules of inheritance are as follows:

(1) A blood group antigen cannot appear in a child unless present in one or other (or both) of the parents.
(2) If one or other parent is homozygous for a particular blood group antigen, it must appear in the blood of the child.

A simple example dependent upon (1) would be the situation in which the mother and putative father were both of group O and the child group A. The A gene of the child must have been inherited from its father who could not, therefore, be group O. The serological test has thereby excluded him from paternity.

An example dependent upon (2) would be a putative father of Rh type CC who must therefore pass C to all his offspring and who could not be the father of a child of type cc. However the application of the second rule cannot be quite so reliably made since homozygosity for a particular gene cannot be so accurately determined; the possibility of a rare allele being passed to the child which goes undetected must be considered. An example of this might be a putative father who was CC^w and a child C^wc; if anti-C^w was omitted from the testing sera the father would appear to be CC (*i.e.* positive with anti-C and negative with anti-c) while the child would appear to be cc (*i.e.* negative with anti-C and positive with anti-c), thus a false exclusion could be obtained.

The greater the number of blood group systems that can be used in cases of doubtful paternity, the greater is the chance of excluding a man if he is not the father of a particular child. If the ABO system alone is considered, there is an 18 per cent chance of excluding paternity but if all the principal blood group systems are included, the chance increases to 62 per cent.

Identification of Samples

It is important to prove that the correct persons have been tested and that there has been no substitution. In some instances a solicitor may be present at the sample taking. When the clients arrive unaccompanied, the serologist must ask for some proof of identity, *e.g.* a driving licence, the signature upon which can be compared with one written at the time of sample taking or a passport. If the putative father and the mother (with child) can be persuaded to be present at the same time, then they are able to identify each other. Posted specimens have to be accompanied by a simple certificate declaring that the blood samples are in fact from the persons whose names appear on the labels.

Sampling. A few ml. of clotted blood from each individual is sufficient. From young babies from whom it is difficult to obtain blood by venepuncture 0·5 ml. to 1 ml. samples taken by heel-prick into heparin or sequestrine are very satisfactory. 2 ml. lithium heparin containers are excellent for blood sampling. Any amount up to 2 ml. can be put into them. Surprisingly, perhaps, 0·4 ml. of blood taken by ear or heel prick into these containers is ample for tests for all the red cell antigens and PGM and the plasma is sufficient for serum grouping, Gm, Gc and haptoglobin typing.

Blood Group Systems Used in Problems of Parentage

These always include tests for ABO (including A_1 and A_2), MNS (occasionally $\bar{s}$) Rh (D, C, C^w, E, $\bar{c}$, and $\bar{e}$) and at least 3 of the following: Fy^a, K, Lu^a, Jk^a, Gm^a. This brings the chance of proving non-paternity, if such is the case, to about 62 per cent.

As well as the above, haptoglobins are added almost routinely and Gc groups and red cell enzymes, such as phospho-gluco-mutase (PGM) are not infrequently included. The combined exclusion rate if all these systems are used is raised to 72 per cent.

Techniques for estimating haptoglobins and Gc groups both of which are genetically inherited serum groups will be found in Chapter 31. The specialised biochemical procedures for detection of red cell enzymes are beyond the scope of this book.

A plan for a full typing of red cells for nine main blood group systems is given in Appendix 1, Procedure No. 3.

It is essential in cases in which an exclusion is found to repeat all the tests with a larger panel of antisera, preparing fresh red cell suspension from the original samples.

Interpretation of Results

Putative fathers are excluded from paternity if results are found which are contrary to one or other or both of the laws of inheritance mentioned earlier in the chapter. The most cast-iron exclusions are those in which it is found that the child possesses an antigen which is absent from the mother and the putative father when all three individuals were tested on the same occasion with the same reagents.

Homozygosity in the putative father for a gene which the child lacks (or *vice versa*) is equally good evidence of non-paternity, provided the serologist is satisfied that the putative father is, in fact, homozygous for the particular gene and does not possess a rare undetected allele. Dosage titrations are often of value here (*see* technique No. 29.1).

The Suitability of the Various Blood Groups Systems for Paternity Testing

ABO Blood Group System

The inheritance of this has been well worked out and is entirely reliable.

The exceedingly few abnormalities as, *e.g.* one apparent mutation where mother was AB and child O, or a case where a B gene was suppressed in one generation (*see* Chapter 30), which have been found are the accumulation of years of work by many serologists and are drawn from many thousands of family studies. They can in no way be said to throw into disrepute the reliability of ABO tests in cases of doubtful paternity.

The results of sub-typing with anti-A_1 are valuable in certain circumstances. An exclusion based on the finding of an A_2 child must be viewed with caution and should not be given much weight unless an exclusion supporting it is found by another blood group system. The evidence for non-paternity is on more reliable grounds if the child reacts with anti-A_1 while the mother and putative father do not. Particularly is it of value to find that a child is A_1 in a case of exclusion based on putative father and mother being group O and child group A.

The rarities and anomalies in the system are unlikely to lead to erroneous conclusions about paternity if red cells are routinely tested with group O serum and sera are tested with A_1, A_2, B and O red cells.

For example, O_h ("Bombay" phenotype) is disclosed by the presence of a powerful anti-H in the serum. A_m patterns as a group O with a missing anti-A and A_x is agglutinated by group O serum only (*see* Chapter 32).

The very rare families in which an AB child has one group O parent, are recognisable by the comparative weakness of the B antigen and the presence of a fraction of the anti-B spectrum of antibodies in the serum (*see* page 363).

MNS

The MN typing of family material has been studied for over 40 years and the results establish beyond doubt its reliability as a tool for the solution of problems of parentage. Nevertheless, the rare MN alleles (*e.g.* N_2, M_g, etc.) must be remembered in a medico-legal context (*see* Chapter 34).

In practice, the possible presence of such rare alleles must be considered wherever the putative father is M and the child N or when the putative father is N and the child M. If, in either of these, the father and the child had, for example, Mg, an entirely opposite interpretation of results would have to be made. The man, far from being excluded from being the father of the child, would be virtually proven to be the father since they both would have this very rare allele. However, M_g has not been found in testing at least 60,000 English blood donors. Moreover, anti-M_g can be obtained fairly readily and should be included in the tests where appropriate. M^k producing no M, N, S or s is of similar rarity to M_g but anti-M^k is not available. "Dosage" titrations may be helpful as confirmatory tests.

The Rh System

This system is of value in excluding paternity but there are sometimes difficulties in connexion with alternative genotypes. Paternity could appear to be excluded by the probable genotypes of the persons tested but there might be a rare alternative genotype on the basis of which there would not be an exclusion. An example taken from an actual paternity problem will help to make this point clear.

Mother—phenotype R_1R_1, *i.e.* C+ D+ E− c−
probable genotype CDe.CDe
Child—phenotype R_1r, *i.e.* C+ D+ E− c+
probable genotype CDe.cde
Putative father—phenotype R_1R_2, *i.e.* C+ D+ E+ c+
probable genotype CDe.cDE

Given that the probable genotypes are the actual genotypes in the above case, the putative father could not be the father of the child. But should the father be of the alternative genotype CDE.cde he could be the father of the child. This genotype is about sixty times less common than CDe.cDE (*see* Table 11.3), so the chance of his belonging to this genotype is less than 1 in 60.

Uncommon Rh alleles, C^x, E^w, etc., must be remembered and if possible sera capable of detecting them used to check any apparent exclusion (*see* Chapter 33).

The Lutheran System

With good anti-Lu^a sera, evidence of non-paternity might be accepted, but owing to the small number of families studied to date, exclusion on this system alone should be regarded with caution.

The Kell System

Tests with anti-K are suitable for paternity work but the frequency of K is such that non-paternity could only be proved in less than 1 per cent of cases.

The Duffy System

The Fy^a antigen can be useful for paternity tests providing a reliable pure anti-Fy^a serum is available for testing. Unfortunately, anti-Fy^a often occurs in a mixture of antibodies and care must be exercised that the serum is specific. Anti-Fy^b is also suitable but the possibility of the presence of Fy^c must not be overlooked.

The Kidd System

This system is sometimes useful but the necessary antisera are not readily available at the present time, mainly because they deteriorate rapidly on storage.

The Lewis System

In view of remarks previously made (*see* Chapter 15), on the inheritance of the Lewis groups, it is not surprising to learn that this system cannot be applied to tests for disputed paternity.

Secretion of A, B and H Substances

The secretor genes can be applied with confidence to problems of parentage, but only the "mating" sese x sese could show an exclusion; *i.e.* if the child were a secretor. Such a mating occurs in 5 per cent of English families.

P Groups

Like secretion, the P system could only be helpful in 4–5 per cent of cases in which the mother and alleged father had no trace of P_1, while the child had a strongly developed P_1 antigen.

Example Case

The following is a case in the authors' experience in which blood grouping achieved a threefold result.

There were two putative fathers, one of whom—Mr. Smith—was described as being the father of the baby's mother (Miss Joan Smith). Thus the question of incest arose.

Tests for ABO, MNS, Rh, Fy^a and Kell groups were made. All the significant results were those relating to the Cc alleles of the Rh system, as shown below:

	Anti-D	Anti-C	Anti-C^w	Anti-E	Anti-c
Mr. Smith	+	+	−	−	−
Mr. Jones	+	Weak	+	−	+
Miss Joan Smith	−	−	−	−	+
Baby John Smith	+	Weak	+	−	+

Mr. Smith (the girl's father) was excluded from paternity since his genotype was CC and that of the baby C^wc.

Mr. Jones was likely to be the father since he and the child both shared the rather infrequent gene C^w. In fact, on probability, Mr. Jones is fifty times more likely to be the father than a random man.

The third totally unexpected finding was that Mr. Smith was, after all, not the father of Miss Joan Smith since she was Rh negative and had cc!

Presentation of Results

Results have to be presented at two levels. First a summary of the findings must be given in sufficient detail to satisfy a second blood grouping expert, because occasionally the legal profession will call upon another blood group specialist to do confirmatory tests.

Secondly, the results must be intelligible to solicitors and the courts who, in respect of blood groups, are in the position of laymen.

It is our practice to sum up the findings in one of two ways—according to whether or not an exclusion of paternity has been found.

(*a*) In cases of exclusion we say "Mr. X has been excluded beyond reasonable doubt from being the father of baby Y".

(*b*) In cases of non-exclusion we say "The blood group findings do not exclude Mr. X from the possibility of being the father of baby Y".

However, with regard to (*b*) on occasions some tact has to be displayed!

When the putative father happens to be the husband or when it is known that the people concerned hope that there will not be an exclusion, it is more appropriate to say "there is nothing in the blood group findings against the paternity of Mr. X".

The Possibility of Proof of Paternity from Blood Groups

The usefulness of blood groups in assisting in proof of non-paternity is now well established and, the Courts accept blood group evidence.

Proof of paternity (*i.e.* determining that only one particular man can be the father of a particular child) is at the present time, impossible. However, assistance towards giving a judgement can be obtained by calculating the chance in a given case of a putative father who is *not* the true father being able to pass on the blood group genes necessary for making him, on blood group evidence, a possible father for the child. If this chance is small enough to be statistically significant then the putative father, who besides having these required genes, is known to the mother, is likely to be the true father of the child.

The usual procedure is as follows:

If, after completion of a blood group investigation upon putative father, mother and child, no exclusion of paternity is evident, the blood group genes which have been shown to be of paternal origin are noted. The chance the putative father has of passing on these genes all together in one single sperm is compared with the chance of obtaining such a sperm from a man in the random population (for, if the putative father is not the true father, he is a randomly selected man from the blood group point of view).

The combined chance of obtaining the necessary genes from the putative father is arrived at by multiplying together either 1 or 0·5 according to whether he is known to be homozygous or heterozygous for the relevant gene. If this is unknown, he is arbitrarily taken to be heterozygous.

The figure for the probability of obtaining the genes from a randomly selected man is calculated by multiplying together the known frequencies of the genes in the appropriate racial population.

The balance of these probabilities gives the odds in favour of paternity. A whole range of results is obtained. If, in testing a family, only common blood group genes are found, or if only one or two genes are known for certainty to come from the father, the odds in favour of paternity would not be significant. Statistical significance begins at the 19:1 level.

The example shown below is illustrative.

Name	ABO	MNS	D	C	$\bar{c}$	E	C^w	K	Fy^a	Hp
Mr. R	A_1	MNS+	+	+	+	−	−	+	+	2–2
Mr. W	A_1B	MS+	+	+	+	−	−	−	+	2–1
Mrs. W	A_2	MS+	+	−	+	+	−	−	+	2–2
Baby W	A_1	MNS+	+	+	+	−	−	+	−	2–2

The results of a blood group analysis in which one of two putative fathers (Mr. W) is excluded from paternity of baby W and the probability of the other (Mr. R) being the father is statistically significant.

Baby W has to receive A_1, N, C (almost certainly as CDe) and K from his father as the mother lacks them all.

In addition, haptoglobin type 2 must be of paternal origin, since the child is homozygous for the gene. Mr. R's probability of paternity is worked out as follows:

	A_1	N	CDe	K	Hp^2	*Probability*
Mr. R.	0·5	0·5	0·5	0·5	1·0	0·0625
Random man	0·21	0·46	0·41	0·05	0·58	0·0012

Balance of probabilities in favour of Mr. R. 52 to 1 (approx).

Thus, in this case the results of a blood group analysis exclude one putative father (Mr. W) and the probability of the other (Mr. R) being the father is statistically significant.

If there is a possibility of another related man being involved in the case, then special calculations may have to be made; the extreme case being where the putative father has an identical twin. On blood grouping evidence the probabilities would, of course, be the same for each twin.

Identification of Stains and Fragments from Individuals

Since the subject of this book is blood group serology we are mainly concerned with the blood-group aspect of the identification of stains from body fluids. However, it must be realised that, in any actual forensic problem, the identification of a stain as being, for example, human blood must precede any attempt to ascertain its groups. These preliminary tests make a claim on material which may already be inadequate in quantity and is always irreplaceable. No criminal who accidentally stains his coat with blood will obligingly offer a repeat sample for the convenience of the laboratory! Thus, techniques which have the merit of requiring small amounts of material for their performance are those of choice providing they satisfy the major criterion of reliability.

For the sake of completeness and clarity, a brief summary of the necessary steps in the identification of a body fluid follows.

Screening Tests

Chemical tests such as the benzidine or Kartlemeyer tests for blood and the acid phosphotase test for seminal fluid are invaluable particularly when the nature of the stain is not obvious to the naked eye, perhaps because of its small size. They have the virtue of not using up an appreciable amount of material and of being so sensitive that there is no point in carrying out serological tests on areas in which these tests are negative. Thus, for example, in the absence of a positive benzidine test, one would not find it worth while to apply any other tests to the suspected stained area.

Critical Tests of Identity

The identification of a stain as blood, unless only too obvious to the naked eye, is by successfully demonstrating the presence of hæmoglobin. This is usually done by the hæmochromogen crystal test or by spectroscopic examination.

Seminal fluid is identified by the examination of a smear for spermatozoa; in addition, an immunological method is sometimes used (Coombs *et al.*, 1963).

Saliva reveals itself by the starch test for amylases together with a histological examination for buccal cells. Vaginal fluid shows squamous epithelial cells but is negative for amylase, and is found in different situations.

Species Identification

This is usually required for a blood stain although on some occasions it may be appropriate to attempt to find the species of origin of other kinds of stain.

The species of origin is determined by using antisera more or less specific for the proteins contained in the serum of the stain. The laboratory must, therefore, possess a collection of reliable antisera capable of making distinctions between various common species, *e.g.*, Man, dog, cat, ox, sheep, chicken, etc. In some countries it may be necessary to make the rather difficult distinction between ape and Man, for which carefully absorbed antisera are required.

In many cases, however, all that is necessary is the establishment of the blood as human, so an anti-human globulin is used first and, if this test (with suitable controls) is positive, the investigation need proceed no further. A negative test may either mean that the blood is other than human or that the proteins in the stain have denatured to the extent of being inactive. At this point tests should be made for other species. Various antisera specific for animal species can be obtained commercially.

There are five main methods by which the antiglobulin may be used:

(*a*) Ring test.
(*b*) Antiglobulin consumption test.
(*c*) Electrophoresis in agar.
(*d*) "Mixed" agglutination.
(*e*) Passive hæmagglutination.

Of these, we propose to describe in detail the anti-globulin consumption test (technique No. 29.2) and the electrophoretic method 29.6. References to some of the other techniques may be found at the end of the chapter.

The anti-globulin consumption test should always be included in the "repertoire" of the laboratory. It is highly sensitive and will detect globulin in dilutions of the order of 1 in 50,000. It is not dependent upon having a clear stain extract or upon optimum proportions of antigen to antibody; nor does it require such highly specific antisera, as the preciptin or mixed antiglobulin methods. It has been used highly successfully on stains some years old. It is not so readily applicable to the detection of proteins other than human since these require red cells sensitised with protein from the particular animal species for which the test is being made.

When it is necessary to test for the protein of species other than human, an electrophoretic method in agar gel is recommended; this method is also excellent for identifying human globulin in stains. Using the same buffer system as for Gc groups, the movement of the gamma globulins is toward the cathode, while albumin and all other globulins move toward the anode. Thus it can be arranged that the non-gamma globulins from a stain to be tested for its species of origin, move towards the gamma type antibody in an anti-species specific globulin (anti-human, anti-cow, anti-pig, etc.). At the point between two wells punched in the gell the reactants meet and a line of precipitate is formed (technique 29.6).

(2) The Grouping of Stains

It will be appreciated that direct agglutination tests are not possible for the detection of antigens in blood stains since the red cells have been destroyed and, in the case of stains from other body fluids, the blood group substances are in soluble form.

Three immunological principles are utilised for stain work:

1. Inhibition or specific absorption (*see also* Chapter 8). Methods using this principle depend on the demonstration of the specific uptake of antibody by the corresponding antigen which is present in the stain (*see* technique No. 29.3).

2. Elution. Antibody is taken by the stain and is then eluted by raising the temperature of the test to 56°C in the presence of fresh red cells to which the eluted antibody becomes attached as the tests are allowed to cool (*see* technique No. 29.5).

3. Mixed agglutination (technique No. 29.4). The mixed cell agglutination principle was devised by Coombs, Bedford and Rouillard (1956) for the detection of antigens in cells such as buccal cells, skin cells and platelets, none of which is suitable for direct agglutination tests. The principle of the reaction is illustrated in Plate 11*a* where it may be seen that an antigen on a tissue cell may be revealed by a mixed agglutination procedure if the same antigen is available on a suitable indicator red cell so that an antibody reacting both with the tissue cell and the red cell is capable of binding them together in a mixed cell agglutination reaction.

Teased out fibres of bloodstained cloth will behave as tissue cells in this connexion, as seen in Plate 11*b* and *c*; (*b*) shows A cells bound onto cloth fibres stained with A blood, after treatment of the fibres with anti-A; (*c*) gives the negative appearance after treating the same stain with anti-B followed by B cells.

A Comparison of the Three Methods

The inhibition technique is the least sensitive and requires more material than the direct methods which can be performed on one thread of material.

Only a reduction in titre of the original serum by more than two dilutions is considered significant so that more than three-quarters of the total antibody content of the test reagent has to be absorbed by a stain to give a significant result.

On the other hand, suitable sera are readily available and do not have to be potent, in fact the very opposite—they have to be diluted to give titres of 16–32. In addition, sera do not have to be so free from cross reactions.

In England, however, the inhibition test has been to a large extent superseded by the direct methods.

The absorption-elution and mixed agglutination methods are easier to consider together.

They are more sensitive than the inhibition method and about equally sensitive to each other. Suitable sera have to be specially selected. Antibodies that are readily eluted and which often have a lower titre are most suitable for absorption-elution whereas high titre immune sera are usually best for mixed agglutination.

Great care has to be taken over the stage of washing the fibres free of unbound antibody particularly for absorption-elution where free clumps are more often found and are indicative of a positive reaction.

The Antigens that are Detectable in Blood Stains

Most of the common blood group antigens can be detected by inhibition technique in stains provided these are fresh and sufficiently large, *e.g.* A, B, H, Rh, Kell, Fy^a. The Gm groups have also been demonstrated (Nielsen and Henningsen, 1963).

Recent research has shown that as well as A, B and H the antigens D, C, E, c, C^w, S, Fy^a and K can be successfully demonstrated in stains by the elution method described at the end of this chapter (technique No. 29.5).

Special selection of antisera is of vital importance.

It is highly probable that there is a critical relationship between

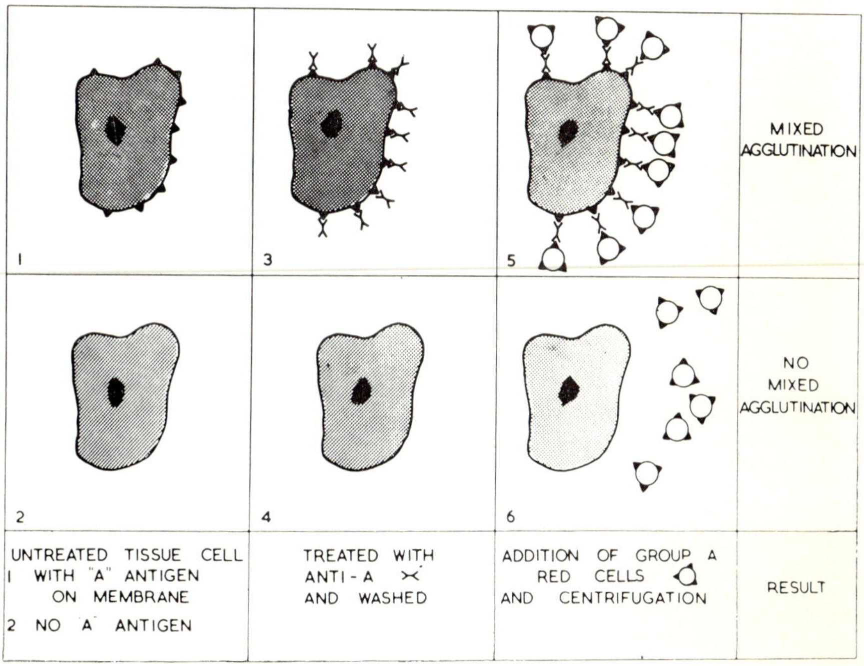

PLATE 11(*a*). Diagrammatic representation of the mixed agglutination reaction for the demonstration of the A antigen on tissue cells.

p. 330

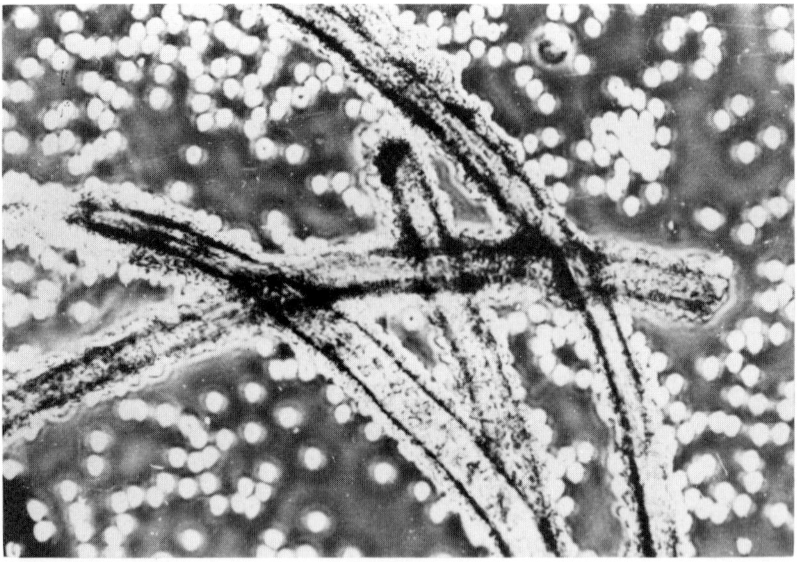

(*b*)

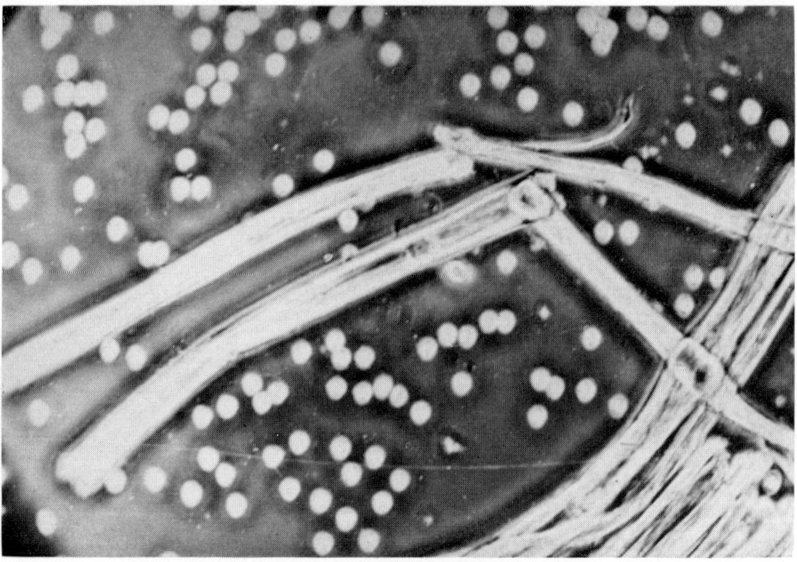

(*c*)

PLATE 11(*b*) and (*c*). Microscopic appearance of a positive (*b*) and negative (*c*) mixed agglutination reaction on blood stained cloth fibres. Phase contrast microscopy ×10 eyepiece; ×40 objective.

(Reproduced from Coombs and Dodd, 1961, by permission)

the required potency of the antiserum and the number of antigenic sites on the red cell for the various antigens. This relationship gains its importance almost certainly because the antigenic sites are not in good shape for the uptake of antibody in blood stains, particularly if these are several weeks or months old.

In the ABO blood grouping of stains, in contrast to the ABO grouping of fresh blood, anti-H (from Ulex) is a most important reagent since it provides a valuable positive reaction which is particularly applicable to O stains in situations (which are many) when it is not possible to test for agglutinins in stains. When there is sufficient material and it is not too old an extract of a stain may show sufficient antibody activity for "cross grouping" to be done. Sometimes papain treated A and B cells may be used with advantage in such tests.

The Grouping of Stains from Other Body Fluids

A, B and H antigens in seminal and salival stains are usually readily detectable and particularly successful results have been obtained with the direct methods described above, using stained teased out fibres. By these methods also it is possible to detect the traces of blood group substances present in the fluids of non-secretors. This is particularly useful from the forensic point of view as otherwise about 20 per cent of the stains encountered could not be grouped.

Mixtures of Stains

In trying to solve actual problems of crime, the serologist very often has to work with mixed stains—*e.g.* blood contaminated with saliva or, more commonly, vaginal fluid mixed with fluid of seminal origin. False results can be obtained if the possibility of mixtures is not realised. For example, a group O secretor man accused of raping a girl who is a group A secretor might be excluded from blame if the serologist wrongly reports that seminal fluid of group A has been identified on the girl's clothing.

Body Fragments

Fragments from individuals, such as skin, dander, muscle fibres, hair, can be successfully typed using ABH antisera. Mixed agglutination is the method of choice for this material.

The Effect of Age and other Adverse Conditions on the Serological Testing of Stains

No rules can be laid down for the effect of the passage of time on the activity of stains. Some fresh stains may deteriorate quickly if adverse conditions obtain, such as dampness, in which bacterial action may flourish. On the other hand, blood group activity may remain in stains many years old. The A, B and H antigens are the most stable.

M and N antigens are usually readily detectable up to 6 months. In experimental stains, kept under laboratory conditions, the Rh antigens D, C, C^w and c have been shown to be active for the same period; but E could only be detected satisfactorily up to 6 weeks. Using anti-S with an a.h.g. titre of 128 clear-cut reactions were obtained by absorption elution on stains up to a period of 6 months (Lincoln and Dodd, 1968).

Contact with soil often reduces activity considerably and, not unexpectedly, harm may be caused by contamination with soap powders, detergents and other chemicals. The substrate may take up antibodies non specifically, therefore controls from adjacent unstained areas form an essential part of any investigation.

Readers who require the forensic aspects of blood grouping in greater detail than space allows here are referred to the Bibliography which follows and also to the relevant chapters in Gradwohl's *Legal Medicine* (2nd ed.).

Technique No. 29.1. Titration technique for revealing antigen–antibody "dosage"

The technique may be required to demonstrate whether or not an antibody produces a "dosage" effect or, given a known dosing antiserum, to find out whether red cells belonging to a particular phenotype are homozygous or heterozygous for a particular blood group gene. This last may be particularly useful in blood grouping in cases of doubtful paternity.

For the sake of clarity, the method is described in relation to c and anti-c; other blood group antigens and antibodies can be similarly investigated using other appropriate red cells and antisera.

Serial dilutions of anti-c are made using the master titre technique (No. 5) and the required number of titrations run out from this, *e.g.* six. Two examples of cde.cde cells are placed in rows 1 and 2 respectively and two examples of CDe.cde or other "single" dose c cells are run into rows 3 and 4. Rows 5 and 6 are used for cells under test.

The dosing phenomena is more usually shown by saline agglutinins but occasionally the effect is well seen when albumin or antihuman globulin methods are used.

At least a fourfold or preferably an eight-fold difference in titre between "single" dose or "double" dose cells should be found before it can be established that the dosage effect is occurring.

The technique is particularly useful in assessing the true genotype of individuals, *e.g.* if red cells thought to be cc behave as double-dose c cells, then they are unlikely to contain a rare antigen such as C^w or C^x.

Technique No. 29.2. Anti-human globulin consumption test

This test detects human globulin. The basis of the method is that human globulin will inhibit the activity of anti-human globulin serum, the inhibition being demonstrated by the failure of the anti-human globulin to agglutinate red cells sensitised by incomplete antibodies. An anti-human globulin serum, giving a titre of 16–32 against strongly sensitised D positive red cells, is suitable. It is mixed with the stain extract and the mixtures left on the bench for at least two hours, or up to 48 hours if the stain is old. The mixtures are then titred and their titres compared with the original titre of the anti-human globulin.

A drop of fluid from each tube, beginning with the most dilute solution, is placed on an opalescent tile. Another row of drops has to be made from the original titre of the anti-human globulin and a further series from a test made of unstained cloth. A drop of D positive red cells, strongly sensitised by incomplete anti-D, is added to each and the mixtures are made uniform with a plastic applicator stick. The tile is rocked gently, left to stand for about five minutes and then read in the normal manner for indirect anti-globulin tests. A reduction in titration value of more than two dilutions is indicative of the presence of human globulin in the extract of the stain being tested.

Technique No. 29.3. Inhibition technique for A, B and H

The anti-A and anti-B chosen should be fairly potent sera which can be diluted with saline just before use to give a titration value of 16–32. Weak antisera not requiring dilution are not so satisfactory. Anti-H (ulex) of about the same titre is included. Equal volume of the stain extract (or finely shredded stained material) and each antiserum are mixed together and left for 1½ to 2 hours at 4°C or, preferably, overnight. The tubes are then centrifuged, the supernatant fluids titrated and the titrations compared with the original titre of the antisera. The original serum has a volume of saline added in place of the extract of the stain. If the antiserum was placed straight onto the stained cloth, then the volume of saline is omitted. A control from an unstained area is included with each set of tests.

The tests are then read in the normal manner for ABO titrations.

The presence of a group specific substance is not considered to be demonstrated unless it can be shown to have brought about a reduction in titre of the original antiserum of 3 or more dilutions.

Technique No. 29.4. Detection of antigens in stains by mixed agglutination

Reagents

Testing Sera. Anti-A and anti-B

These must be monospecific reagents. High titre "immune" sera are particularly excellent but standard grouping sera are often suitable. It must be emphasised, however, that sera must be specially selected and not all high titre sera are equally good. The sera are heated at 50°C for half-an-hour before use. They are also centrifuged as a method of clarification.

Anti-H

The plant lectin, obtained by making a saline extract of gorse seeds (ulex europeus) works well.

Sera may be used neat or, if the titre allows, at dilutions of about 1/5.

Diluents. Diluents and washing fluids are more satisfactory if they contain a little protein—a 1 in 200 solution in saline of heat inactivated normal rabbit serum, absorbed free of antibodies, for A, B and O red cells is suitable or, alternatively, a 1 in 200 solution of bovine albumin.

Red Cell Indicator System. This consists of a 1 per cent solution of the appropriate washed red cells in diluent. For anti-H it is advisable to use papain-treated indicator cells of group O.

Glassware. Some workers prefer to use siliconised tubes to reduce the tendency of the fibres to stick to the glass. Alternatively, polythene tubes may be used but the fibres are not so clearly visible owing to the more opaque nature of the tube. The transfer of fibres is facilitated by using siliconised pipettes. Serologists who normally use one graduated pipette for all operations should note that there is more danger of contaminating one aliquot of fibrils with another than there is of contaminating one antiserum with another through insufficient rinsing of the pipette.

Method

Small pieces are cut out from the blood-stained cloth and, with sharp scissors, cut into lengths of about 0·2 cm. They are then manipulated under a dissecting microscope and the individual fibres teased apart. (Stainless steel dissecting needles are convenient but must be continually sharpened.) The operation is carried out in a few drops of saline or protein diluent.

Another good method of separating the fibres is to place the cut portions of cloth in a siliconised tube covered with a little saline. When the saline has soaked into the segments, they are broken into fibres by inserting a close-fitting glass rod and twirling it in the tube. The bundles of fibres break up by the turbulence induced.

When the fibres are teased sufficiently, they are transferred to 50 × 10 mm. tubes and washed once in diluent. Two or three drops of the appropriate antiserum is then added and the fibres are incubated in the antiserum for some hours or overnight (according to the age of the stains) preferably using a mild agitation by revolving the tubes on a machine such as a Rotatest for some part of the time. At the end of the incubation period, they are carefully washed three or four times in the diluent to free them from uncombined antibody. Many modifications may be adopted for the final stage of the test which, in essence, consists of bringing the indicator red cells into contact with the serum-treated fibres and mounting the product for microscopical examination.

A satisfactory procedure is as follows:

Two or three drops of indicator cell suspension are added to the tubes and left to rotate for about 30 minutes. The fibres are gently drawn up into a capillary pipette and placed on a microscope slide. A cover glass is placed on top and the preparation is sealed with paraffin wax. Viewing takes place under the microscope with dark field, phase contrast or even ordinary illumination. Magnification of ×100 or ×400 may be used. A typical positive appearance is denoted by the coating of the fibres by the indicator cells (*see* Plate 11). Sometimes another kind of positive is encountered in which the indicator cells have tended to break away from the fibres, forming large agglutinated masses. This appearance is often seen with anti-H when papain-treated indicator cells are used. The negative appearance is of uncoated fibres against a background of free (unagglutinated) indicator cells.

When recording results, it is advisable to make two readings and to adopt some suitable symbols for denoting strength of reaction.

Reading (*a*) is of the mixed agglutination proper, *i.e.* the degree to which the indicator cells are bound onto the fibres. Tapping the coverslip with a pointed instrument sometimes facilitates this reading.

Reading (*b*) is of the degree of agglutination of the background indicator cells. Providing the controls of unstained material are negative, showing that washing has been adequate, agglutination of cells unattached to fibres is also indicative of a specific reaction having taken place between the antigen of the stain and the particular antiserum.

Technique No. 29.5. Detection of antigens in stains by absorption-elution

Choice of red cells for use as indicator cells

Cells should not be more than 48 hours old. They are washed three times and ½–1 per cent suspension is made in albumin diluent (1 in 100 bovine albumin). With the exception of A and B antigens, they should as far as possible be from donors homozygous for the antigen it is desired to detect, but at the same time should not react with any unwanted antibody which might also be present in the test serum. For the detection of Rh antigens red cells are papain treated.

Choice of antisera

For A and B, anti-A and anti-B grouping sera, undiluted or suitably diluted are used. H is detected by undiluted anti-H lectin. For M and N, sera have to be specially chosen. About 50 per cent of anti-M sera and 20 per cent of anti-N sera are found satisfactory.

For Rh (D, C, E, c, C^w, e) high titre antisera are usually essential with titres preferably at least 1,000 by enzyme technique.

For Fy^a, K, etc., titres of 128 or more by antiglobulin technique are required. All sera, being used in tests in which the absorption stage takes place at 37°C for long periods, should have a small quantity of sodium azide added.

Method

A thread of blood stained cloth 2–3 mm. long is teased out into individual fibres, using thin pointed glass rods or dissecting needles.

When Rh, Fy^a, K antigens are being detected, a slightly larger piece of stained material is used (*e.g.* 3 × 3 mm.). It is not teased out. Each piece of cloth is placed in a 6 × 1 cm. plastic or glass tube. Some workers prefer to carry out the whole procedure using welled slides. An unstained portion of similar size and material is included as a negative control as well as stains of known groups as both positive and negative controls.

Two volumes of appropriate antiserum are added to each tube and they are capped and incubated for the required length of time at the required temperature (4°C for A, B, H, M and N) (37°C for S, K, Fy^a and Rh).

All tests, except M and N are usually most satisfactory if incubated overnight. M and N tests often cross react too strongly if left for more than several hours at 4°C.

After incubation the serum is removed from each tube and the cloth is sucked dry using a pipette attached to a water pump. Care is taken to use a fine bore pipette so that the material is not lost in the pump.

For A, B, H, M and N the tubes are then filled with ice cold saline and allowed to stand at 4°C until the cloth has settled at the bottom of the tube. It is not usually necessary to centrifuge. Warm saline is used for Rh and other antibodies. The washing process is repeated five times. The last wash is made in albumin diluent.

One or two drops of albumin diluent are then added to each tube and they are placed in a water bath at 56°C for ten minutes, the tubes being gently agitated occasionally. At the end of the elution period, the tubes are removed from the water bath and the appropriate indicator red cells added with as little delay as possible.

Where papain treated cells are used, one drop of $\frac{1}{2}$–1 per cent suspension is added, the tubes are left at 37°C for 1 hour and then read with the microscope.

Where anti-human globulin is being used to detect the eluted antibody, four drops of a 2 per cent suspension of cells is added and after one hour's incubation at 37°C the supernatant fluid and piece of cloth is removed from each tube.

It may be necessary to squeeze the piece of cloth with forceps against the side of the tube.

The cells are then washed three times before being tested with anti-human globulin reagent on a white tile.

Certain modifications may increase the sensitivity of the tests. For example, the anti-globulin test may be performed on enzyme treated red cells (papain) and a spinning anti-globulin technique may be used if desired.

Technique No. 29.6. Special identification of blood stains by electrophoresis in agar

Materials

The buffers and agar used are the same as those given for Gc typing.

The agar is prepared and stored in the same way (*see* technique No. 31.4).

Reagents

Anti-human globulin and other anti-globulins specific for various animal species, *e.g.* cow, pig, chicken, sheep. These can be obtained from Burroughs-Wellcome.

Method

The agar is poured onto microscope slides or a suitable sized glass plate. Glass surfaces must be grease free.

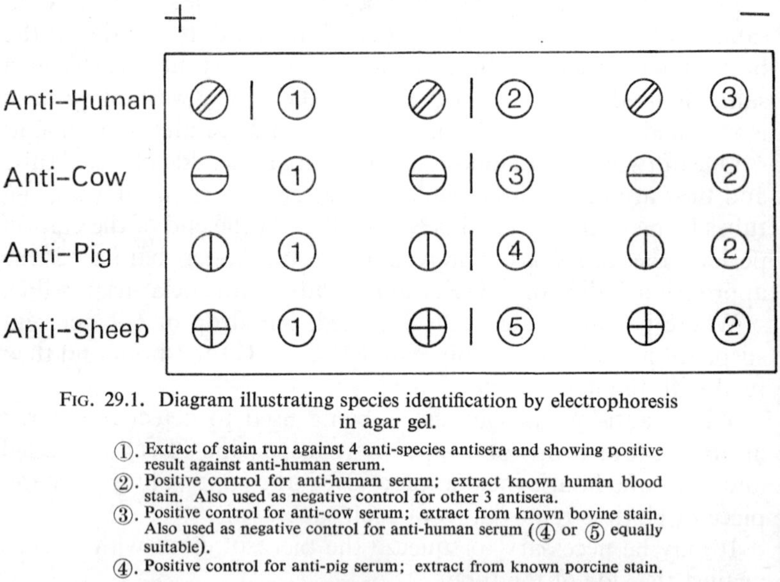

FIG. 29.1. Diagram illustrating species identification by electrophoresis in agar gel.

①. Extract of stain run against 4 anti-species antisera and showing positive result against anti-human serum.
②. Positive control for anti-human serum; extract known human blood stain. Also used as negative control for other 3 antisera.
③. Positive control for anti-cow serum; extract from known bovine stain. Also used as negative control for anti-human serum (④ or ⑤ equally suitable).
④. Positive control for anti-pig serum; extract from known porcine stain.
⑤. Positive control for anti-sheep serum; extract from known ovine stain.

After the gel has set, small wells are punched in the gel in pairs, *see* Fig. 29.1. They should be approximately 1·5 mm. in diameter and 5 mm. apart. They should be accurately placed along the line of electrophoretic movement. The stain to be tested is extracted with gel buffer and a drop placed by means of a fine pipette in the cathodic well of a pair. The antiserum is placed in the anodic well. Controls consisting of extracts of known stains of appropriate age and species are included with each batch of tests. Electrophoresis is performed at 5 V./cm. for 15–20 minutes.

If the antigen extracted from the stain corresponds to the antiserum against which it is tested, a line of precipitation forms between two wells where the reactants meet.

Comment

The test is very sensitive and will detect globulin* in whole blood diluted to 1 in 20,000 to 1 in 30,000.

The extract of the stain to be tested does not have to be clear or fat free.

The same technique can be used for the identification of seminal fluid or saliva with suitable prepared antisera.

* Only the non-gamma globulin in the stain is detected since, in the nature of the test, the gamma globulin is migrating in the *same* direction as the antibody in the anodic well and therefore cannot meet and react with it.

BIBLIOGRAPHY

Bibliography on "Immunology in connection with body fluids and tissues." (1962), *Medicine, Sci., Law*, **2,** 497.

COOMBS, R. R. A., BEDFORD, D., and ROUILLARD, L. M. (1956), "A and B blood group antigens on human epidermal cells demonstrated by mixed agglutination." *Lancet*, **1,** 461.

COOMBS, R. R. A., and DODD, BARBARA (1961), "Possible application of the principle of mixed agglutination in the identification of blood stains." *Medicine, Sci., Law*, **1,** 359.

COOMBS, R. R. A., RICHARDS, C. B., and DODD, BARBARA (1963), "Serological identification of seminal stains." *Medicine, Sci., Law*, **3,** 65.

CULLIFORD, B. J. (1964), "A new method for Precipitin Reactions on Forensic Blood, Semen and Saliva Stains." *Nature, Lond.*, **201,** 1092.

FIORI, A. (1962), "Detection and identification of blood stains." *Methods of Forensic Science*, Vol. 1, p. 252. Ed. F. Lundquist. J. Wiley & Sons, New York/London.

FIORI, A., MARIGO, M., and BENCIOLINI, P. (1963), "Modified absorption-elution method of siracusa for ABO and MN grouping of blood stains." *J. forensic Sci.*, **8,** 419 (July); *contd.* 5353 (October).

GRADWOHL, R. B. H. (1968), *Legal Medicine*, pp. 167–220, 2nd edition. Ed. Camps. Bristol: John Wright & Son, Ltd.

KIND, S. S. (1960), "Absorption-elution grouping of dried blood smears." *Nature (Lond.)*, **185,** 397.

KIND, S. S. (1963), "Some properties of ABH antisera considered in relation to blood group grouping." *J. forensic Med.*, **10,** 51.

LINCOLN, P. J., and DODD, BARBARA E. (1968), "The detection of the Rh antigens C, C^w, c̄, D, E, e and the antigen S of the MNSs system in bloodstains." *Medicine, Sci., Law*, **8,** 288.

NICKOLLS, L. C., and PEREIRA, MARGARET (1962), "A study of modern methods of grouping dried blood stains." *Medicine, Sci., Law*, **3,** 49.

NIELSEN, J. C., and HENNINGSEN, K. (1963), "Experimental studies on the determination of the Gm groups in blood stains." *Medicine, Sci., Law*, **3,** 49.

PEREIRA, MARGARET (1963), "The identification of MN groups in dried blood stains." *Medicine, Sci., Law*, **3,** 268.

STYLES, W. MCN., DODD, BARBARA E., and COOMBS, R. R. A. (1963), "Identification of human blood stains by means of mixed anti-globulin reaction on separated cloth fibrils." *Medicine, Sci., Law*, **3,** 257.

SWINBURNE, LAYINKA M. (1962), "The identification of skin." *Medicine, Sci., Law*, **3,** 3.

WEITZ, B. (1952), "The antigenicity of sera of man and animals in relation to the preparation of specific precipitating antisera." *J. Hyg.*, **50,** 275.

WIENER, A. S., GORDON, EVE B., and EVANS, ANAIS (1958), "The value of anti-H reagents (ulex europeus) for grouping dried blood stains." *J. forensic Sci.*, **3,** 493.

Section 6—Non-red Cell Blood Group Systems

"*I'm a gnu, a g*-nother *gnu*!"
Michael Flanders, Donald Swann, At The Drop of a Hat

Chapter 30

LEUCOCYTE AND PLATELET ANTIGENS AND ANTIBODIES

Leucocytes and Platelet Antigens and Antibodies

Interest in blood group antigens and antibodies has widened to include leucocytes and platelets.

The field is a relatively new one and workers are still feeling their way with regard to the reliability and suitability of various techniques and the conclusions that can be drawn from results obtained. Interest is focused on antibodies which are specific for leucocytes and platelets and their possible clinical significance and on the antigens which red cells and white cells may have in common, *e.g.* antigens of ABO and Rh systems, etc.

The authors have little personal experience of methods for the detection of leucocyte and platelet antigens and antibodies. The following brief survey is intended merely to furnish a starting point for those intending to study the subject more deeply and to give others a glimpse of a complex topic.

Leucocytes

Serological tests with leucocytes present problems which are absent from the corresponding tests with erythrocytes. For example, it is not easy either to obtain concentrated suspensions of leucocytes or to overcome the spontaneous clumping to which leucocytes are prone. Moreover, leucocytes must be relatively free from platelets and red cells otherwise the results of tests may be invalidated.

It is possible to obtain leucocyte suspensions either from defibrinated blood (Dausset and Nenna, 1952) or from blood collected into sequestrine (Engelfriet and Van Loghem, 1961). In both methods the white cells are separated from most of the red cells by increasing the red cell sedimentation rate by the addition of macromolecular substances such as polyvinylpyruolidine (P.V.P.) or dextran.

A method of preparing lymphocyte suspensions from whole blood after sedimentation of the red cells with dextran has been described by Batchelor and Chapman, 1967.

However, the method of separation influences the subsequent agglutination reaction. When blood is defibrinated the reaction occurs in serum; platelets and fibrinogen are absent although complement, Ca^{++} and Mg^{++} ions are still present. There may be some injury to the leucocytes. When anticoagulants are used, platelets and fibrinogen are present, Ca^{++} and Mg^{++} ions are removed and the action of complement is usually inhibited. The leucocytes are more intact.

Leuco-agglutination tests are influenced by external factors more readily than red cell tests, *e.g.* amount of fresh serum present, the presence of Ca^{++} and Mg^{++} ions, pH, viability of cells. A detailed study of such factors, together with techniques for antibody detection, is contributed by Dausset *et al.*, to *Immunological Methods* (1964) to which reference should be made.

Leuco-agglutinins

These antibodies, like agglutinins for red cells, cause direct clumping of leucocytes. They occur often in the sera of patients who have had multiple transfusions or in the sera of pregnant women. They are practically never naturally occurring. They are best detected in test serum inactivated at 56°C which is then mixed with an equal quantity of leucocyte suspension. Experience is needed in reading the tests because there is almost always some agglutination of the negative controls particularly if incubation is prolonged. However, the true positives are usually readily distinguishable from the weaker, indeterminate reactions of the controls. It is claimed (Lalezari and Bernard, 1964) that leucocytes prepared by a Polybrene method, remain in homogenous supension on prolonged incubation at 37°C so that a leuco-agglutinin detection test of increased sensitivity, because of the possibility of increased incubation time, can be performed.

Leucocyte Incomplete Antibodies

The existence of these, as would be expected, cannot be shown by direct agglutination, so indirect methods have to be devised. Several of these are in use and they each have their exponents.

One of these, the anti-globulin consumption test, is described in detail in *Immunological Methods* by Dausset. This method is based on the fact that cells which have taken up globulin will neutralise anti-human globulin if mixed with it, as can be shown by testing the anti-human globulin both before and after neutralisation, against red cells sensitised by an incomplete antibody, which for convenience is almost always incomplete anti-D. We describe this technique in a different context (*see* Chapter 29, technique No. 29.2).

A second method used is that of mixed agglutination (Chalmers *et al.*, 1959). We describe the forensic application of this method also in Chapter 29 (technique No. 29.4).

There is no doubt that most incomplete leucocyte antibodies are auto-immune antibodies although this fact is sometimes difficult to establish. Papain has been used to distinguish between them.

The Clinical Significance of Leucocyte Antibodies

Leucocyte antibodies are produced as a result of multiple transfusion and they can cause transfusion reactions, the main characteristic of which is pyrexia although the reaction may sometimes be quite severe and shock-like.

The role played by leucocyte antibodies in pathological states, particularly those involving leucopenia is not altogether clear because so many of these states are treated by transfusion, thereby inducing the formation of leucocyte antibodies.

Jensen (1964) has studied leuco-antibodies in pregnant women and has found complete leuco-agglutinins in 2 per cent of the primigravidæ and 16 per cent of multigravidæ. Incomplete leucocyte antibodies were considerably more infrequent than the complete form which is rather contrary to the findings in respect of transfusion immunisation. He did not find any connexion between the presence of leuco-agglutinins and miscarriages, stillbirths, congenital malformations or neonatal deaths, although he did record an increase in the incidence of premature deliveries in the current pregnancy among women with leuco-antibodies in their serum. The role of leucocyte antibodies in tissue transplants is discussed below.

Leucocyte Groups

Sera with leucocyte agglutinins formed during pregnancy have been used to work out the antigens present in leucocytes, other than those common to both leucocytes and red cells (van Rood and van Leeuwen, 1963). The inheritance of these has been found to be even more complicated than that of red cell antigens. Moreover some of the antigens are not very strong. A number of workers in this field have confirmed the existence of at least twelve leucocyte antigens which appear to be the strongest ones. These include the now well-known Mac antigen of Dausset (1958), the first to be discovered.

Interest in leucocyte antigens has much increased since it was realised that some of these antigens are relevant in histocompatibility tests in connection with organ transplants, particularly kidney. Indeed compatibility, or near compatibility with regard to leucocyte groups is of greater importance than compatibility of red cell antigens. Within the context of transplants, with the exception of the ABO groups, red cell antigens are ignored in matching donors and recipients. The importance of some of the leucocyte antigens has been demonstrated by skin graft experiments. Recipients lacking a particular leucocyte antigen (X) were immunised by intradermal injection of leucocytes containing X. After immunity had been established and antibodies formed, skin grafts both from an X positive and an X negative individual were transplanted on the immunised individual. If the antigen X is important for transplants it is to be expected that the skin graft from the X positive individual will have a significantly shorter survival than the skin graft from the X negative individual. Readers who would like to study the subject in more depth are recommended to read van Rood 1966; van Rood *et al.* (1967).

The main system of leucocyte antigens important for histocompatibility is now termed HL-A. It is one of the most complicated genetical systems known in man. As its genetics is getting better known it has been possible to subdivide the systems into at least two sub-loci each of which governs multiple alleles. Some alleles are commonly inherited together after the pattern of the Rh system. Some of the antigens recognised have not yet received an official place in the HL.A nomenclature, which at the moment extends from HL.A1 to HL.A8.

A recent assessment of the HL.A position can be found in the Proceedings of the Symposium Transplantation Antigens and Tissue Typing (1969).

Antigens Common to Leucocytes and Erythrocytes

A number of workers have tested leucocytes for the well-known blood group antigens with varying success and in some cases controversial results. It seems to be fairly well established that A and B antigens are present on leucocytes when they are present in the corresponding erythrocytes. This has been particularly well shown by Gurner and Coombs (1958) using the mixed cell agglutination technique. However, results of tests for other blood group antigens such as D, M, N, Lutheran, etc., are not so conclusive. It would seem that the indefinite nature of the results may be due to the low content of antigens other than A and B in leucocytes. In fact, the amount of A and B in leucocytes is probably also not great but the strength of their antigens in part makes up for this.

Dausset using the anti-human globulin consumption technique claims to have demonstrated the antigen D in leucocytes. On the other hand, Coombs using the mixed cell agglutination method failed to find D. Tests for other antigens on the whole seem to be weak and inconclusive.

Platelet Antibodies

Platelet antibodies exist both as cold and warm antibodies. Their properties and reactions are comparable with those of leucocytes. They are found after multiple transfusion or pregnancy and there is a good deal of cross reaction with leucocyte antigens.

They have considerable clinical significance as idiopathic thrombocytopenic purpura is associated with a high incidence of auto-antibodies for platelets and thrombocytopenia secondary to some drugs is the result of antibodies being formed to platelets which have been modified by the drug.

A number of different immunological principles have been invoked for the demonstration of platelet antibodies, such as mixed agglutination, antiglobulin consumption, the use of tanned red cells and complement fixation.

Pearson *et al.* (1964) favours complement fixation after making a comparative study of the various techniques.

Using these techniques platelets have been shown to possess many of the antigens which are found in red cells and also to have platelet groups which do not correspond to known red cell blood group systems.

Transfusion of platelets is a tedious procedure owing to their labile nature, but is in certain cases well worth while. The failure to obtain consistently good results may be partly due to lack of information about platelet groups; it has been noted that the first platelet transfusion is usually the most effective for controlling hæmorrhage in any given patient. Platelets should if possible be transfused as fresh whole blood, preferably from donors with thrombocytosis. The blood is collected into plastic bags or siliconised bottles using ACD or EDTA as anticoagulant and immediately transfused; if this is not advisable or possible platelet-rich plasma prepared from blood similarly collected and immediately transfused is the second method of choice.

The whole subject of platelets, platelet antibodies and their relation to certain types of hæmorrhagic disease is too complex to be dealt with in a general textbook. At the end of this chapter we have included a separate bibliography which, while not completely comprehensive, will give a fairly complete picture to anyone studying the subject. The "review" papers give very detailed references, while the individual papers describe the various techniques mentioned above in sufficient detail for those wishing to use them.

BIBLIOGRAPHY

ASHHURST, D. E., BEDFORD, D., and COOMBS, R. R. A. (1956), "Examination of human platelets for the ABO, MN, Rh, Tj[a], Lu and Le systems of antigens by means of mixed erythrocyte-platelet agglutination." *Vox Sang.*, **1,** 235.

BATCHELOR, J. R. and CHAPMAN, B. A. (1967), "Genetic background and transplantation antigens." *Symp. Tissue Org. Transplant.* (*suppl. J. clin. Path.*, **20,** 415).

CHALMERS, D. G., COOMBS, R. R. A., GURNER, R. W., and DAUSETT, J. (1959), "The mixed antiglobulin reaction in the detection of human isoantibodies against leucocytes, platelets and Hela cells." *Brit. J. Hæmat.*, **5,** 225.

COOMBS, R. R. A., MARKS, J., BEDFORD, D. (1956), "Specific mixed agglutination. Mixed erythrocyte and platelet anti-globulin reaction." *Brit. J. Hæm.*, **2,** 84.

CRONKITE, E. P., and JACKSON, D. P. (1959), "Use of platelet transfusions in hemorrhagic disease." *Progress in Hæmatology*, Vol. II, 239.

DAUSSET, J., and NENNA, A. (1952), "Presence d'une leuco-agglutinine dans le serum d'un cas d'aggranulocytose chronique." *C. R. Soc. Biol.* (*Paris*), **146,** 1539.

DAUSSET, J., COLOMBANI, J., et EVELIN, J. (1958), "Présence de l'antigène Rh (D) dans les leucocytes et les plaquettes humaines." *Vox Sang.*, **3,** 266.

DAUSSET, J., COLOMBANI, J., and OKOCHI, K. (1964), "Leucocyte and platelet agglutination." *Immunological Methods*, 539. Ed. J. F. Ackroyd. Blackwell Scientific Publications, Oxford.

DAUSSET, J., and COLOMBANI, J. (1964), "Detection of anti-leucocyte and anti-platelet antibodies by the anti-globulin consumption test." *Immunological Methods*, 575. Ed. J. F. Ackroyd. Blackwell Scientific Publications, Oxford.

DAUSSET, J. (1958), "Iso-leuco-anticorps." *Act. Hæmat.*, **20,** 156. Transplantation Antigens and Tissue typing (1969), ed. Elves and Nisbet.

ENGELFRIET, C. P., and VAN LOGHEM, J. J. (1961), "Studies on leucocyte iso- and auto-antibodies." *Brit. J. Hæm.*, **7,** 223.

GURNER, B. W., and COOMBS, R. R. A. (1958), "Examination of human leucocytes for the ABO, MN, Tj[a], Lutheran and Lewis systems of antigens by means of mixed erythrocyte-leucocyte agglutination." *Vox Sang.*, **3,** 13.

HARRINGTON, W. J., MINNICH, V., and ARIMURO, G. (1956), "The autoimmune thrombocytopenias." *Progress in Hæmatology*, Vol. I, 166.

JENSEN, K. G. (1964), "Leucocyte antibodies in serums of pregnant women. Serology and clinic." *Vox Sang.*, **9,** 315.

KISSMEYER-NIELSEN, F. (1953), "Demonstration of platelet antibodies by hæmagglutination of antigen coated tanned erythrocytes." *Vox Sang.*, **3,** 123.

LALEZARI, P., and BERNARD, G. (1964), "Improved leucocyte antibody detection with prolonged incubation." *Vox Sang.*, **9**, 664.

MUSTARD, J. F. (1956), "Platelets in stored blood." *Brit. J. Hæm.*, **2**, 17–24.

PEARSON, HOWARD A., SHULMAN, R., MANDER, V. J., and CONE, T. E. (1964), "Isoimmune neonatal thrombocytopenic purpura. Clinical therapeutic considerations." *Blood*, *XXIII*, 154.

STEFANINI, M., CHATTERJEA, J. B., DAMESHEK, W., ZANNOS, L., and PEREZ-SANTIAGO, E. (1952), "Studies on platelets II. The effect of transfusion of platelet-rich polycythemic blood on the platelets and hemostatic function in 'idiopathic' and 'secondary' thrombocytopenic purpura." *Blood*, **7**, 53.

STEFANINI, M., DAMESHEK, W., CHATTERJEA, J. B., ADELSON, E., and MEDNICOFF, I. (1953), "Studies on platelets IX." *Blood*, **8**, 26.

STEFANINI, M., PLITMAN, G. I., DAMESHEK, W., CHATTERJEA, J. B., and MEDNICOFF, I. B. (1953), "Studies on platelets XI. Antigenicity of platelets and evidence of platelet groups and types in men." *J. Lab. and Clin. Med.*, **42**, 723–738.

TULLIS, J. L. (1956), "Identification and significance of platelet antibodies." *New Eng. J. of Med.*, 255, 541.

VAN LEEUWEN, A., EERNISSE, J. G., and VAN ROOD, J. J. (1964), "A new leucocyte group with two alleles—leucocyte group five." *Vox. Sang.*, **9**, 431.

VAN ROOD, J. J., and VAN LEEUWEN, A. (1963), "Leucocyte grouping. A method and its application." *J. clin. Invest.*, **42**, 9.

VAN ROOD, J. J. (1966), "Leucocyte groups and histocompatibility." *Vox Sang.* (*Bard*), **11**, 276.

VAN ROOD, J. J., VAN LEEUWEN, A., BRUNING, J. W. (1967), "The relevance of leucocyte antigens for allogeneic renal transplantation." *Symp. Tissue Org. Transplant.* (*suppl. J. clin. Path.*, **20**, 504).

CHAPTER 31

SERUM ALLOTYPES

THE development of more and more refined methods for the separation of serum proteins has made possible the discovery of differences between individuals which follow inherited patterns. These serum proteins can be grouped together into systems which are just as authentically blood group systems as those involving the red cell antigens which form the principle subject of this book. Like the red cell antigen systems some of them began with the discovery of a simple antibody and its corresponding antigen; and subsequently other related alleles were found and it was realised that the systems were much more complicated than was at first apparent.

Some of these serum components and the techniques for their identification are beyond our present scope; these are therefore dealt with quite shortly and details of methods are not given. The following systems are included: (1) Gm. (2) Inv. (3) haptoglobins. (4) Gc. (5) Ag. (6) Lp. (7) Serum transferases. We have chosen to describe three of these systems, *i.e.* Gm, haptoglobins and Gc groups in more detail than the others since they are used fairly extensively in the investigation of cases of doubtful paternity. Details of techniques for the identification of allotypes of each of these three are given.

Gm typing will be most familiar to students of red cell types since Gm allotypes can be identified by methods similar to those used for red cell typing. Haptoglobins are usually determined by means of starch gel electrophoresis in agar. A summary of the salient features of serum allotypes will be found in Table 31.1. For a detailed review *see* Series Hæmatologica, Vol. 1, 1968.

Gm Groups

These owe their identification to an observation by Grubb (1956), Grubb and Laurell (1956) following the discovery that the serum of a small proportion of people, mostly sufferers from rheumatoid arthritis would, in quite high dilution, agglutinate D positive cells previously sensitised by incomplete anti-D. Grubb noticed that this agglutination could be inhibited by the

Table 31.1
Summary of Serum Allotypes

System	Globulin fraction	Principle Genes	Phenotypes	Method of detection
Gm	IgG (heavy chains)	Gm^a (Gm 1) Gm^b (Gm 5)	Gm(a+b−) Gm(a+b+) Gm(a−b+)	Inhibition of agglutination of globulin coated red cells by anti-Gm
Inv	IgG, IgA, IgM (light chains)	InvL Inv(a)	Inv(a+1−) Inv(a+1+) Inv(a−1+)	Inhibition of agglutination of globulin coated red cells by anti-Inv
Gc	α_2	Gc^1 Gc^2	Gc 1–1 Gc 2–1 Gc 2–2	Immuno-electrophoresis in agar
Ag	β_1 lipoprotein	Ag^a Ag	Ag(a+) Ag(a−)	Agar gel precipitation
Lp	β_1 lipoprotein	Lp^a Lp	Lp(a+) Lp(a−)	Agar gel precipitation
Haptoglobins	$\alpha 2$	Hp^1 Hp^2	Hp 1–1 Hp 2–1 Hp 2–2	Starch gel electrophoresis
Transferrins	$\beta 1$	Tf_C Tf_B Tf_D	C BC CD	Starch gel electrophoresis

serum of about 60 per cent of Swedish people. This ability to inhibit is inherited as a Mendelian dominant character.

Further investigations showed that it was probable that the inhibitor was located in the gamma globulin fraction of the serum. Hence the name Gm (a+) for the phenotype of the inhibitory sera and Gm (a−) for that of the non-inhibitory sera. The difference between Gm (a+) and Gm (a−) is not absolute but the inhibitory power of Gm (a+) is normally at least ten times that of Gm (a −) and the two can nearly always be readily distinguished. An "intermediate" type may be encountered but it is rare. For the successful determination of Gm types, both the rheumatoid arthritic and anti-D sera have to be specially selected. Only a proportion of each are suitable, for instance, in one experiment only 6 out of 66 high titred incomplete anti-D sera were found to be suitable for coating red cells and the useful sera were from Gm (a+) people.

Other Gm Types

Harboe and Lunderall (1959) discovered in the serum of one patient with rheumatoid arthritis an agglutinating substance which was inhibited by some but not all sera of phenotype Gm (a+) and by none of the sera of phenotype Gm (a−).

Among Norwegians, 26 per cent contained this agglutinating substance while 74 per cent did not do so. These positive were said to be of type Gm^x while the substance was termed anti-Gm^x. Gm^x like Gm^a is carried on to the red cells by means of the incomplete anti-D serum since only the anti-D sera from individuals who are Gm^x + will do for the detection of Gm^x.

A further allele of Gm, Gm^b antithetical to Gm^a* was found (Harboe 1959). The anti-D used to disclose this allele was from an individual of type Gm(a− x−). The rheumatoid arthritic serum was selected from 65 such sera as being the only one which agglutinated red cells coated with this particular anti-D. When this system was used to test the inhibitory power of random sera, 97 out of 119 (81·5 per cent) were positive. All of 46 Gm(a−) types gave inhibition of agglutination; this fact, with others, including family studies, led to the conclusion that the new inhibitory substance was part of the Gm system.

The Gm antigens are all related in heavy chains of IgG globulins and are not found in IgA or IgM. To date, at least 23 different Gm variants have been discovered including some racial differences (Steinburg *et al.*, 1960). Current evidence indicates that the

* Gm^b is not a true allele to Gm^a; in some races they are inherited together.

known Gm antigens are controlled by genes from at least three different cistrons.

The terminology for the Gm system was revised in 1965 by a committee of the World Health Organisation. Gm^a became Gm(1); Gm^b, Gm(5); Gm^x, Gm(2).

Gm Typing

Selection of Suitable Reagents. It is strongly recommended that beginners obtain a known anti-Gm typing serum, preferably anti-Gm^a, from an experienced laboratory, together with a selected anti-D for use with it. Otherwise the worker must select by trial and error from among rheumatoid arthritic sera (R.A.), with high titres by the Rose–Waaler technique, using red cells coated with anti-D from a number of different sources.

Anti-D for Coating Red Cells

Only a few anti-D sera are suitable and these will be found among those of high titre.

The red cells used are preferably of genotype CDe.CDe or CDe.cDE and must be of group O. They are coated in the proportion of 0·4 ml. packed cells with 5 ml. of anti-D diluted according to the titre of the original serum. The cells are incubated with the serum for $\frac{3}{4}$ to 1 hour at 37°C and then washed three times. They should give strong rapid agglutination with an anti-human globulin reagent.

Anti-Gm Sera

Rheumatoid arthritic (Ragg) sera suitable for typing come usually from patients with long histories of the disease. The sera should be treated at 63°C for 10 minutes as this destroys the R.A. factor and prevents agglutination of saline controls.

Particularly satisfactory reagents can be prepared from the occasional healthy donor who possesses anti-Gm antibodies (Snagg).

Rheumatoid agglutinators (Ragg) are less specific than the anti-Gm sera from normal persons (Snagg) in that they are often inhibited by high concentrations (*e.g.* $\frac{1}{2}$–$\frac{1}{4}$) of serum negative for the corresponding Gm factor. They also tend to be less sensitive than Snagg sera and are inhibited by only low dilutions of sera containing their specific Gm factor. Other sources of satisfactory anti-Gm sera are rabbits or monkeys immunised with human gamma globulin. These anti-Gm sera show a specificity and sensitivity similar to the Snagg type of antibodies.

A known Gm^a positive (preferably a heterozygote giving a "single dose" positive) and a Gm^a negative are included with each batch of tests.

Anti-Gm^a reagents are more easily obtained than anti-Gm^b and anti-Gm^x both from rheumatoid and normal donors. Different examples of anti-Gm^b sera sometimes show slight differences in specificity.

Screening of Sera for Gm Antibodies

Each serum to be tested is diluted 1 in 5 with saline.* Equal volumes of this and a 2 per cent suspension of the sensitised red cells are mixed, left at room temperature for 1 hour and read for agglutination. Strong positives can be titrated. Normal uncoated group O cells mixed with each serum is an essential control since a serum may contain an atypical antibody which would agglutinate the test cells. It will be appreciated that only cells coated with anti-D from a Gm^a positive individual will detect the presence of anti-Gm^a antibodies. Similarly anti-Gm^b will have to be looked for with Gm^b sentitised cells and anti-Gm^x with Gm^x sensitised cells.

Technique No. 31.1. Gm typing using anti-Gm^a

Equal volumes of serum to be Gm^a-typed and anti-Gm^a each diluted 1 in 5 are mixed and left at room temperature for about 30 minutes. The mixtures are then run out onto a tile and a drop of sensitised D positive cells added to each. They are rocked and read as for direct anti-globulin tests (*see* technique No. 10.3b).

Controls

(1) The test cells + anti-human globulin.
(2) The test cells + anti-Gm^a.
(3) The test cells with each test serum at a dilution of 1/5.

Technique No. 31.2. The dis-agglutination technique for Gm typing

This method is often used in preference to technique No. 31.1. Drops of anti-Gm^a $\frac{1}{5}$ are delivered on to a tile allowing one drop for each serum to be Gm typed plus controls. A drop of Gm^a sensitised red cells is added to each, immediately mixed and the tile is rocked gently until agglutination of the sensitised cells is well developed. Then an equal drop of each serum to be typed is

* If serum is used undiluted, the high protein concentration tends to cause agglutination of the sensitised cells.

added to the agglutinated red cells and the mixture is thoroughly stirred. The agglutination disperses and is only reformed if the test sera lack the corresponding Gm^a component. The controls required are the same as those for technique No. 31.1.

Inv Groups

In 1960, Ropartz *et al.* described Inv, a second system of inherited antigens in which, so far, three distinct types have been recognised Inv(1), Inv(a) and Inv(b). The Inv antigens in contrast to those of the Gm system are related to the light chains of the globulin molecule and are found associated with IgG, IgA and IgM globulins. No linkage has been detected between Gm and Inv. Inv antibodies also occur in the sera of patients with rheumatoid arthritis and in a few normal sera. Patients who have received multiple transfusions are sometimes a source of both Gm and Inv antibodies.

Haptoglobins

These are hæmoglobin-binding proteins found with the α_2 globulins (*see* frontispiece). Their major function appears to be the prevention of loss of hæmoglobin, and thus of iron, from the body. They can be separated by means of starch gel electrophoresis and characteristic patterns obtained (Smithies, 1955). These patterns are the result of two genetically inherited components called for convenience Hp1 and Hp2. Most individuals can be classified into one of three types: Hp1-1, Hp2-1, Hp2-2. The appearance of each type after starch gel electrophoresis is shown in Plate 12. In developing the bands after electrophoresis, the hæmoglobin binding capacity of haptoglobin is utilised and the fact that benzidine forms a blue coloured compound in the presence of hæmoglobin. The three main groups are easily distinguishable. Hp1-1 forms a single thick band which lies next to the free hæmoglobin on its cathodic side. Hp2-1 and Hp2-2 both form a cluster of lines well to the cathodic side of the Hp1-1 band and they are readily distinguishable from each other. The Hp1 component of the Hp2-1 type occupies the same position as the corresponding band of the Hp1-1 but is not so pronounced. This band is absent from Hp2-2. Hp2-1 has in addition a broad band lying at the extreme anodic side of its cluster. This band stains more intensely than any of the Hp2-2 bands. It is of interest to note that the Hp2-1 pattern is different from that obtained by mixing haptoglobins of the two homozygous types. This is in contrast to the Gc groups described below. A few rare variants have

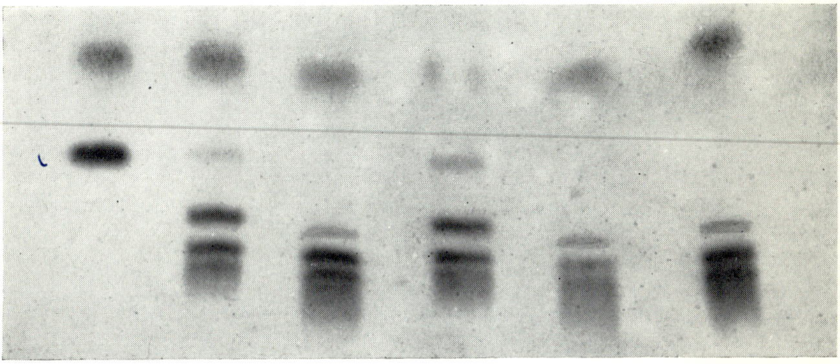

Hpl–1 Hp2–1 Hp2–2 Hp2–1 Hp2–2 Hp2–2

PLATE 12. Photograph of haptoglobin patterns in starch gel.

[*To face p.* 352

been observed. Hp2-1 (modified) is found in about 10 per cent of negroes. This resembles the normal Hp2-1 in the mobilities of the components but there is relatively more of the fast moving component as in Hp1-1 and relatively less of the components in the slower moving cluster. Another rare variant HpCa has zones similar to those of both Hp2-1 and Hp2-2, and Hp2-2 components being present in greater concentration than the Hp2-1 components.

Haptoglobin components are not fully developed at birth and it is recommended that in testing for this system in cases of doubtful paternity the infants should be at least 4–6 months old. Haptoglobins are occasionally absent from healthy adults and also from individuals in whom a hæmolytic process is taking place.

Technique No. 31.3. The determination of haptoglobin types

Reagents

The starch for the gel is "Starch hydrolysed" obtained from the Connaught Laboratories, Toronto.

Tris-citrate buffer for gel pH 8·6–8·8

0·076M Tris is made by dissolving 9·19 g./litre H_2O.

0·005M citric acid is made by dissolving 1 g. citric acid/litre H_2O.

These solutions are mixed in equal parts.

Poulik's borate buffer for electrophoresis bath. pH 7·8–8·0.

0·30M boric acid is made by dissolving 18·5 g acid/litre H_2O.

0·05M sodium hydroxide is made by taking 50 ml. 1N, NaOH and making up to 1 litre with H_2O.

A mixture containing 2 parts (or 600 ml.) of boric acid and one part (or 300 ml.) of NaOH should produce a sufficient quantity of solution at the correct pH. Each pH must be checked carefully using a pH meter. The borate buffer can be used for several "runs" but must be taken out of the bath and filtered between each "run" and the pH checked.

Preparation of benzidine solution for development of Hp bands

5 ml. glacial acetic acid is diluted with 5 ml. distilled water in a test tube. Approximately 25 mg. benzidine and 200 mg. barium peroxide are added and the whole mixed. With experience these amounts may be judged by eye. It will be found that the powders do not completely dissolve. The solution is freshly prepared

immediately before use. Great care must be exercised in the handling of benzidine; the powder must not be inhaled and when applying the solution to the tests rubber gloves must be worn. All benzidine contaminated glassware and perspex must be carefully washed separately in plenty of running water and must not be added to the general pool of dirty glassware.

Preparation of starch gel

The gel is prepared by making a 13 per cent solution of starch in the gel buffer; 150 ml. of starch solution makes a mould of 14 × 12 cm., suitable for about six samples.

The starch–buffer mixture is gently heated in a buchner flask over a blue flame with continuous shaking. The solution first becomes very viscous and then, as boiling point is approached, it becomes fluid again. *Gentle* heating should be continued for 1–2 minutes. The flask is then evacuated at about 500 mm. Hg for 30 seconds to boil and de-gas the solution. A water pump if reliable, or a high vacuum pump may be used. Afterwards the starch solution is quickly poured into a suitable mould and left to set in a draught free atmosphere at room temperature. A piece of perspex about $\frac{1}{2}$–1 cm. in thickness, upon which a frame may be constructed with perspex rods, forms a suitable mould. The gel should cover an area of about 14 × 12 cm. and be about 7 mm. thick. When the gel is set it may be covered lightly with polythene or other wrapping to prevent drying, and placed at 4°C for 4–6 hours or overnight.

Application of samples to the gel

The samples, to which a little hæmoglobin is added to make them pink (hæmolysed red cells from the donors of the serum samples may be used), are taken up into pieces of 3M Whatman paper (about 4 × 4 mm.). The papers should be thoroughly impregnated with the test serum but any excess serum should be drained of; if the papers are too wet there may be diffusion and blurring of the bands.

The gel is then cut through its whole depth and across the width about 2 cm. from the end that is intended for the cathode. The cut off piece is gently moved so that the impregnated papers can be inserted in a row at right angles to the surface and at such a depth that they do not project above the surface level of the gel. A distance of approximately 5 mm. should be left between each specimen. The slit is then closed and the preparation is then ready for electrophoresis.

Electrophoresis

This is carried out at 6 V/cm. measured across the gel, for 2–3 hours in the bath buffer described above. For wicks, three layers of surgical gauze are suitable. These are stretched across the width of the gel at each end and should make good even contact, overlapping the gel by about $1\frac{1}{2}$ cm. The free ends should dip well under the buffer solution in the bath. The whole wicks are immersed in the buffer solution before being placed in position. Care must be taken that they do not become dry during the run. The voltage across the gel is checked using an avometer and adjustment to the voltage reading on the power supply made to maintain the correct voltage across the gel. A reading of 200 V on the power pack will probably be found suitable. It is usual to maintain constant voltage on the power supply.

Slicing and staining of gel

At the end of the run the gel is sliced horizontally. A dermatome such as the Allen and Hanbury's Improved dermatome is suitable; the blade should pass steadily through the gel in one movement along its length. A piece of perspex of about half the thickness of the gel placed at each side parallel to its length is of assistance in making a clean cut at the right depth. The sliced gel is opened like a book and the freshly made benzidine solution is painted on in generous amount. The hæmoglobin bands should begin to appear after a few seconds and be fully developed within a few minutes. Reading should take place immediately the bands are clearly seen as there is gradual fading after 5–10 minutes. The appearance is as in Plate XII.

Alternative staining method.

Phenolphthalein staining for haptoglobins

Phenolphthalein becomes colourless in alkaline solution but in the presence of hydrogen peroxide and an oxidising agent such as the peroxidase of haemoglobin a deep pink colour develops. It is therefore suitable for staining the various haptoglobin components as these are conjugated with haemoglobin.

Reagent

2 g. of phenolphthalein and 20 g. of potassium hydroxide are boiled slowly in 100 ml. of distilled water, using a reflux condenser and adding 10–20 g. of powdered or granulated zinc during the process. Boiling is continued until the solution becomes colourless; this takes one hour approximately. When cool the solution

should be apportioned out into dark bottles and some of the zinc added to keep the solution in the reduced form. A part of this stock solution is made up for use as required by adding an equal volume of methyl alcohol and 2 volumes of hydrogen peroxide (10 volume strength). It is painted generously over the starch gel.

The Gc System

This system was discovered by Hirschfeld (1959). He recognised three different precipitation patterns in the α_2 globulin of human serum, by a method of immuno-electrophoresis. Family studies showed the patterns to be genetically controlled and two simple codominant genes were postulated. The gene Gc^1 gives in double

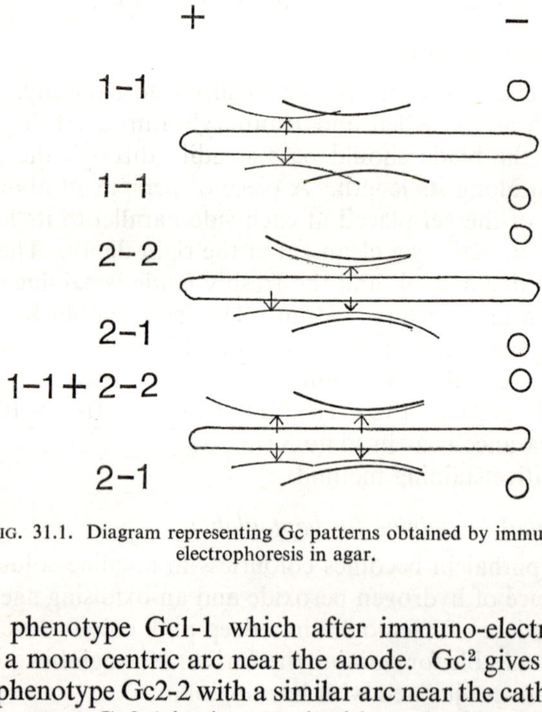

FIG. 31.1. Diagram representing Gc patterns obtained by immuno electrophoresis in agar.

dose the phenotype Gc1-1 which after immuno-electrophoresis shows as a mono centric arc near the anode. Gc^2 gives in double dose the phenotype Gc2-2 with a similar arc near the cathode while the heterozygote Gc2-1 is characterised by a double arc similar to a bird's outstretched wings. These patterns are shown diagrammatically in Fig. 31.1. The heavy line of the α_2 macroglobulin is shown also as this forms an essential marker.

The distribution of Gc genes is fairly uniform among Caucasians. Gc^1 has a frequency of 0·73 and Gc^2 0·27. Family studies have shown the system to be a reliable genetic marker and a useful tool in cases of doubtful paternity in which the system offers about a 15 per cent chance of excluding a man wrongly accused.

Gc exclusions are checked by mixing the critical serum which demonstrates the exclusion with an equal quantity of a serum of known Gc type, e.g., Gc 1–1 can be checked by mixing with an equal quantity of a known 2–2. This will run as a Gc 2–1 when tested by the usual technique. Similarly Gc 2–1 can be mixed with a Gc 2–2 or 1–1 to give a 2–1 with asymetric lines towards either the 2 or 1 position.

Technique 31.4. The determination of Gc types

Preparation of buffer solutions

	for agar	*for tank*
Barbituric acid (diethyl)	3·32 g.	13·8 g.
Sod. veronal (sod. barbitone)	21·02 g.	87·6 g.
Calcium lactate	3·07 g.	3·84 g.
Dist. H_2O	2 litres	10 litres
1 per cent merthiolate	2 ml.	10 ml.

The pH of the buffers must be checked; they should give a pH reading of 8·6. With the addition of merthiolate they may be stored in a cool place for weeks. Tank buffer can be used for more than one electrophoretic run if it is removed from the bath, filtered and the pH checked.

Preparation of agar

The following are convenient quantities.

6 gm. agar (Oxoid or Difco) are added to 300 ml. dist. H_2O and melted in a boiling water bath, with occasional stirring. It is important that the agar is *completely* dissolved. 200 ml. agar buffer and 100 ml. dist. H_2O are mixed and warmed to 60°C and then added to the melted agar. Finally 6 ml. of merthiolate is added. The agar is then bottled and stored at room temperature.

Preparation of agar slides

An appropriate quantity of prepared agar is melted in a boiling water bath. A thermometer is inserted into the agar. It will be found that the agar is completely melted at about 90°C.

The microscope slides or glass must be absolutely grease free and are therefore polished with spirit immediately before use.

The melted agar is quickly distributed across the slides using a convenient graduated pipette (*e.g.* 10 ml.), allowing about 3 ml.

of agar per slide. The operation must be carried out on a completely level surface, for example on a levelling table. The slides are left for 30 minutes on the bench before use. It is recommended that they are poured immediately before being required, and not stored overnight.

Punching holes and trough

The manufacturers of electrophoresis equipment will supply a punch especially designed for punching out the circular wells and troughs required for Gc determinations. Alternatively, the pattern can be punched by hand, using a pipette for the circular wells and two safety razor blades bound, one on each side of a microscope slide for the trough between the wells. By whichever method, two circular wells (2 mm. in diam.) are punched about ¾ in. from the cathodic end of the slide (*see* Fig. 31.1). Then a longitudinal basin or trough is cut in a central position. The distance between each well and the central trough should be 4–5 mm. The centres of the circular wells are removed by suction. The same pipette as that used for punching the holes, attached to a water suction pump is convenient. The trough, which has been outlined, is not cut out at this stage.

Setting up the tests

Serum samples to be tested are placed one in each circular well using a fine pipette. Care must be taken not to overfill. Controls of known Gc types, 1-1, 2-2, and 2-1 are included with each run. It is advisable to mix an equal quantity of amido schwarz with one of the controls as this facilitates the assessment of how far the samples have run during the course of the electrophoresis. A good deal of trial and error may be required before the optimum conditions for the electrophoretic run are found. Wicks consisting of two layers of Whatman paper No. 3 may be used. Care must be taken that these are pressed evenly along the length of the tray holding the microscope slides or along the glass plate if this is used in preference to slides. The wicks must be well immersed in the tank buffer before use and must not be allowed to become dry during the run. 6–7 v./cm. across the gel for 1½–2 hours will probably be found to be satisfactory running conditions.

After electrophoresis, the central trough in each slide is opened by removing the agar strip in the centre. This can be effected with a short metal or wooden stick after cutting the agar at each end of the trough. Each trough is then filled with anti-Gc serum and the slides are placed in a moist chamber at 37°C for 18–24 hours. (Anti-Gc sera may be obtained commercially, but it is recommended that those with suitable facilities and expertise should attempt to produce their own antisera in rabbits.) They are then read against a dark background using oblique light. Special viewing boxes can be constructed for this purpose. The Gc lines are those which lie nearest to the trough.

A permanent record can be made by photographing the results immediately or the slides may be stained as follows:

Staining of Gc tests

There are a number of methods of which the following is one which has given satisfactory results.

Slides are left for some hours in a saline bath and then overnight under distilled water. Damp filter paper is then pressed firmly on top of the slides and they are left to dry for about six hours in the incubator at 37°C. They are cleaned with cotton wool or tissue moistened with water and stained for 3 minutes in 1 per cent amido black. Excess stain is removed by washing in hot running tap water after which the slides are placed in 2 per cent acetic acid for one hour and dried.

Comfirmation tests

Results may be checked by mixing equal quantities of two sera and repeating the electrophoresis. For example if type Gc1-1 is mixed with Gc2-2 the resulting electrophoretic pattern will be that typical for Gc2-1. Moreover if Gc2-1 is mixed with Gc1-1 the resulting Gc2-1 pattern will show a stronger than normal Gc1 arc. The converse being true if Gc2-1 is mixed with Gc2-2.

Ag System

In 1961 Allison and Blumberg found that sera from certain individuals who had received many transfusions, formed iso precipitins against donor serum proteins. Only a certain proportion of human sera formed precipitates in agar gel against such a serum from a multi-transfused individual. The "new" polymorphism was found to be associated with β-lipoproteins and the system was termed Ag and the first found antibody anti-Ag. The technique for detection of Ag antisera and antibody is by agar gel diffusion and micro diffusion tests on microscope slides can be made satisfactory. As usual further research showed the system to be a complicated one and it is now thought that there are five antibody specificities. These have been called anti-Ag(x), anti-Ag(a_1), anti-Ag(z) and anti-Ag(t) with corresponding antigens Ag(x), Ag(y), Ag(a_1), Ag(z) and Ag(t).

Not all the theoretically possible various combinations of these antigens have been found. The combinations observed could be accounted for by postulating complex genes similar to the Rh system.

Lp System

This is also a β-lipoprotein variant but it is independent of Ag. Berg (1963) immunised rabbits with purified human β-lipoprotein. After appropriate absorption an antibody was left which divided the population into two types Lp(a+) and Lp(a−). The method of detection is by precipitation after double diffusion in agar (Berg, 1963).

Serum Transferrins

These are iron binding proteins composed of β_1 globulins of which there are a number of variants. There are also racial differences. A few Caucasians have a faster migrating variant B, while approximately 12 per cent of negroes have been found to be heterozygous for a slow moving variant D. The different types are detectable by starch gel electrophoresis (Giblett, 1962).

BIBLIOGRAPHY

ALLISON, A. C., and BLUMBERG, B. S. (1961), "An isoprecipitation reaction distinguishing human serum protein types." *Lancet*, **1**, 634.

BERG, K. (1963), "A new serum type system in Man—the Lp system." *Acta path. microbiol. scand.*, **9**, 369.

BRANDTZAEG, B., FUDENBERG, H., and MOHR, J. (1961), "The Gm (r) serum group." *Acta genet.*, **11**, 170.

GIBLETT, E. R. (1962), "The plasma transferrins," in *Progress in Medical Genetics*. Second Edition. New York: A. G. Steinberg, Grune and Stratton.

GRUBB, R. (1956), "Agglutination of erythrocytes coated with 'incomplete' anti-Rh by certain rheumatoid arthritic sera and some other sera." The existence of human serum groups. *Acta path. microbiol. scand.*, **39**, 195.

GRUBB, R., and LAURELL, A. B. (1956), "Hereditary serological human serum groups." *Acta path. microbiol. scand.*, **39**, 390.

HARBOE, M. (1959), "A new hæmagglutinating substance in the Gm system, Anti-Gm^b." *Acta path microbiol scand.*, **47**, 191.

HARBOE, M., and LUNDERALL, J. (1959), "A new type in the Gm system." *Acta path. microbiol. scand.*, **45**, 357.

HIRSCHFELD, J. (1959), "Immuno-electrophoresis demonstration quantitative differences in human sera and their relation to haptoglobins." *Acta path. microbiol. scand.*, **47**, 160.

ROPARTZ, C., LENOIR, J., and RIVAT, L. (1961), "A new inheritable property of human sera; the Inv factor." *Nature, Lond.*, **189**, 586.

SMITHIES, O. (1955), "Zone electrophoresis in starch gels; group variations in the serum proteins of normal human adults." *Biochem. J.*, **61**, 629.

STEINBERG, A. G., GILES, BRENDA G., and STAUFFER, RACHEL (1960), "A Gm-like factor present in Negroes and rare or absent in Whites. Its relation to Gm^a and Gm^x." *Amer. J. Hum. Genet.*, **12**, 44.

Section 7—Intricacies of the Blood Group Systems —Rare alleles, modifying genes, modern genetic theory and pathways of inheritance

"Curiouser and curiouser"
Lewis Carroll, ALICE IN WONDERLAND

CHAPTER 32

ABO BLOOD GROUPS

IN this chapter we propose to deal shortly with four topics:

(1) ABO variants.
(2) ABO inheritance, in particular with regard to the synthesis of the blood group substances.
(3) Antibody molecules of more than one specificity.
(4) Differences in antibodies of the same general specificity.

(1) ABO Variants

As early as 1935 ABO variants were beginning to be described and the number found has steadily increased, particularly in the past few years when constant searches through large numbers of blood samples have been rewarded.

The rare variants can be divided on genetic grounds into three categories:

Those resulting from rare alleles occurring at the A or B loci.
Those caused by rare genes modifying in some respect the expression of the common A and B genes.
Acquired antigens producing an apparent ABO variant.

Rare Alleles

A_3. Blood of sub-type A_3 can be recognised by its characteristic appearance after agglutination by anti-A serum (Friedenreich, 1936). An even distribution of small clumps is seen accompanied by large numbers of unagglutinated red cells. One is reminded of the "mixed blood" picture which occurs when, for example, a mixture of group A and group O red cells is treated with anti-A serum. In fact, the suggestion that A_3 blood is in reality a mosaic of A_2 and O has been made; however, the free cells have been shown to take up anti-A and also to be agglutinated by certain group O (anti-A plus anti-B) sera. Moreover, if they are separated from the agglutinated cells and mixed with a further volume of the original anti-A serum, a proportion of them are agglutinated, a "mixed blood" picture almost identical with the original being obtained.

Secretors belonging to sub-group A_3 have A substance in their saliva. A_3 persons do not usually have anti-A_1 agglutinins in their sera. On the other hand, A_3B persons often have anti-A_1 occasionally active at 37°C and may have anti-A also at low temperatures. The conclusion that A_3 is an allele at the ABO locus is in accordance with the results of family studies.

A_{int}. This is a type of A acquiring the name "intermediate" from its weak reaction with anti-A_1.

It is commoner in Negroes than in Whites. Although the variant might be thought to be intermediate between A_1 and A_2, on account of its behaviour with anti-A_1 it has been found to have more H than has A_2 and therefore does not fit in the intermediate position.

A_{end}. (Weiner, Sanger and Race, 1959). This very weak A was found in two generations of a family and behaved like a weak A_3. But unlike A_3 the saliva contained H but no A.

A_{el}. (Reed and Moore, 1964.) The A in the red cells can only be demonstrated by elution; secretor saliva contains H but no A.

A_{bantu}. (Brain, 1966.) This kind of A, occurring in 4 per cent of Bantu A samples, gives a pattern of agglutination like A_3, but the saliva of secretors contains H but no A and anti-A_1 is commonly present in the serum.

Ag. (van Loghem *et al.*, 1957.) This very rare variant (two cases described) gives even weaker reactions than A_3, giving negative or ± agglutination with anti-A (group B) sera and (+) "mixed blood" appearance with anti-A + anti-B (group O) sera. The red cells, however, contain a strong A antigen as shown by absorption and elution experiments. In the one case where the Ag individual was a secretor the saliva was comparable with that of an A_2 secretor. The serum had no anti-A or anti-A_1. It is possible that Ag should be included in the sub-group Am (*see* below). One of the two cases described had a myeloblastic leukæmia and no abnormality had been detected when he was tested two years previously. The abnormality of his cells may therefore be associated with the disease. The second case, however, was a healthy donor.

A_X. This variant is by no means as strictly defined as A_3 and for that reason has collected, since its discovery by Fischer and Hahn in 1935, several different names, *e.g.* A_4, A_5, A_Z and A_O. Broadly the cells can be distinguished by the fact that they give negative or weak reactions with anti-A sera, negative with anti-B but positive reactions with especially chosen group O sera (anti-A + anti-B). The percentage of group O sera with which they react varies from example to example, some being agglutinated by almost all, others by as little as 10–20 per cent of sera. Fortunately it is possible to select O sera which will detect all A_X samples; sera where the anti-A component is immune are particularly effective. There is little or no A group specific substance in the saliva. The serum usually contains anti-A_1 agglutinins and may also contain agglutinins which react with A_2.

The variation, especially in antigen strength of the red cells from individual to individual which occurs even in members of one family, raises a doubt as to whether A_X is a rare allele at the ABO locus or whether it is the result of modifying genes and should be more properly included in the section below. It is indeed probable that some examples of the A_X phenotype are due to an allele at the ABO locus and others to the action of suppressor genes. Families in which A_X children have occurred when the parents were both group O and one in which an A_2B man transmitted an A_X gene may well belong to the latter category.

B_V. Variants at the B locus are even rarer than at the A. B_V is a sub-group originally discovered by Mäkela and Mäkela (1955) and later studied by Boorman and Zeitlin (1959), which almost certainly arises from a very rare allele. The reactions with anti-B serum are weak compared with standard group B cells. The sub-group is similar to A_X in that it reacts more strongly with O sera than with the anti-B of group A sera. It is not, however, reacting with the same component as the A_X. The cells do not react with anti-B serum prepared in a rabbit, and there is no reaction between B_V cells and human anti-B sera completely absorbed with rabbit cells. The serum contains anti-B agglutinins reacting with all normal group B cells, though not with B_V cells. This anti-B reacts with only a fraction of the B substance found in group B secretors. The anti-A component of the serum agglutinates A_X cells, in this respect behaving like a group O rather than a group B serum. The saliva contains what appears to be a fraction of the normal B blood group substance reacting with a fraction of the anti-B in normal sera.

B_3. Moullec *et al.* (1955) has described an allele at the B locus which he has called B_3, characterised by a weaker reaction with anti-B serum together with free cells similar to that given by A_3 with anti-A serum. Unlike A_3 where secretors have plenty of A substance, two B_3 secretors had no B substance in their saliva. The serum did not contain any anti-B. Some families classified as B_3 whose saliva contained B are described by Bhatia *et al.* (1965).

B_W. Levine *et al.* (1958) described this variant occurring in several members of one family. The red cells gave a "mixed blood" appearance with anti-B and with group O serum similar to that given by A_3 with anti-A. B_W secretors secreted B substance in their saliva. There was no anti-B in their serum. Family studies suggest that B_W is an allele at the ABO locus rather than the effect of suppressor genes.

B_X. The cells of this sub-group behave as O, being unagglutinated by anti-B and by anti-A + anti-B (group O) sera (Yokoyama *et al.*, 1957). The serum and saliva, however, contain B group specific substance. The serum contains no anti-B. This may be an allele at the B locus or may be due to suppressor genes. If the latter, it has been suggested that they may be the Yy genes responsible for the A_m phenotype (*see* below). The B_X family does not suggest that the gene responsible is recessive however and yy in the Am family in which B occurs has no suppressive effect on the B antigen.

B_k. An unusual subgroup of B (B_k) has been described by Jacobowicz *et al.* (1961), the behaviour of which was in some respects analogous to A_2. This was seen in absorption and elution tests in which B_k cells were not very effective in absorbing anti-B from group O or group A sera, although anti-B taken up on B_k cells was readily eluted. B_k, like A_2, reacted very strongly with anti-H. Individual differences within group B would seem to be detectable by lectins (Ottensoon *et al.*, 1963).

AB with anti-B. A patient with apparently normal A_1B red cells whose serum contained anti-B was described by Seyfried *et al.* (1963).

The anti-B agglutinated the patient's own red cells below 37°C with optimum reactions at 4°C; in addition, it was neutralised by her own saliva. However, it did not behave as a normal isoagglutinin since it was not very potent and yet was not easily absorbed.

It is important to note, in studying the A and B variants, the absence of antibodies specific for them. There is, for example, no anti-A_m or anti-A_x. In fact when A_x cells were injected into rabbits in an attempt to produce a specific antibody, only a normal anti-A appeared. The notable exception is A_1 for which there is the corresponding antibody anti-A_1. But even this antibody cross reacts under certain conditions with A_2 cells.

This absence of specific antibodies is almost certainly due to the fact that although there are a number of different A and B variants produced by slightly different A and B genes, or caused by suppressor genes, there is, in chemical terms, no great difference in the antigen expressed on the red cell. The differences in behaviour of the variants in agglutination tests are also possibly due to differences in quantity, distribution and spatial arrangement of the antigen molecules on the red cell, all of which factors are under genetic control.

The variation in agglutinating ability of different anti-A sera with A_3, A_x, A_m, etc., is probably largely influenced by the physico-chemical properties of the anti-A antibodies they contain. There is evidence, for example, that A_m cells are susceptible to agglutination by high titre "immune" O sera with a high IgG content, whereas agglutination of A_x cells is facilitated by IgM antibodies. The cross reacting antibodies of group O sera probably play a large part in the agglutination of A_x, particularly when these are IgM. A selected immune group O serum in the author's laboratory agglutinated A_x cells to a titre of 256 and A_m to 64 by saline technique.

Genes Modifying the Expression of the A and B Genes

To explain some of the ABO variants it is necessary to postulate the existence of modifying genes which are only being detected by their effect on the expression of the ABO genes.

Bombay bloods. The most striking example of such genes is found in the "Strange case of the Bombay Bloods", first described by Bhende *et al.* (1952). Levine *et al.* (1955) described a family (shown in Fig. 11) which illustrates the way in which this rare phenotype arises. The parents of the propositus are first cousins. The propositus has handed on her mother's B gene to her own daughter but lacks expression of the gene in her own red cells or her saliva. In fact with anti-A and anti-B grouping sera, the propositus behaves as group O, but the agglutination expected of normal group O cells with anti-H serum is missing and a powerful anti-H is present in her serum. With "immune" anti-B from O serum there is weak agglutination. A further significant feature is that the mating of two apparent non-secretors (Le^a positive) has given rise to a daughter who is a secretor and has Le^b.

Levine and his associates believed that the best explanation for all the unusual findings in this family was given by postulating a rare gene x which in homozygous state suppresses both the ABO phenotype and the ABH secretion. If this was so, it followed that there probably existed a common gene X possessed by almost all

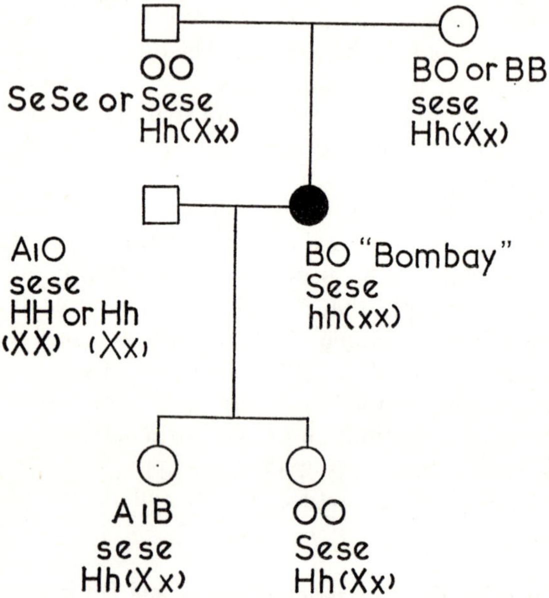

FIG. 32.1. Family study showing gene interaction resulting in suppression of blood group substance B (from Levine *et al.* (1955) modified).

people which in either single or double dose played a part in the synthesis of A and B substances. The Xx genes are now considered to be the genes which control the production of H and are, therefore, now called Hh. The "Bombay" propositus in Fig. 32.1 is a non-secretor in spite of the fact that she has the Se gene, because she is homozygous hh and therefore lacks H. (*See* also below (2).)

A$_m$. The characteristics of this variant are as follows:

(*a*) Absence of agglutination with anti-A sera (from group B or group O). One example at least, however, was consistently agglutinated by group O sera where the anti-A was immune.

(*b*) The red cells of some examples absorb anti-A (from group B) others do not do so.

(*c*) Saliva contains A and H substances.
(*d*) Anti-A and anti-B are consistently absent from the serum.

A number of authors have described variants which fit into this category and can be classed as A_m. Weiner *et al.* (1957), who present the most complete family studies, consider that it is due to the recessive effect of a modifying gene (y). They show quite conclusively that the genotypes of their two A_m propositii are in reality A_1O and A_1B, from a consideration of the ABO groups of their parents and siblings. Although in both cases there were children the ABO groups of these gave no further information. Perhaps in a future case it will be shown that the A_m gives rise to a normal A child as would be expected if A_m is indeed due to a recessive gene y. If the presence of the modifying gene does account for this rare A variant, it must only be affecting A since in the families studied no effect on H or B was noted (in only one case was B present but there it appeared to be quite normal). How the genes Yy should be viewed in the light of the scheme for the synthesis of blood group mucopolysaccharides described below is, at the present time, not clear.

A^b. Andersen (1960) has described a weak B antigen which may be the result of a modifying gene on another locus than ABO. In some ways it is similar to the acquired B antigen described below in that the B antigen is only found in association with A. In one particular family (Pe) the A^b occurs in 3 generations (*see* Fig. 32.2). Two of the group O's (I_1 and I_2) lack anti-B suggesting that they may be carriers of the modifying gene. The $A_1{}^b$ serum contained a weak anti-B which was neutralised in the normal way by B substance, the $A_2{}^b$ sera contained no anti-B. The saliva of the secretors investigated contained B substance. It is possible that one case of A^b described by Andersen may be of the acquired B-type and he suggests that the inherited type such as in the Pe family could be due to a genetically determined enzymatic process, while the acquired is the result of an enzyme introduced into the organism from the outside. Andersen (1961) induced O cells to behave as cells of group B by treatment with E coli 086.

Seyfried *et al.* (1964) describe a similar family in which the propositus was A_2B with anti-A_1 and anti-B in the serum. Eight out of 67 anti-B sera did not react with the red cells, and the name BSL was given to the apparent B antigen. The inheritance was unusual in that A_2B children arose from a group O parent. This occurred in two generations suggesting therefore that the antigens were inherited together and the genotype of the individuals was probably A_2BO and thus it is doubtful whether BSL is an allele of B and inherited separately.

Further families where A and B appear to have been inherited on the same chromosome have been reported by Yamaguchi *et al.*

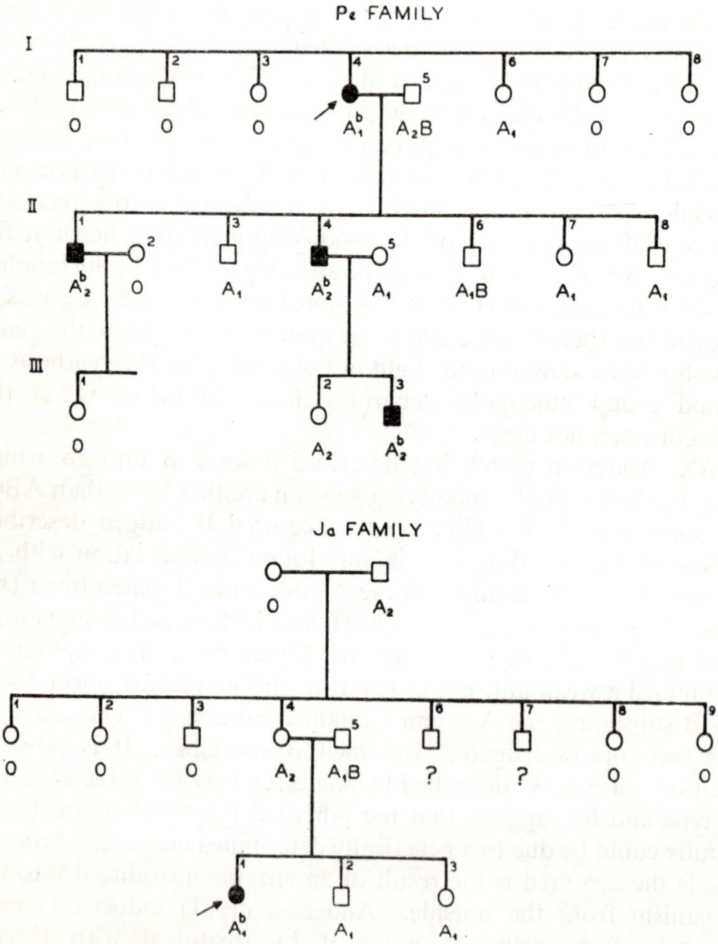

FIG. 32.2. Two families showing an inheritable B-like character in persons of group A (after Andersen, J. (1960), *Blood*, **16**, 1163).

(1965) and (1966), Yasuda *et al.* (1966) and Madsen and Heistö (1968).

Ah. This rare type of A was described by Levine *et al.* (1961). The Ah cells were agglutinated by anti-A and anti-Le^a but not by anti-A_1 or anti-H. The serum contained potent anti-H and anti-A_1. The authors considered that the Ah was produced by the action of a suppressor gene, an allele of X other than x. More recently Jakobowicz *et al.* (1965) have described the partial expression of A in a group AB which has some of the features of Ah but is not identical with it. Unlike Ah, the cells were Le(a−). These authors do not consider that their family possesses a recessive modifying gene (like Xx) because rather too many unrelated people would have to be heterozygotes. They tend to favour the presence of a sex-linked gene Xa which, when coupled with a second X (Xa or X), would affect the biochemical pathway leading to the full production of A material.

Other variants of A which are unnamed by their discoverers, but which are possibly inherited, have been described by Moore *et al.* (1961) and Jakobowicz and Noakes (1963).

Acquired Antigens Producing an ABO Variant

During the past years evidence has accumulated to show that under certain conditions, possibly connected with old age and/or disease, persons who belong to group A_1 and who have no B gene can acquire a B-like antigen so that their cells type as AB with anti-B in the serum.

The B-like antigen varied in strength from one case to another and also in samples taken at different times from the same case. Saliva was not examined in all cases but of those tested none secreted B substance although some were secretors of A and H. The anti-B in their serum appeared to be quite normal. It did not react with the acquired B of the individual's own cells.

Usually the patient was old, and often suffering from cancer which fact, however, may have been the reason for the blood grouping.

The phenomenon has not been encountered in the testing of young healthy persons, *e.g.* blood donors.

This phenomenon has so far mainly been found in persons of phenotype A_1. The absence of a group O and the rarity of group A_2 acquiring a B antigen is statistically significant. A number of authors have described modified A antigens associated with disease. These are summarised by Gold (1964) who himself noted several cases of modified A in leukæmic patients.

Marsh (1960) has shown that it is possible to change group A_1, A_2 and O red cells *in vitro* by the action of a bacterial filtrate of powerful activating properties (which included a T changing factor), so that the red cells acquire a B antigen.

So far neither this nor a similar organism producing a B antigen has been demonstrated in the blood *in vivo*, but it is certainly feasible that such an organism may be the causative factor and that it is only a matter of time before one will be found. The acquired or pseudo-B acquired by A_1 cells *in vivo* differed slightly from that produced by the bacterial enzyme *in vitro*.

It is possible (*see* above) that one case of the variant A_g may have arisen as the result of a disease process (myeloblastic leukæmia), this, however, did not appear to be accompanied by an acquired antigen, and certainly the A_g cells were not agglutinated by anti-B sera.

Acquired or "pseudo B" is of importance within the context of forensic blood grouping. Blood from bodies which have undergone putrefaction often acquire a B-like antigen of bacterial origin.

(2) ABO Inheritance, in particular with regard to the Synthesis of the Blood Group Substances

Modern theories as to the mode of inheritance of the antigens of the ABO system owe much to the biochemist.

It is fortunately not necessary in routine work for the blood group serologist to know the exact chemical composition of the antigens and antibodies with which he works; we shall give, therefore, merely a very short summary of the results of a tremendous volume of biochemical work and then spend a little longer discussing the way in which these studies have influenced modern thought on the subject of inheritance of blood groups in general and the ABO and Lewis groups in particular.

It will be remembered that blood group substances are found in saliva and other body fluids. In secretors the ABH substances depend on blood group; *i.e.* A secretors have A and H, B secretors, B and H, AB secretors, A, B and a small amount of H, O secretors H only and non-secretors have no appreciable ABH substance. All but about 6 per cent of the population (*see* end paper) have Le^a group specific substance. Non-secretors of ABH have the greatest amount with the exception of those non-secretors who are le.le— and have no Lewis substance at all.

To study the chemical composition of these substances it is necessary to purify them. Purified blood group substances can be prepared from saliva, gastric mucin and especially from some pseudo-mucinous cysts, the latter giving the best yield.

The studies of biochemists, notably of Morgan and Watkins (for review *see* Watkins, 1966 and Morgan and Watkins, 1968) and of Kabat, have shown that A, B, H and Lewis substances are all glycoproteins with a high percentage of carbohydrate. Average molecular weights range from 3×10^5 to 1×10^6. A single secretion contains a family of molecules all closely related in structure and composition. They probably consist of a large number of relatively short oligosaccharide chains attached at intervals to a peptide backbone. Pure preparations of A, B, H and Le^a substances have the same five sugars, D-galactose, L-fucose, N-acetyl-D-glucosamine, N-acetyl-D-galactosamine and N-acetylneuraminic acid and the same fifteen amino acids.

Some quantitative differences are seen: for example, compared with other blood group substances, Le^a has a lower fucose content and A a greater concentration of N-acetyl-galactosamine. Differences in specificity are determined by which of the sugars occupy the terminal positions on the side chains of the macromolecule. Thus, it is characteristic for the molecule having A specificity to have a terminal N-acetyl-D-galactosamine residue joined in α glycosidic linkage to the next sugar. The various A antigens are probably partly reflecting different spatial arrangements and partly different distribution of these on the red cell surface.

B specificity is associated with a terminal D-galactose joined in α linkage to the next sugar. L-fucose is involved in both H and Le^a specificity, thus showing that the nature of the terminal sugar alone is not responsible for these specificities, but the way it is linked to the next sugar and other factors must be involved as well.

Recently, research into the chemical nature of the Le^b character has been carried out (Marr, Donald, Watkins and Morgan, 1967). It had long been realised that, although anti-Le^a and anti-Le^b sera almost always gave antithetical reactions, they were not recognising products of allelic genes Le^a and Le^b. The biochemical studies mentioned above support the conclusion that the Le^b determinant is an interaction product of the H and Le genes. Thus, it is not necessary to postulate the existence of a separate Le^b gene to account for Le^b activity.

Some of the most important later work on blood group substances has been directed to the identification and characterisation of α-N-acetyl-D-galactosaminyl transferase formed as the enzymic product of the A gene and an α-D-galactosyl transferase associated with the B gene. Such transferases have been isolated from stomach mucosal linings and the submaxillary glands of people of the appropriate blood group (Race *et al.*, 1968; Hearn *et al.*, 1968).

According to recent theories of inheritance (Crick, 1958) genetic material consists of deoxyribonucleic acid (DNA) which is arranged in such a way as to provide "information" for the exact arrangement of amino-acids for a given protein. This would mean that proteins are the only direct results of gene action.

The fact that the difference between A, B, H and Le^a substances is not in their protein structure but in the carbohydrate portions of the molecule, suggests that the blood group substances are not the direct product of the gene but that the blood group genes produce protein enzymes which act at a late stage upon a basic glycoprotein to give it blood group specificity In fact, good experimental evidence has now been produced for the existence of enzymes known as transferases, present in salivary glands and stomach mucosal linings, which are capable of fulfilling this required function (Race *et al.*, 1968; Hearn *et al.*, 1968). It then becomes necessary to postulate genes whose function it is to control the production of the basic glycoprotein. It is interesting that as early as 1952 Wiener and Wexler suggested that blood group genes only influenced a late stage in the development of blood group substances because approximately equal amounts of glycoprotein were present in non-secretors and secretors.

Other supporting evidence has gradually accumulated, notably the fact that more than one blood specificity can occur on one molecule. For instance group AB persons have A molecules, B molecules and AB molecules (Morgan and Watkins, 1956).

At the same time that the biochemists were thinking that blood group substances were produced by the action of more than one set of genes, serologists were approaching the same conclusion from another direction. It will be remembered that to explain the "Bombay bloods" (*see* above) Levine *et al.* postulated that these were homozygous for a rare gene x which in homozygous state suppresses the ABO phenotype and the ABH secretion. They also concluded that x almost certainly had a common allele X whose presence in single or double dose was necessary for the production of A, B and H substances. It has now been decided to call these genes Hh as they determine the production of H substance. In fact this nomenclature was proposed in 1955 when Watkins and Morgan suggested that "Bombay bloods" were hh. The work of Ceppellini on the relationship of the ABO and Lewis systems also suggested that a series of genes were concerned in ABO and Lewis inheritance.

Both Watkins and Morgan (1959) and Ceppellini *et al.* (1959) have outlined theories, starting from their separate viewpoints but closely influenced by each others' observations and opinions, of the way in which the ABO and related blood group substances

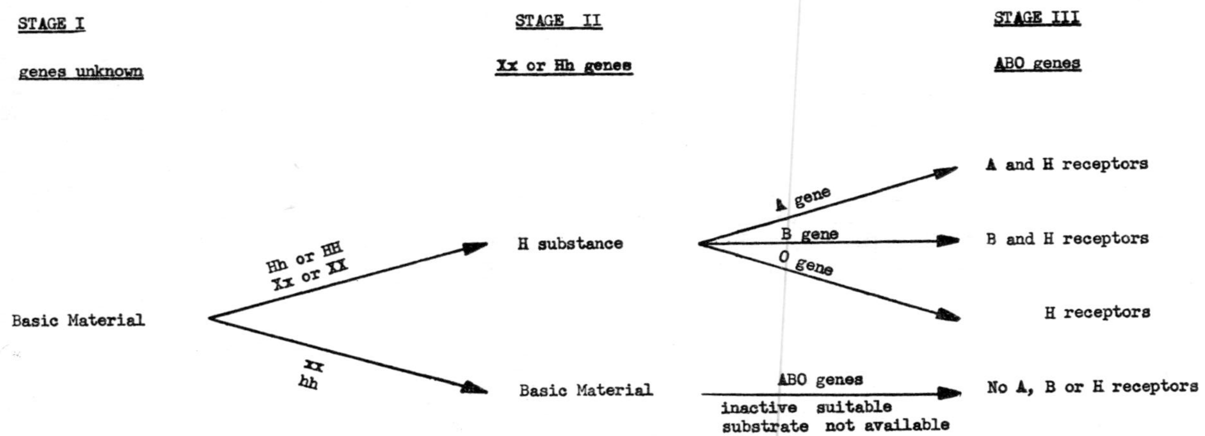

FIG. 32.3. Stages in the production of the blood group receptors of red cells.

are genetically controlled and synthesised. Their theories are substantially the same, agreeing in all essentials.

It is suggested that a common precursor blood group substance exists which is converted through a series of stages to the final highly specific blood group products. The conversions are almost certainly effected by specific enzymes, the synthesis of which is controlled by the genes.

The position postulated for red cells is shown in Fig. 32.3. The Hh genes are thought to control the development of H substance which is then acted upon by the ABO genes. The O gene is inactive in the conversion of H substance and the rare genotype hh being unable to convert basic material to H results in blood of the "Bombay" type. It seems fairly certain that the A_1, A_2 and B genes are not equally effective in the conversion of H. Moreover, there is always some H remaining unchanged. It is considered that the A_1 gene, either in single or double dose (AA or AO) converts the preformed H substance to A with a fair degree of efficiency. The A_2 gene is thought to bring about a similar conversion but to do it less effectively so that more H remains unchanged. This would account for the observed phenomenon that A_2 reacts almost as strongly as O with anti-H sera. The B gene in either single or double dose (BB or BO) converts H to B substance but here again some residual H remains unchanged. In AB individuals since the A and B genes both act on the H substrate very little unconverted H remains, as indeed is found experimentally.

None of the stages in the formation of blood group substances on the red cell (and probably in tissue cells as well) is affected by the secretor status of the individual. The Lewis types of red cells are not considered at this stage as it is now postulated that they arise from Lewis antigens in the plasma becoming attached to the red cells.

The second diagram (*see* end paper) shows the extension of the theory needed for the blood group substances in saliva and other body fluids. For the production of these substances the same genes operate as are effective for red cells but, in addition, the Lewis and the secretor genes have to be fitted into the picture.

In 1932 Schiff and Sasaki showed that the ability to secrete A, B or H substances in saliva was inherited as a Mendelian dominant and the genes concerned were called S and s (now called Se and se). At one time the fact that all Le^a positive individuals were non-secretors of A, B and H suggested that Le^a could be equated with se but it was later realised that both the secretor and

Lewis genes were needed to explain some of the other phenotypes found, *e.g.* the Le^{a-b-}non-secretor.

The genes Le, H, Se, A and B are transforming genes which control certain stages in the conversion of the precursor substance to the specific products secreted. The genes le, h, se and O can in this connexion be thought of as inactive genes or amorphs as they play no part in the conversion of the precursor substance (they may, however, have other functions). It is considered that the genes normally act in the order shown and that if the conversion step to H is missing (hh genotype) this constitutes a block to the action of ABH genes. The precursor substance, which is produced as the result of genes of which we at present know nothing, except that they appear to be universally present in man, is a macromolecular glycoprotein with all the peptide chains completely synthesised and with most of the carbohydrate chains already integrated in the molecule. This precursor substance should, according to the theory, be found in the secretions of persons of the genotype lele, *i.e.* those individuals who are non- secretors of A, B, H, Le^a or Le^b. When saliva from such an individual was investigated it was found to contain a glycoprotein which was very similar to the active blood group substances. The exact differences between the precursor substance and the Le^a, Le^b, A, B and H substances to which it can be converted are obviously of great importance in understanding how serological specificity is determined but for our present purpose it is enough to state that the chemical differences found between these substances support the theory that they are derived from the same basic precursor substance by a series of transforming genes.

A few concrete examples may be of value here.

Group A secretor

(*a*) *Red cells.*

Basic substance produced by genes unknown.

Basic substance converted to H by gene H (either Hh or HH).

H substance partially converted to A by gene A (AA or AO).

Result.—Red cells have A and H receptors and combine with anti-A and anti-H.

(*b*) *Saliva.*

Basic substance produced by genes unknown.

Basic substance converted to Le^a by gene Le(LeLe or Lele).

Le^a substance partially converted to H and Le^b by genes H and Se (HH or Hh and SeSe or Sese).

H substance partially converted to A substance by gene A (AA or AO).

Result.—Saliva contains blood group substances A, H and Le^a and Le^b.

Group O secretor Le^{a-b-}

(*a*) *Red cells.*

Basic substance produced by genes unknown.

Basic substance converted to H by gene H.

O gene has no conversion effect on H.

Red cells have H receptors.

(*b*) *Saliva.*

Basic substance produced by genes unknown.

Basic substance not modified by Lewis genes—genotype lele).

Basic substance converted to H by genes H and Se (genotype HH or Hh and Sese or SeSe).

H substance not converted by O gene.

Saliva contains H substance only.

(*Note*: It will be realised that most group O secretors will be Le^{a-b+} and will have H, Le^a, and Le^b substances in their saliva.)

Group B non-secretor

(*a*) *Red Cells.*

Basic substance produced by genes unknown.

Basic substance converted to H by gene H.

H substance partially converted to B by gene B.

Red cells have B and H receptors.

(*b*) *Saliva.*

Basic substance produced by genes unknown.

Basic substance converted to Le^a substance by gene Le.

Le^a substance not converted by secretor genes—genotype sese (whatever Hh genotype).

ABH genes have no effect on Le^a substance.

Saliva contains Le^a substance only.

Group B non-secretor, Bombay type

(*a*) *Red cells.*

Basic substance produced by genes unknown.
No conversion of basic substance—genotype hh.
B gene unable to convert as no H substance available.
Red cells have no B or H receptors.

(*b*) *Saliva.*

Basic substance produced by genes unknown.
Basic substance converted to Le^a by Le.
Le^a substance not converted to H or Le^b by gene Se because blocked by hh
Saliva contains Le^a substance only.

(3) Antibody Molecules of More than One Specificity

Group O sera as well as containing anti-A and anti-B antibodies very frequently contains antibodies which cross react with both A and B red cells.

They are quite simple to demonstrate by preparing eluates from A and B red cells using group O sera as the source of antibody. Eluates from A cells as well as giving the expected agglutination with A cells also agglutinate cells of group B and conversely eluates from B cells agglutinate A cells as well as B. Further evidence of cross reactivity can be obtained by inhibition tests. Absorption of group O serum with group A cells or A group specific substance will often result in a reduction in titre against B cells while absorption with cells or substance of B specificity reduces the titre against A cells.

Immune sera are the best source of cross-reacting molecules.

The exact nature of these antibodies has been an interesting and controversial problem for some years. At one time (Dodd, 1952) it was considered that some antibody molecules in group O sera have both anti-A and anti-B combining sites giving a molecule with two different specificities. In support of this is the fact that eluates from A cells (first exposed to certain group O immune sera) after the addition of A substance agglutinate specifically cells of group B. Similarly eluates from B cells (which have been exposed to group O immune serum) agglutinate group A cells specifically after the addition of B substance.

It is almost certain that IgG antibodies have only two combining sites; if each of these had a different specificity agglutination of red cells could not occur unless the cells used contained both A and B antigens. However, it is known that cross-reacting antibodies do not require the presence of both A and B in order to be capable of causing agglutination.

An alternative theory (Koeckert, 1920; Wiener, 1953) postulates that another antibody "anti-C" exists in group O sera and that A, B and AB individuals have a common antigen C on their red cells.

A third theory, largely due to Kabat (1956) considers that these antibodies are of a more primitive type than ordinary anti-A and anti-B molecules and are directed to chemical groupings, which the A and B antigens have in common.

It is possible that antibodies cross react not because they are of a more primitive type but because they become highly specific for a greater number of determinants on the antigen molecules which stimulate their production.

A fact which has clearly emerged from a study of these antibodies, is that they always show a preference for the antigen that has stimulated their production (Dodd, 1952). Thus, if A is the stimulating antigen so that anti-A is the immune antibody, then the cross-reacting molecules react more strongly with A cells than with B and if B is the stimulating antigen the opposite effect occurs and the antibodies react more strongly with B than A.

A recent theory (Dodd, Lincoln and Boorman, 1966) takes into account the similarity of the A and B active structures. These structures differ only in the replacement of the N-acetylamino group ($NH.CO.CH_3$) at carbon 2 in the terminal sugar of the A structure by an OH group at carbon 2 on the B structure.

It is envisaged that cross-reacting antibodies are produced with receptors directed towards common determinants of the antigen molecule *including* the carbon 2 site. Thus two types of cross-reacting antibodies are formed according to whether A or B has been the stimulating antigen. When produced in response to A they will combine very firmly with, for example, A_1 with the maximum number of determinants, less firmly with other subgroups of A, *e.g.* A_3, A_x, A_m and also less firmly with B; while cross reacting antibodies produced in response to antigen B will be firmly attached to B and more weakly to A.

This would account for the fact mentioned above that these antibodies react preferentially with the antigen which stimulated their production.

Cross-reacting antibodies have been shown to exist in both agglutinin and incomplete forms (Dodd, 1957) and to pass across the placenta more easily than anti-A and anti-B antibodies

(Unger and Wiener, 1954). They have also been studied in relation to certain animal red cells: opossum, rat, hamster, guinea pig, pig and rabbit (Owen, 1954 and Dodd, 1958), and in this way variations of specificity among cross-reacting antibodies have been revealed.

(4) Differences in Antibodies of the Same General Specificity

By now it will have been appreciated that anti-A and anti-B antibodies display heterogeneity in a number of different ways. Many investigations have clearly demonstrated marked heterogeneity both in physical and chemical properties and in serological specificity. In fact, it is found, not surprisingly, that anti-A and anti-B antibodies follow the pattern which emerges from the general field of modern immunology in which it is shown that a whole spectrum of antibody molecules varying in molecular size, specificity and in affinity for the corresponding antigen, etc., arises following the stimulus afforded by a single antigen.

Evidence that anti-A and anti-B molecules are not all exactly alike has been obtained from experiments with animal red cells. For example, the existence of human anti-B molecules of differing specificities has been obtained by absorption experiments with the B-like antigen which is widely distributed in the animal kingdom. The major earlier work on this subject was that of Friedenreich and Witt (1933). More recently Owen (1954) noted a number of different human anti-B fractions using the B antigen of opossum, rat, hamster and rabbit; and Dodd (1957 and 1958) carried out absorption and elution experiments using the red cells of human group B, rabbit, pig and guinea pig.

For example, nearly all human anti-B sera can be shown, by repeated absorption with rabbit red cells (which have a B antigen), to contain rabbit reacting anti-B and non-rabbit reacting anti-B; the proportions of the two fractions vary considerably in individual sera, some sera containing a great deal of rabbit reacting anti-B while others contain very little. An extension of the number of animal species used for the experiments uncovers further differences, not only in the anti-B population of human sera but in the B antigen of the various animals.

Studies on human anti-A sera using pig cells having an A antigen has disclosed an intriguing further difference between "immune" and "natural" human anti-A (Winstanley *et al.*, 1957). Human sera devoid of hæmolysin for human group A cells do not react with the A antigen on pig cells. On the other hand, human anti-A sera of the so-called "immune" type having hæmolysin activity for group A cells, do interact with the A antigen on group A pig cells. The antigen concerned on the pig red cells has been designated A^p and thus A^p must be recognised as a component of the A antigen on human red cells and the hæmolysin occurring in human "immune" anti-A sera must be anti-A^p in specificity.

In a later paper, Konugres and Coombs (1958) showed that the anti-A^p of immune anti-A sera corresponded with that fraction of incomplete anti-A which fails to be inhibited by A substance in the partial neutralisation test (technique No. 25.5).

Quite a different approach to the study of heterogeneity of anti-A and anti-B molecules has been made by Wurmser and co-workers (Filitti–Wurmser *et al.* (1954)). They have made thermodynamic studies and show differences in thermodynamic properties of the anti-B from individuals of different ABO genotype, *i.e.* OO, AA and AO. Their results apply to agglutinins and not to any form of immune anti-B molecules. Moreover, they find a striking homogeneity of the isoagglutinins in a given serum. Their work has been caıefully described, albeit with some strong criticisms, by Kabat (1956). There are obviously many technical difficulties but nevertheless a pattern of results emerges which must surely have some significance even if not fully understood.

More recently Filitti–Wurmser and Jacquot–Armand (1960) working with immune antibodies of both anti-A and anti-B specificities have shown by thermodynamic experiments that there is heterogeneity in these immune antibody populations as shown by their combination with the corresponding antigen. This is in contra-distinction to the homogeneity displayed by the "natural" agglutinins.

The glimpse given in this chapter of the new work on the ABO groups should dispel any idea that this is an old-fashioned blood group system from which we have nothing new to learn. However, lest the modern complexities should cause despondency, let it be said that given care and good reagents it is just as straightforward as it ever was to determine the correct ABO group of the majority of persons.

BIBLIOGRAPHY

Andersen, J. (1960), "An inheritable B-like character in persons of blood group A." *Blood*, **16**, No. 2, 1163.

Andersen, J. (1961), "Production of B character on human erythrocytes by hæmosensitization with purified Escherichia coli O 86 substance." *Nature*, **190**, 730.

Bhatia, H. M., Undevia, J. V., and Sanghui, L. D. (1965), "Second Indian family of weak B (B_3)." *Vox Sang.*, **10**, 506.

Bhende, Y. M., Deshpande, C. K., Bhatia, H. M., Sanger Ruth, Race, R. R., Morgan, W. T. J., and Watkins, Winifred M. (1952), "A new blood-group character related to the ABO System." *Lancet*, i, 903–904.

BOORMAN, KATHLEEN E., and ZEITLIN, R. A. (1958), "A sub group of B." *Proc. VII Congress of the International Society of Blood Transfusion*, 716–720. S. Karger, Basle and N. York.

BRAIN, P. (1966), "Subgroups of A in the South African Bantu." *Vox Sang.*, **11,** 686.

CEPPELLINI, R., DUNN, L. C., and INNELLA, F. (1959), "Analisi Genetica formale dei Caratteri Lewis Con particolare Riguardo alla Natura Epistatica della specificita Serologica Le^b." *Folia Her. et Path.*, **8,** 261–296.

CRICK, F. H. C. (1958), "Symposium on the biological replication of macro-molecules." *Soc. Exp. Biol.* XII–138.

DODD, BARBARA E. (1952), "Linked anti-A and anti-B antibodies from group O sera." *Brit. J. exp. Path.*, **33,** 1–18.

DODD, BARBARA E. (1957), "Further studies of antibody molecules having both A and B specificity." *Trans. 6th Congress of the European Society of Hæmatology.* S. Karger.

DODD, BARBARA E. (1958), "Further evidence for the heterogeneity of the anti-AB molecules of group O sera." *Proc. Seventh Congress International Society of Blood Transfusion.* S. Karger.

DODD, B. E., LINCOLN, P. J., and BOORMAN, K. E. (1967), "The cross-reacting anti-bodies in Group O Sera, immunological studies and a possible interpretation of the observed facts." *Immunology*, **12,** 39.

FILITTI-WURMSER, S., JACQUOT-ARMAND, Y., AUBEL-LESURE, G., and WURMSER, R. (1954), "Physico-Chemical study of human iso-hæmagglutination." *Ann. Eugen.*, **18,** 183.

FILITTI-WURMSER, S., JACQUOT-ARMAND, Y. (1960), "Étude Quantitative de L'Hétero-généité des Agglutinines anti-A ou anti-B immunes des sérums humains." *Rev. D'Hémat.*, **15,** No. 1. 25.

FISCHER, W., and HAHN, F. (1935), "Ueber auffallende Schwäche der gruppenspezi-fischen Reaktionsfähigkeit bei einem Erwachsenen." *Z. Immun. Forsch.*, **84,** 177–188.

FRIEDENREICH, V., and Witt, S. (1933), "Ueber B-Antigen und B-Antikörper bei Menschen und Tieren." *Z. Immun. Forsch.*, **78,** 152.

FRIEDENREICH, V. (1936), "Eine bisher unbekannte Blutgruppeneigenschaft (A_3)." *Z. Immun. Forsch.*, **89,** 409.

GILES, CAROLYN M., MOURANT, A. E., and ATABUDDIN, A. H. (1963), "A Lewis negative 'Bombay' blood." *Vox Sang.*, **8,** 269.

GOLD, R. (1964), "Modified A antigen in three cases of acute leukæmia and one case of 'pre-leukæmia'." *Sangre*, **9,** 131.

HEARN, VERONICA M., SMITH, ZEENAT G., and WATKINS, W. M. (1968), "An α-N-Acetyl-D-galactosaminyl transferase associated with the human blood group A character." *Biochem. J.*, **109,** 315.

JACOBOWICZ, R., SIMMONS, R. T., and WHITTINGHAM, S. (1961), "A subgroup of group B blood." *Vox Sang.*, **6,** 706.

JACOBOWICZ, R., and NOAKES, J. E. (1963), "A further example of an unnamed variant of blood group A." *Med. J. Aust.* (May), **4,** 657.

JAKOBOWICZ, R., SIMMONS, R. T., GRAYDON, J. J., CONSTANTOULAKIS, M., and EHRLICH, M. (1965), "Partial expression of A in group AB and group A members of a Greek family, not conforming with previously reported examples." *Vox Sang.*, **10,** 552.

KABAT, E. A. (1956), *Blood Group Substances: Their Chemistry and Immuno-chemistry* (Academic Press, New York).

KOECKERT, H. L. (1920), "A study of the mechanism of human isohemagglutination." *J. Immunol.*, **5,** 529–537.

KONUGRES, ANGELYN, and COOMBS, R. R. A. (1958), "Studies on human anti-A sera with special reference to so-called 'immune' anti-A. Identification of the antibody detected by Witebsky's 'partial neutralisation' tests as anti-A^P and the occurrence of the A^P antigen on human and animal red cells." *Brit. J. Hæmat.*, **4,** 261.

LEVINE, P., ROBINSON, ELIZABETH, CELANO, M., BRIGGS, OLIVE, and FALKINBURG, L. (1955), "Gene interaction resulting in suppression of blood group substance B." *Blood*, **10,** 1100–1108.

LEVINE, P., CELANO, M. J., and GRISET, T. (1958), "Bw. a new allele of the ABO locus." *Proc. VI Cong. Int. Soc. Blood Trans.*, 132–135.

LEVINE, P., UHLER, M., and WHITE, JANE (1961), "A_h an incomplete suppression of A resembling O_h." *Vox Sang.*, **6,** 561.

LOGHEM, J. J. van., DORFMEIER, HANNY, and HART, MIA, V. D. (1957), "Two A antigens with abnormal serological properties." *Vox Sang.*, **2,** 16–24.

MADSEN, GRETHE and HEISTÖ, H. (1968), "A Korean family showing inheritance of A and B on the same chromosome." *Vox Sang.*, **14,** 211.

MÄKELÄ, O., and MÄKELÄ, PIRJO (1955), "A weak B containing anti-B." *Ann. Med. exp. Fenn.*, **33,** 33–40.

MARR, ANNE M. S., DONALD, A. S. R., WATKINS, WINIFRED M., and MORGAN, W. T. J. (1967), "Molecular and genetic aspects of human blood-group Le^b specificity." *Nature, Lond.*, **215,** 1345.

MARSH, W. L. (1960), "The Pseudo B Antigen. A Study of its Development." *Vox Sang.*, **5,** No. 5, 387–396.

MOORE, B. P. L., NEWSTEAD, P. H., and JOHNSON, J. (1961), "A weak example of the blood group antigen A." *Vox Sang.*, **6,** 151.

MORGAN, W. T. J., and WATKINS, W. M. (1956), "The product of the human blood group A and B genes in individuals belonging to group AB." *Nature, Lond.*, **177,** 521.

MORGAN, W. T. J., and WATKINS, WINIFRED M. (1969), "Genetics and Biochemical Aspects of Human Blood Group A-, B-, H-, Le^a- and Le^b-specificity." *British Medical Bull.*, **25,** No. 1, 30.

MOULLEC, J., SUTTON, ELAINE, and BURGADOR, M. (1955), "Une variante faible de l'agglutinogène de groupe B." *Rev. Hémat.*, **10,** 574–582.

OTTENSOOSEN, F., LEON, N., and SATO, M. (1963), "Individual differences within the B group detected by lectins." *Vox Sang.*, **8,** 724.

OWEN, R. D. (1954), "Heterogeneity of antibodies of the human blood groups in normal and immune sera." *J. Immunol.*, **73,** 29.

RACE, CAROLINE, ZIDERMAN, DIANE, and WATKINS, WINIFRED M. (1968), "An α-D-Galactosyl transferase associated with blood group B character." *Biochem. J.*, **107,** 733.

REED, T. E., and MOORE, B. P. L. (1964), "A new variant of blood group A." *Vox Sang.*, **9,** 363.

SCHIFF, F., and SASAKI, H. (1932), "Der Ausscheidungstypus, ein auf serologischem Wege nachweisbares Mendelndes Merkmal." *Klin Woch*, **34,** 1426–1429.

SEYFRIED, H., WALEWSKA, I., and GILES, C. M. (1963), "A patient with apparently normal A_1B red cells whose serum contains anti-B." *Vox Sang.*, **8,** 273.

SEYFRIED, H., WALEWSKA, I., and WERBLINSKA, B. (1964), "Unusual inheritance of ABO group in a family with weak B antigens." *Vox Sang.*, **9,** 268.

UNGER, L. J., and WIENER, A. S. (1954), "Studies on the C antibody of group O serum with special reference to its role in hemolytic disease of the newborn." *J. Lab. Clin. Med.*, **44,** 387.

WATKINS, W. M., and MORGAN, W. T. J. (1955), "Some observations on the O and H characters of human blood and secretions." *Vox Sang.*, **5, 1** (Old Series).

WATKINS, W. M., and MORGAN, W. T. J. (1959), "Possible genetical pathways for the biosynthesis of blood group mucopolysaccharides." *Vox Sang.*, **4,** No. 2, 97–119.

WATKINS, WINIFRED M. (1966), "Blood-group substances." *Science*, **152,** 172.

WEINER, W., LEWIS, H. B. M., MOORES, PHYLLIS, SANGER, RUTH, and RACE, R. R. (1957), "A gene y, modifying the blood group antigen A." *Vox Sang.*, **2,** 25–37.

WEINER, W., SANGER, RUTH, and RACE, R. R. (1959), "A weak form of the blood group antigen A: an inherited character." *Proc. 7th Congr. int. Soc. Blood Transf.* 720.

WIENER, A. S. (1953), "The blood factor C of the ABO system, with special reference to the rare blood group C." *Ann. Eugen.*, **18**, 1.

WIENER, A. S., and WEXLER, I. B. (1952), "The mosaic structure of red blood cell agglutinogens." *Bact. Rev.*, **16**, 69.

WINSTANLEY, D. P., KONUGRES ANGELYN and COOMBS, R. R. A. (1957), "Studies on human anti-A sera with special reference to so-called 'immune' anti-A." *Brit. J. Hæmat.*, **3**, 341.

YAMAGUCHI, H., OKUHO, Y., and HAZAMA, F. (1965), "An A_2B_3 phenotype blood showing atypical mode of inheritance." *Proc. Jap. Acad.*, **41**, 316.

YAMAGUCHI, H., OKUHO, Y., and HAZAMA, F. (1966), "Another Japanese A_2B_3 blood group family with the propositus having O-group father." *Proc. Jap. Acad.*, **42**, 512.

YASUDA, J., AMANO, H., MATSUNAGA, K., and HAYAMA, K. (1966). Paper presented at the 14th Congress of Japan Society of Blood Transfusion.

YOKOYAMA, M., STACEY, S. M., and DUNSFORD, I. (1957), "Bx a new sub-group of the blood group B." *Vox Sang.*, **2**, 348–356.

CHAPTER 33

Rh GENES AND ANTIGENS; THE PRESENT POSITION

IN this chapter we deal firstly with further Rh antigens and secondly with a reappraisal of the Fisher theory of inheritance. The two subjects are very closely connected so that to some extent the first merges into the second.

We also discuss the D antigen with special reference to those D^u individuals who have produced anti-D antibodies.

The study of LW, an antigen related to Rh, but segregating independently of it has shown that the development of the Rh antigens, like the ABH antigens, is complex and requires the postulation of basic substances from which Rh and LW are derived.

Further Rh Antigens

C^w. This antigen was detected when a patient who was R_1R_1 (CDe.CDe) made an antibody against transfused blood which was apparently of the same antigenic make-up namely R_1R_1 (CDe.CDe) (Callender and Race, 1946). The antibody agglutinated the blood of about 3 per cent of the population all of whom were C positive. The antigen responsible for the stimulation was named C^w, the full genotype of the transfused blood being C^wDe.CDe and the corresponding antibody, anti-C^w. A number of anti-C^w sera have since been found and, in addition, the curious fact has come to light that the majority of anti-C sera have the specificity anti-C + anti-C^w (similarly anti-CD sera are mostly anti-D + anti-C + anti-C^w in specificity). Since the frequency of the C^w antigen is low (3 per cent), it would seem that the antigen C can stimulate the production of anti-C^w. Anti-C^w can cause a transfusion reaction and hæmolytic disease of the fœtus. C^w is an allele at the C locus.

C^x. Another rare form of C is C^x (Stratton and Renton, 1954). This is an allele at the C locus and the specific antibody anti-C^x has been found. This antibody was responsible for a case of hæmolytic disease of the newborn. The antibody is very rare and unlike anti-C^w is not normally found in anti-C sera.

c^v. C^u. Other forms of C found, are c^v and C^u. These differ from C^w and C^x in that they were not discovered through the finding of specific antibodies, but they were differentiated according to their behaviour with anti-C and anti-c sera. Both of them are agglutinated by some anti-C sera but not others.

It is possible that C^u is a real allele of C similar to D^u, but it is also possible to interpret it as being a depressed C, written (C). c^v is not a true allele, it is rather the expression of C in the R_zr (CDE.cde) phenotype which gives weak reactions with many anti-C plus anti-Ce and the latter component does not react with R_zr cells (*see* further under compound antigens).

D^u. We have dealt at some length with the subject of D^u in Chapters 11 and 12 as this Rh subtype is quite common and affects routine Rh typing. It was originally defined as a cell which reacted with some but not all anti-D sera in saline and albumin tests, but was positive with all anti-D sera by anti-human globulin technique. Such cells are also positive with most anti-D sera if they are first enzyme treated. Individuals of this type are regarded as Rh positive; they do not make anti-D. The type of D^u whose possessor can make anti-D is that which actually lacks part of the D complex. Such cells if negative with a particular anti-D are negative by all techniques including antihuman globulin. These are better thought of, not as D^u, but as another sub-type of D (*see* below).

D-subtypes

As mentioned above it is possible to find a few persons whose red cells are positive for D yet whose sera contain antibodies which are specific for D except that they are negative with a very few D positive persons including the individuals in whom the antibodies are found. Very often, although not always, the red cells of the D positive individuals are of the D^u type.

Tests with the various examples of these anti-D sera in parallel reveal differences between them in that they do not all give the same pattern of reaction; in fact, the results indicate that the D antigen is a complex one and these antibodies are specific for different parts of it. It is when a part of the D antigen is missing in a particular individual that an antibody to the missing fraction may be formed. Four different fractions with corresponding antibodies have been named Rh^A, Rh^B, Rh^C, Rh^D by Wiener and his co-workers (Wiener *et al.*, 1957; Unger *et al.*, 1959; Unger and Wiener, 1959; Sacks *et al.*, 1959.) In 1964 a further agglutinogen which was Rh positive but lacked all four factors Rh^A Rh^B Rh^C and Rh^D was described. The serum of this case contained an anti-Rh antibody which reacted with all Rh positives except the cells of the patient herself. In addition a variant form of Rh^A termed $Rh\alpha$ has been described (Unger and Wiener, 1959). Most D positive individuals possess all the fractions and so do not form the antibodies. There are some racial variations; for instance Rh^A is absent to a greater extent in negroes (8 out of 877 tested compared with 0 out of 942 whites). It is found, not surprisingly, that ordinary anti-D sera from Rh negative people contain mixtures of these antibodies directed towards special groupings of the D molecule. It is, of course, necessary to carry out absorptions with red cells known to lack one or more of the fractions A, B, C or D in order to reveal the presence of the corresponding antibody in an anti-D serum. Once the antibodies, anti-D^A, etc., have been obtained in a pure form, they can be used to detect the presence or absence of the various factors in D positive individuals. So far it is found that there is much variety in the antibody mixtures which occur, but anti-Rh^B is a component of most anti-D sera.

Tippett and Sanger (1962) studied eighteen persons who appeared to be D positive or D^u and showed that they fell into six classes of D antigen. Since that time Dr. Tippett has studied a further 36 cases and still the majority fall into the six original classifications. The table (No. 33.1) summarises her findings. Most of the anti-D antibodies made by such people are weak and need to be tested by papain or ficin methods.

Categories I to IV would probably be typed as Rh positive in routine tests, while categories V and VI would appear to be D^u.

Any apparent anti-D in a D or D^u positive individual should be investigated by a specialist laboratory. In addition to the six categories found by Dr. Tippett it could be that the antibody was really anti-LW (*see* below). Category V persons have the antigen known as D^w, (*see* below). Category IV persons are also Gonzales, (Go^a) positive.

Of recent years a new concept of a gene has arisen; it is now no longer thought of as a single simple entity but as having many mutational sites. The gene locus as envisaged today comprises a finite section of a chromosome and contains the information necessary to control a particular chemical reaction, or set of reactions. Within the gene locus, smaller units can be identified, these are the mutational sites and are the smallest portions of genetic material which are not divisible by recombination.* A mutation occuring at any one of its many sites affects the expression of a whole gene locus. We have seen that sub groups of D exist where a small part of the D antigen complex is missing and

* For definition see Glossary.

Table 33.1

Subdivision of the D antigen—(After Tippett and Sanger 1962, and Tippett 1963)

Category	Reactions with anti-"D" sera found in						Remarks
	Rh negatives	Cat. II	Cat. III	Cat. IV	Cat. V	Cat. VI	
I	+	+	+	+	+	+	The anti-D in the two members of this group is weak
II	+	−	+	+	+	+	
III	+	+	−	+	+	+	Cells prob. Rh^d serum; prob. anti-Rh^D
IV	96%+	−	W	−	+	+	Contains and segregates with Go^a
V	74%+	+	−	+	−	some − some W some +	Prob. identical with D^W
VI	35%+	some + some −	−	−	−	−	May be heterogenous
"Normal" D Pos. cells	+	+	+	+	+	+	
"Normal" D Neg. cells	−	−	−	−	−	−	

that these persons may make anti-D antibodies whose specificity differs only marginally from the more usual anti-D antibodies. These almost certainly arise as the result of small mutations at one or more of the sites which make up the D gene. Gonzales (Go^a) segregates with category IV as mentioned above and it is tempting to think of it as an allele at the small mutational site of the part of D missing in Category IV, although this may not be the true explanation.

D^W. In 1962 an antigen Wiel was discovered in the Rh system. It has been shown to be part of the D segment of that system and has now been designated D^W. It is rare in whites but not uncommon in negroes.

E^u and E^w. E^u was described in 1950 by Ceppellini *et al.* It is an allele at the E locus and gives rise to an E antigen which is agglutinated by some anti-E sera but not others. Several families with E^u have been studied and they have all given the same pattern of reaction with a given set of antisera which suggests, although the number of examples is small, that E^u is a more uniform variant than D^u. No anti-E^u has been found.

The allele E^w was discovered by the finding of an antibody which had been the cause of hæmolytic disease (Greenwalt and Sanger, 1955). The mother was CDecde and the father C^wDecDE^w while the affected child was $CDecDE^w$. E^w is characterised by being agglutinated by some anti-E sera and not others but in contrast to E^u a specific anti-E^w exists. The allele is very rare, although a further example has now been found.

hr^s. An antibody was found in the blood of a Bantu woman which reveals more than one kind of hr″ (Shapiro, 1960). He called the antibody anti-hr^s. Her cells, and as found later those of a number of other negroid types, lacked a component of the hr″(e) antigen. This component has been given the name hr^s and the antibody anti-hr^s. This antibody which was present in a pure form in the propositus is contained in most, if not all, anti-hr″(e) sera and seems to be the major or even the only component of some sera. Errors may arise in anti-hr″(e) typing, if an anti-hr″(e) which is pure anti-hr^s is used for typing a blood which is hr″(e) positive but lacks the component hr^s.

e^s. This is an allele of e found in negroid bloods. The antiserum was originally called anti-VS.

e^i. A new allele of e has been found in a Chibcha Indian tribe.

ET. Vos and Kirk (1962) found a naturally occurring antibody in the serum of an Australian aborigine which reacted with E positive white persons but not with all E positive Australian aborigines thus showing that some of them lack the ET component.

r^G. A few individuals have been found whose red cells are negative with anti-sera C,* C^W, C^X, D and E, but positive with anti-CD (Allen and Tippett, 1958; Kevy *et al.*, 1959). The cells are also positive with anti-sera c, e and ce, although the strength of the reaction is only slightly higher than would be expected of persons heterozygous for the corresponding antigens. It is not certain whether G is reacted upon by anti-C that is made in D positive persons. The antigen responsible, called G, is obviously a member of the Rh system, but how exactly it fits into the scheme of things is not yet clear. However, its discovery does explain two well known anomalies. Eluates containing anti-G made from cells of the rare type r^G after they have been in contact with anti-CD react with any blood containing D or C antigens and thus suggest that all bloods having C or D have G. Thus G is most likely to be the antigenic factor which causes the production of "anti-CD" in C−D− persons, and furnishes an explanation of why "anti-CD" is fairly common in persons of type C−D− whereas C is known to be poorly antigenic in persons of type C−D+.

G also affords an explanation of why "anti-CD" may occasionally be found in the serum of sensitised Rh negative women whose husbands are C−. These sera are in fact anti-D + anti-G *see also* below.

r^M. This unusual gene complex is related to r^G in that the propositus was thought to be Rh negative until her cells were found to react with anti-CD sera. However, the reactions are generally weaker than those of G, also the gene seems to give rise to some C and E (Tippett *et al.*, 1961). The new Rh antibody anti-VS (*see* below) does not react with r^Mr or r^Gr red cells.

V. This factor was discovered by means of the serum of a patient who had received multiple transfusions (De Natale *et al.*, 1955). It was thought at first that the corresponding antigen was confined to negroes, but it has now been shown to be present, rarely, in whites.

Recent work makes it almost certain that anti-V is detecting a compound antigen (*see* below) made when c and e^s (which is a fraction of e found in negroid blood and not to be confused with hr^s which is a factor lacking in some negroid bloods), are inherited from the same parent, *i.e.* in the "cis" position. Thus anti-V is better called anti-ce^s.

* A few anti-C sera gave positive reactions, *see* Kevy *et al.*, 1959; Tippett *et al.*, 1961.

f. In 1953 the finding of an antibody which reacted with the gene complexes cde and cDe led to the postulation of a Ff locus on the Rh chromosome, with f occurring mainly in the complexes Cdef and cDef. More recently (*see* below) it has been considered that anti-f is really anti-ce directed against a compound ce antigen formed when c and e are inherited together (cis position). The picture is now further complicated by the fact that the gene complex Dc-reacts with the anti-f (anti-ce) serum.

Gene Complexes Showing Supression

Some of the gene complexes shown below were originally thought to be due to a small deletion at the Rh locus. They are now thought of as showing suppression. When one or more antigens are "suppressed" however the expression of the others appears to be enhanced possibly because more "basic" substance from which Rh antigens are made is available. These interesting subtypes are listed here and also considered below under Theories of Inheritance.

D – –. A peculiar Rh genotype was described in 1951 (Race *et al.*, 1951) which was designated – D –, – D – now written D – – D – –. As this implies, the cells were not agglutinated by anti-C, anti-c, anti-E, or anti-e sera. They were, however, agglutinated by anti-D sera; in fact they reacted in a saline medium with serum containing incomplete anti-D antibodies. It was postulated that the D – – was an example of a gene deletion some generations back and the homozygous D – – D – – was the result of intermarriage; the parents were half second cousins. Further examples of this rarity have since been encountered, perhaps the most interesting being in a group of 117 Metis occupying a Reserve near old Fort Edmonton, of whom seven were shown to be homozygous D – – D – – and fourteen heterozygous, *e.g.* D – – CDe (Buchanan and McIntyre, 1955).

C^wD –. This Rh gene complex was found many times in a Canadian family (Gunson and Donohue, 1957). The strength of the D was similar to that of D – –.

Dc–. Tate *et al.* (1960) have described this gene complex in which there is no evidence of any E–e activity. The complex gives rise to antigens D, (more in amount than usually corresponds to one D gene) c, (less than usually corresponds to one "c" gene) and f, (less than usually corresponds to one dose).

– – – or d – –. This chromosome characterised by its failure to react with Rh antisera D. C, c, E and e was described in 1958 by Henningsen.

It is now thought that most people lacking Rh antigens are not really examples of the – – –/– – – phenotype as they lack LW also and can pass on normal Rh genes to their children. They are called Rh_{null} and will be discussed together with LW. It is possible however that the – – –/– – – phenotype does exist—(Ishmori and Hasekura (1967)). The heterozygous form of – – – as was found by Henningsen has been found in at least two other cases.

–D+G–. Stout *et al.* (1963) described a family where the Rh phenotype R_2rG– occurred in four members (3 generations). This is most unusual, most D positive persons being also G positive.

r^L. Metaxas and Metaxas-Bühler (1961) give this name to an Rh gene complex which is distinguished by the possession of markedly weak c and e antigens. It occurred in a mother and her son. There were no other observable differences between its activity and that of a normal cde chromosome product. r^L can be designated d(c)(e).

RN. This complex has weak C and e antigens and could be written (C)D(e). It was found in a Negro family and differs in its reactions from the (C)D(e) cells described below.

(C)D(e). This complex has been found in the main in Northern European families, six propositi were described by Broman *et al.* (1963) and others have been found since.

(c)D(E) or (c)d(e). This was found by Kornstad and Øyen (1967) in a woman of phenotype R_1R_2.

(C)D–. Found by Salmon and Sy Baba and reported by Race and Sanger in Blood Groups in Man (page 210). The D in this case was unusual also, corresponding to Tippett's subtype IV. The propositus was homozygous, formed Rh antibodies and was successfully transfused with D – – D – – blood.

Theories of Inheritance

Over the years there has been a gradual awareness that the individual Rh genes sometimes affect each other and may vary in their expression according to their partners.

A difference in the C and E antigens of the red cells of individuals whose genotypes contain the same Rh genes but in different combinations was shown by Race *et al.* (1954) when C and E were in the cis* position, the antigen C was inhibited and when C and E were in the trans* position, E was inhibited. Only certain antisera made this distinction; when other sera were used the antigens

* For definition *see* Glossary.

C and E appeared to be present in about the same strength in all the different genotypes tested.

Another striking example of what has been termed position effect is cited by Ceppellini *et al.* (1955). Individuals who appeared to be of the genotype $CD^{u}e$. Cde did not in fact have a D^{u} gene but a normal D which could not express itself properly in the presence of Cde. This was realised when it was noted that on segregation away from Cde the apparent $CD^{u}e$ chromosome behaved as a normal CDe.

Rosenfeld and Haber (1958) have suggested that some at least of these position effects are accounted for by the production of antibodies to compound antigens. For example, it is supposed

Rh Compound Antigens

Compound antigen	Name of antibody	
	Original	*Present*
Ce	anti-rh_1	anti-Ce
CE	Jarvis (also contains anti-Ce)	anti-CE
ce	anti-f	anti-ce
cE	not yet identified	
Ce^{s}	not yet identified	
ce^{s}	anti-V	anti-ce^{s}

that when C and e are in the cis position (as in C*de*.cdE and CD*e*.cDE) they combine to produce a compound antigen, Ce. On the other hand, when C and e are in the trans position the compound antigen is not formed. The antibody corresponding to the Ce antigen is anti-Ce. This antibody, however, does not behave as does a mixture of anti-C + anti-e which will agglutinate C and e wherever these are found; on the contrary it will only agglutinate the red cells of individuals who have C and e in the cis position. In standardising Rh antisera it is important to test whether they are of this type.

It is now thought that the antigen originally designated f is the compound antigen formed by the genes ce when they are in the cis position. This is consistent with the original observation that anti-f reacted with cde, cDe and $cD^{u}e$, but not with, for example, cells of the genotype CDe, cDE where c and e are in trans.

Furthermore the antigen V and the R′ of negroes (R'^{s}) now become comprehensible. The R′ of negroes is characterised by its failure to be agglutinated by the type of anti-C which is mainly anti-Ce in specificity. This negative reaction was unexpected since the negro R′ chromosome was thought to have both C and e in the cis position and therefore should make the compound antigen Ce.

A relationship between V and negro R′ was discovered by Sanger *et al.* (1960) by means of a serum which only agglutinated blood samples which were V+ or R′s. Absorption and elution experiments showed that almost certainly only one antibody is responsible for reactions with V and R′s.

The reactions obtained with anti-V and anti-VS (R'^s) can be explained by postulating the existence of an allele of E, e^s, which is much commoner in negroes than in Caucasians and that anti-VS is anti-e^s. This explains why anti-Ce which is an antibody for the compound antigen Ce does not react with those negroid cells of type Ce^s (*see* Table above). Anti-V is on this theory anti-ce^s

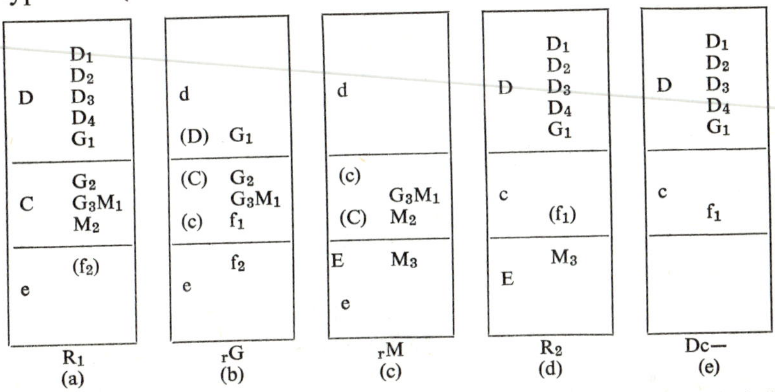

FIG. 31.1. Diagrammatic representation of some Rh chromosomes showing the hypothetical subdivisions of the cistrons. ( ) denotes that this portion, although present is not capable of giving rise to the complete antigen and so the red cells will not react with the corresponding antibody.

reacting with the compound antigen ce^s formed when c and e^s are on the same chromosome.

On the other hand it should be noted that Shapiro does not agree with this explanation and has demonstrated two antibodies defining two factors hr^V and hr^H in several sera thought to be anti-VS (e^s) but that another so called anti-VS serum was pure anti-hr^H (Hernandez).

It is probable that the antigens G and M are also compound antigens arising not from interaction of whole genes but from those portions of the D and C genes which are adjacent. This was first suggested as a possibility by Race and Sanger in 1959. Boorman and Lincoln (1962) expanded this idea and showed that it would explain many of the observed reactions of these antigens. Figure 33.1 shows their diagrammatic representation of (*a*) R_1, (*b*) r^G, (*c*) r^M, (*d*) R_2, and (*e*) Dc-genes.

Table 33.2 shows the known reactions of r^G and the expected reactions according to the theory; r^G will be expected to be negative with anti-D, not because D does not include the antigen G, but that any sera which are mixtures of anti-D and anti-G will be classed as anti-CD sera because, anti-G reacts with R′r cells.

Table 33.2

Comparison of the Observed Reactions of r^G with Rh anti-sera

Anti-serum	Observed reaction	Theoretical reaction
Anti-D	Negative	Negative
Anti-C	Positive with some sera; negative with others.	Positive or negative depending on whether serum contains anti-G
Anti-E	Negative	Negative
Anti-c	Negative	Negative
Anti-e	Negative (one was positive)	Positive
Anti-f	Positive (one was said to be negative)	Positive
Anti-CD	Positive	Positive
Anti-DE	Negative	Negative

Table 33.3

Comparison of the Observed and Theoretical Reactions of r^M with Rh anti-sera

Anti-serum	Observed reaction	Theoretical reaction
Anti-D	Negative	Negative
Anti-C	Some negative, some positive	Positive or negative depending on whether serum contains anti-"M"
Anti-E	Positive	Positive
Anti-c	Negative	Probably negative
Anti-e	Probably weakly positive	Probably weakly positive
Anti-f	Negative	Negative
Anti-CD	Weakly positive	Weakly positive
Anti-DE	Positive	Positive

Such sera can sometimes be separated into anti-D and anti-G, so that an apparent anti-CD serum where the stimulus is known to be R_2 (*e.g.* an R_2r child) or R_0 can often be used to provide an anti-G reagent. Anti-G blocks the reaction of anti-D and anti-C but not of anti-E, which is again consistent with G being a compound antigen produced by portions of the C and D cistron. If anti-f is thought of as anti-ce then it should be negative with r^G, but it is in fact positive and this is the main reason why, Boorman and Lincoln considered that f is a similar antigen to G and is produced by a portion only of the c and e cistron.

In the case of r^M (Fig. 33.1(c) and Table 33.3) the suggestion is that the M antigen arises from sites at the C, E junction. The similarity of r^M and r^G suggest that M and G share the same locus between them with quite possibly some overlap as shown in Fig. 1(b) and (c).

A further consideration was the possibility of f being analogous to r^G and r^M and being formed, not by the whole ce cistron but by the part nearest to the ce junction. This idea offers an explanation for r^G being f positive and r^M being f negative. It also helps to explain what has been one of the major problems of the modern theories of inheritance namely how the Rh gene complex Dc– (Tate *et al.*, 1960) can give rise to the antigen f albeit in about half the normal single dose. This small amount of "f" could well be produced by the "f" portion of the c gene (Fig. 31.1(e)).

Suppression of Rh Antigens

We have noted above the existence of samples of blood lacking one or more of the Rh antigens (*e.g.* D – –). When D – – was found in 1950 by Race and Sanger they concluded that the most likely explanation was that it resulted from a small deletion. Now their alternative theory that it could be a suppression is thought to be more feasible.

The inheritance of D – – gene presents some difficulty as there are too many cases of consanguinity among parents of D – – D – –, homozygotes and also too many of their siblings are also D – – D – –.

The D antigen resulting from the gene D – – is stronger than normal and reacts with some incomplete anti-D sera in saline. It is sometimes possible to detect D – – heterozygotes by this test although cells may react in this way and not have a D – – antigen.

D – – persons are of course particularly liable to be immunised and they produce complex antibodies—sometimes the antibody cannot be separated and appears to be directed against CcEe or as the Americans have called it, Hr_0, a Rhesus factor they say all other cells share. C^wD – and cD – have also been described. There is also one possible – – –/– – – in Japan and several – – – heterozygotes in Europe. More persons are known who lack any Rh antigen but these lack also the related antigen LW.

There are several families known in which, while a C antigen (for instance) is present, it is weaker than usual. These weak forms may well be examples of alleles at the corresponding loci.

LW. LW is the name most people now give to the antigen detected in 1940 by Landsteiner and Wiener using anti-rhesus monkey sera prepared in guinea-pigs.

It was only gradually that it was realised that the animal serum was detecting a different antigen from that detected by anti-Rh sera.

In 1942 Fisk and Foord pointed out that newborn babies were all positive with anti-"Rh" guinea-pig serum although they could easily be typed as Rh positive or Rh negative using human sera.

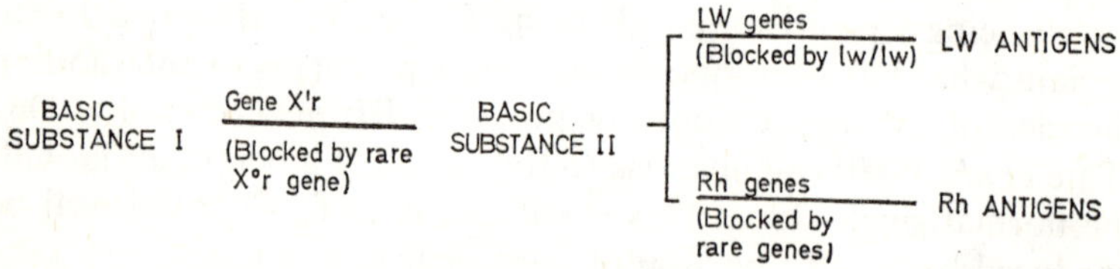

FIG. 33.2.

In 1952 Murray and Clark produced apparent "anti-D" antibodies in guinea-pigs in response to heat extracts of human Rh negative cells.

In 1961 Levine and his colleagues confirmed this but showed that the antibody was not anti-D as it still agglutinated red cells blocked with human incomplete anti-D.

Human "anti-D" sera have been found from which the antibody could be completely absorbed by Rh negative cells. The families of two women who had such "anti-D" antibodies were extensively studied. They revealed that these D-like antibodies were anti-LW and that LW was genetically independent of Rh. In 1961, Vos and colleagues reported finding an aboriginal woman with no Rh antigens ---/---. This condition is now called Rh_{null}, as she was later shown to lack LW antigen also. Figure 33.2 is a diagram of the sort of reasoning that is needed to explain this phenomenon.

It envisages an original basic substance (1) which is acted on by a gene called by Levine X′r to produce a second basic substance (2) which is then available to be converted to LW by the LW gene and to Rh antigens by the Rh genes. The gene X′r is considered to have a rare allele X^0r which is a "silent" gene in that it does not convert substance (1) to substance (2) so no LW or Rh antigens can be formed.

Rh_{null} Disease. A type of haemolytic anaemia which resembles

Hereditary Sphercytosis (Acholuric Jaundice) commonly accompanies the Rh_{null} condition of the red cells. There is a haemolytic anaemia with reticulocytosis and increased red cell osmotic fragility. The anti-globulin test is negative.

The Place of the Rh System in Modern Genetics

Recent genetical work on other biological material, *e.g.* bacteria and moulds, has produced the conception of a gene being a minute length of chromosome with many, perhaps hundreds of mutational sites. Moreover, crossing over can happen as a rare occurrence between these sites. The modern name for gene is cistron. The new facts that have accumulated about Rh genes and antigens would fit well into the cistron idea of a gene, although at the moment it is not known how many cistrons are involved. Whether two mutational sites (loci) belonging to the same or separate cistrons is defined by the cis-trans test. Suppose two different genes combine to produce one character but can only accomplish this if they have segregated together (cis position) then they are said to be non-complementary and to have their sites within the same cistron. If, however, the genes can still produce their compound character when they have originated from opposite chromosomes they are said to be complementary and to have their sites on separate cistrons. Evidence of this nature is obtained from a study of the behaviour of anti-ce and anti-Ce in the Rh system. As already indicated compound antigens and therefore compound antibodies are produced when ce and Ce are in the cis position, but not when they are in the trans position. These facts by definition put C and E into the same cistron which almost certainly contains many C and E sites.

BIBLIOGRAPHY

ALLEN, F. H., and TIPPETT, P. A. (1958), "A new Rh blood type which reveals the Rh antigen G." *Vox Sang.*, **3** (N.S.), 321.

BOORMAN, K. E., and LINCOLN, P. J. (1962), "A suggestion as to the place of r^G and r^M on the Rh system." *Ann. Hum. Genet.*, **26**, 51.

BROMAN, B., HEIKEN, A., TIPPETT, PATRICIA A., and GILES, CAROLYN M. (1963), "The D(C)(e) gene complex revealed in the Swedish population." *Vox Sang.*, **8**, 588–593.

BUCHANAN, D. L., and MCINTYRE, J. (1955), "Consanguinity and two rare matings." *Brit. J. Hæmat.*, **1**, 304.

CALLENDER, SHEILA T., and RACE, R. R. (1946), "A serological and genetical study of multiple antibodies formed in response to blood transfusion by a patient with lupus erythematosus diffusus." *Ann. Eugen. Lond.*, **13**, 102–117.

CEPPELLINI, R., DUNN, L. C., and TURRI, M. (1955), "An interaction between alleles at the Rh locus in man which weakens the reactivity of the Rh_0 factor (D^u)." *Proc. Nat. Acad. Sci. Wash.*, **41**, 283–288.

CEPPELLINI, R., IKIN, ELIZABETH W., and MOURANT, A. E. (1950), "A new allele of the Rh gene E." *Boll. Ist. Sieroter Milanese*, **29**, 123.

CHOWN, B., LEWIS, MARION, KAITA, H., and PHILIPPS, SYLVIA (1964), "The Rh antigen D^W (Wiel)." *Transfusion*, Vol. 4, No. 3 (May–June).

DE NATALE, A., CAHAN, A., JACK, J. A., RACE, R. R., and SANGER, RUTH (1955), "V, a new Rh antigen common in negroes, rare in white people." *J.A.M.A.*, **159**, 247.

GREENWALT, T. J., and SANGER, R. (1955), "The Rh antigen E^W." *Brit. J. Hæm.*, **1**, 52.

GUNSON, H. H., and DONOHUE, W. L. (1957), "Multiple examples of the blood genotype C^wD–/C^wD– in a Canadian family". *Vox Sang.*, **2**, No. 5, 320–331.

HENNINGSEN, C. (1958), "A new 'deleted' Rh-Chromosome." *Nature, Lond.*, **181**, 502.

ISHIMORI, T., and HASEKURA, H. (1967), "A Japanese with no detectable Rh blood group antigens due to silent Rh alleles or deleted chromosomes." *Transfusion, Philad.*, **7**, 84.

KORNSTAD, L., and ØYEN, R. (1967), "An Rh gene complex producing weak c and E antigens." *Vox Sang.*, **13**, 417.

KAITA, H., LEWIS, MARION, and CHOWN, B. (1964), "The Rh antigen E^W." *Transfusion*, Vol. 4, No. 2 (March–April).

KEVY, S. V., SCHMIDT, P. J., and LEYSHON, W. C. (1959), "A second example of the blood type rh^G." *Vox Sang.*, **4**, 257–266.

LANDSTEINER, K., and WIENER, A. S. (1940), "An agglutinable factor on human blood recognised by immune sera for rhesus blood." *Proc. Soc. exp. Biol., N.Y.*, **43**, 223.

LAYRISSE, M., LAYRISSE, ZULAY, and GARCIA, E. (1961), "New Rh phenotype, $Dcce^ie^if$, found in a Chibcha Indian tribe." *Nature*, Vol. 191, No. 4787 503–504 (July 29).

LAYRISSE, M., LAYRISSE, ZULAY, GARCIA, E., and PARRA, J. (1961), "Genetic studies of the new Rh chromosome Dce^if (Ro^i) found in a Chibcha tribe." *Vox Sang.*, **6**, 710–719.

LEVINE, P., CELANO, M. J., WALLACE, J., and SANGER, RUTH (1963), "A human 'D-like' antibody." *Nature*, **198**, 596.

METAXAS, M. N., and METAXAS-BÜHLER, M. (1961), "An Rh gene complex which produces weak c and e antigens in a mother and her son." *Vox Sang.*, **6**, No. 2, 136.

PONTECORVO, G. (1959), *Trends in genetic analysis*, p. 36. Columbia Univ. Press, N. York.

RACE, R. R. (1948), "The Rh genotypes and Fisher's theory." *Blood*, **3**, suppl. 2, 27–42.

RACE, R. R. (1960), "The genetics of Rh." *VIII Congress of the Int. Nat. Soc. Blood Trans., Tokyo*.

RACE, R. R., MOURANT, A. E., LAWLER, SYLVIA D., and SANGER, RUTH (1948), "The Rh chromosome frequencies in England." *Blood* 3, **689**, 695.

RACE, R. R., SANGER, R. (1960), "Consanguinity and certain rare blood groups." *Vox Sang.*, **5**, 383–385.

RACE, R. R., SANGER, RUTH, and LAWLER, SYLVIA D. (1948), "Allelomorphs of the Rh gene C." *Heredity*, **2**, 237.

RACE, R. R., SANGER, RUTH, and LAWLER, S. D. (1960), "The Rh antigen called c^V a revocation." *Vox Sang.*, **5**, 334.

RACE, R. R., SANGER, RUTH., LEVINE, P., MCGEE, R. T., LOGHEM, J. J. van, HART, MIA v. d. and CAMERON, C. (1954), "A position effect of the Rh blood group genes." *Nature, Lond.*, **174**, 460.

RACE, R. R., SANGER, RUTH, and SELWYN, J. G. (1951), "A possible deletion in a human Rh chromosome; A serological and genetical study." *Brit. J. Exp. Path.*, **32**, 124.

RACE, R. R., and TAYLOR, G. L. (1943), "A serum that discloses the genotype of some Rh positive people." *Nature, Lond.*, **152**, 300.

RACE, R. R., TAYLOR, G. L., BOORMAN, KATHLEEN E., and DODD, BARBARA E. (1943), "Recognition of Rh genotypes in man." *Nature, Lond.*, **152**, 563.

ROSENFIELD, R. E., and HABER, GLADYS V. (1958), "An Rh blood factor rh (Ce) and its relationship to hr (ce)." *Amer. J. Hum. Genet.*, **10**, 474–480.

ROSENFIELD, R. E., VOGEL, P., GIBBEL, NATALIE., SANGER, RUTH., and RACE, R. R. (1953), "A new Rh antibody, anti-f." *Brit. Med. J.*, **i**, 975.

ROSENFIELD, R., HABER, GLADYS V., and DEGNAN, TH. J. (1964), "Rh alleles $R^{-10,20}$, and new evidence for $R^{2,4}$." *Vox Sang.*, Vol. **9**, No. 2, p. 168.

SACKS, M. S., WIENER, A. S., JOHN, ELSA F., SPURLING, CARROLL L., and UNGER, L. J. (1959), "Isosensitization to the new blood factor Rh^D with special reference to its clinical importance." *Ann. Int. Med.*, **51**, 740–747.

SALMON, and SY BABA (1968). Personal communication to Race and Sanger—reported by them in *Blood Groups in Man.* Fifth Edition.

SANGER, R. (1960), "Rh antigens." *Rh conference, Princetown., U.S.A.*

SANGER, R., NOADES, J., TIPPETT, P., JACK, J. A., and CUNNINGHAM, C. A. (1960) "An Rh antibody specific for V and R'^s". *Nature, Lond.*, **186**, 171.

SHAPIRO, M. (1960), "Serology and Genetics of a new Blood Factor hr^s." *J. For. Med.*, **7**, 96.

SHAPIRO, M., and PATH, F. C. (1964), "Serology and genetics of a 'new' blood factor: Hr^H." *Journal of Forensic Medicine*, Vol. 11, No. 2 (April–June), pp. 52–66.

SCHMIDT, P. J., and HOLLAND, P. V. (1969), "Rh_{null} disease." *XII International Congress on Blood Transfusion Abstracts*, 145.

STOUT, T. D., MOORE, B. P. L., ALLEN, F. H. Jr., and CORCORAN, PATRICIA (1963), "A new phenotype –D+ G– (Rh: 1,–12)." *Vox Sang.*, **8**, 262–268.

STRATTON, F., and RENTON, P. H. (1948), "Rh genes allelo morphic to D.' *Nature, Lond.*, **162**, 292.

STRATTON, F., and RENTON, P. H. (1954), "Hæmolytic disease of the newborn caused by a new Rh antibody, anti-C^X." *Brit. Med. J.*, **i**, 962.

SUSSMAN, L. N., and WIENER, A. S. (1964), "An unusual Rh agglutinogen lacking blood factors Rh^A, Rh^B, Rh^C, and Rh^D." *Transfusion*, Vol. 4, No. 1 (Jan–Feb.)

TATE, HERMINE, CUNNINGHAM, C., McDADE, MARY G., TIPPETT, PATRICIA A., and SANGER, RUTH (1960), "An Rh gene complex Dc–." *Vox Sang*, **5**, 398–402.

TIPPETT, PATRICIA, and SANGER, R. (1962), "Observations on subdivision of the Rh antigen D." *Vox Sang.*, **7**, 9–13.

TIPPETT, PATRICIA A., SANGER, RUTH, DUNSFORD, I., and BARKER, M. (1961), "An Rh gene complex r^M, in some ways like r^G." *Vox Sang.*, **6**, 21–33.

UNGER, L. J., and WIENER, A. S. (1959), "A new antibody anti-Rh^c resulting from isosensitisation by pregnancy with special reference to heredity of new Rh-Hr agglutinogen, Rh^2." *J. Lab. and Clin. Med.*, **54**, 835–842.

UNGER, L. J., and WIENER, A. S. (1959), "Observations on blood factors Rh^A, Rh^L, Rh^B, and Rh^C." *Amer. J. Clin. Path.*, **31**, 95–103.

UNGER, L. J., WIENER, A. S., and WEINER, L. (1959), "New antibody (anti-Rh^B) resulting from blood transfusion in Rh positive patient." *J.A.M.A.*, **170**, 1380–1383.

WIENER, A. S. (1943), "Genetic theory of the Rh blood types." *Proc. Soc. Exp. Biol., N.Y.*, **54**, 316–319.

WIENER, A. S., GEIGER, J., and GORDON, E. B. (1957), "Mosaic nature of Rh_0 factor of human blood." *Exper. Med. and Surg.*, **15**, 75–82.

Chapter 34

YET FURTHER COMPLEXITIES: ANOTHER LOOK AT MNSs̄, P, KELL, LUTHERAN, KIDD AND OTHER SYSTEMS

Blood group systems almost always appear to be uncomplicated when they are first discovered. The usual sequence is the finding of a single antibody detecting an antigen on red cells, followed by the finding of a second antibody antithetical in its reactions to the first.

It is postulated therefore that the two antibodies are detecting antigens produced by a pair of allelic genes (*e.g.* M and N, Fy^a and Fy^b, Jk^a and Jk^b, etc.). The ABO system was an exception and was probably the least simple at the point of its discovery.

Experience has shown that the simple beginnings have been followed by further discoveries which have laid bare complexities which have not always been easy to unravel. This state of affairs lasts until with the appearance of further findings a system seems to crystallise and to take its final form—an unwise conclusion to draw as the history of several of the systems described below will illustrate. The P system, to take but one example, has already developed in four main stages: in 1927 the discovery of a single antigen (although varying in strength) and its corresponding antibody; in 1955 the recognition that the antigen Tj^a belonged to P; in 1959 an extension to include P^K and in 1965 a further extension to include Luke.

As new antibodies are found each necessitates careful investigation including family studies to determine whether it is part of one of the known systems or quite independent of them.

Our knowledge of blood groups therefore is always in an exciting state of fluidity, although fortunately enough is known about most of them to enable us to deal safely with their clinical application.

Families with rare genes or displaying unusual genic effects, although in some respects collectors pieces, have yet contributed vitally to the understanding of various blood group systems. There are now a number of examples. The rare "Bombay" bloods together with the meticulous biochemistry, notably of Morgan and Watkins, have confirmed a basic design underlying the structure of the ABO system (*see* Chapter 32). Some of the rare antigens described in this chapter would seem to suggest a similar design for other systems although biochemical confirmation is as yet lacking.

Antigens which segregate with a well recognised system but are not alleles at the same locus are always a puzzle (*see* those associated with MNSs). These may be phenotypic associations as well as genic ones.

Another factor which is reasonable to consider as a cause of odd reactions is the possible steric effect that antigens may well exert one upon another on the surface of the red cell. Realising that about 1,000,000 antigens sites are reserved for the A_1 antigen, up to 35,000 for D and 60,000 for c on each red cell, as well as unknown numbers for countless other antigens, it would be scarcely surprising to find occasional interference with normal reactions. Perhaps the relationship between Luke and the ABO system is due to interaction at the red cell surface (*see* page 407) or perhaps even more striking is the effect of A_1 on Le^b where the majority of anti-Le^b sera do not detect Le^b on A_1 cells but the occasional anti-Le^b serum is found to react as well with A_1 Le(b−) as with O Le(b+) cells.

Rare MNSs Alleles and Associates

The complexity of the MNSs system is obvious from a glance at Tables 34.1, 2 and 3. In itself it can form a life study. In attempting to arrange the variants we have followed Race and Sanger in adopting two broad categories. Variants which are almost certainly the products of alleles at the MN or Ss loci are shown in Table 34.1. These are characterised by their failure to react with some or all of the regular anti-MNSs antisera. In many cases the specific antibody has been found. The second category (34.2) is composed of antigens closely associated with the MN and Ss loci but not, in the main, affecting the expression of the M, N, S, s antigens with which they are associated. They are detected by the finding of specific antisera and family studies then reveal that the gene for the rare antigen in question is segregating with the MNSs gene. The Miltenburger group of antigens really belongs in Table 34.2 but because it is more complex we have given it a table of its own (34.3).

Alleles at the MN and Ss Loci

U or S^u. In 1953 an antibody was described by Wiener *et al.* which agglutinated the red cells of 1,100 white persons tested but was negative with twelve out of 989 New York Negroes; the antibody was called anti-U. It was later shown by Greenwalt *et* *al.* (1954) that blood samples negative with anti-U were also negative with anti-S and anti-s. Anti-U therefore began to be thought of as anti-S plus anti-s or more accurately anti-Ss as absorption and elution failed to separate the components. The reactions, however, do not fit completely those expected of anti-Ss since some S–s– samples are positive with anti-U although the strength of the reaction varies considerably. The anti-body is probably quite readily produced in S–s– individuals, it has been shown to have considerable clinical significance. In spite of little understood complexities it is generally considered that the absence of S and s is due to an allele at the Ss locus and that the symbol S^u is therefore appropriate.

Mg. This is an exceedingly rare allele, except in Switzerland. It is selected for a short description owing to its great interest and the fact that it has a specific antibody which is by no means as rare as the antigen. The antigen Mg does not react with anti-M or anti-N. The Mg propositus (Allen *et al.*, 1958) was a patient requiring blood and by chance the serum of his selected donor contained anti-Mg.

When Mg pairs with M, a single dose M reaction is obtained on typing with anti-M and a negative reaction with anti-N; blood of type MgN appears to be NN but gives only a single dose reaction with anti-N sera. The presence of Mg could theoretically give rise to false exclusions in cases of doubtful paternity; it is unlikely to do so in practice however, both on account of its rarity and the fact that anti-Mg should always be fairly readily obtainable for the confirmation of relevant results. Among English people, 23 examples of anti-Mg were found out of 703 individuals tested, although tests on 61,128 English donors did not reveal a single example of the Mg antigen! In Switzerland, however, the frequency of Mg is 0·153 per cent and this has enabled family studies to be carried out even to the finding of one family in which each parent had Mg and a child was produced who was homozygous for Mg and, of course, negative with both anti-M and anti-N (Metaxas *et al.*, 1966).

Other Alleles

The other alleles summarised in Table 34.1 are all rare with the exception of M_1 and T_m.

M^c is an interesting antigen, intermediate between M and N as shown by the fact that it reacted with 25 out of 27 anti-M sera and 5 out of 28 anti-N sera. M^k (Metaxas and Metaxas-Bühler, 1964) is considered to be an allele at the MN locus because it does not produce any M, N or Mg antigen. The background may however be more complicated than this as M^k is always associated with an absence of Ss antigens also. A human anti-M^k has not so far been found but a weak anti-M^k has been produced by the injection of M^k cells into rabbits. The discovery of further examples of M^k and two "new" alleles M^z and M^r are illustrative of the rewards which may be expected through testing large numbers of blood samples with "dosing" anti-M and anti-N sera. (Metaxas *et al.*, 1968.) These workers selected a pair of human sera (anti-M and anti-N) which would only agglutinate red cells of type MM and NN and these were used in conjunction with normal rabbit anti-sera. Any cell sample whose reactions with the rabbit sera were M+N− or M−N+ and which were not agglutinated by the appropriate "dosing" serum, was presumed to be heterozygous at the MN locus and to possess one of these rare alleles. In their investigation on 3,895 blood donors (Swiss) 15 such samples were found and in each of these a rare allele was demonstrated: Mg in six cases, M^k in five and one example each of M^c, M^z, M^r and N_2 (*see* Table 34.1).

Associated Antigens (*see* Table 34.2)

Of the antigens associated with MN, Hu and He have been known for many years. Anti-Hu was produced in rabbits after injection with the blood of a negro, Mr. Hunter (Landsteiner, Strutton and Chase, 1934). All blood samples giving positive reactions belonged to groups N or MN. Another negro antigen, He, was found by Ikin and Mourant (1951). Anti-He was made in rabbits also.

The other rare antigens shown in Table 34.2 were brought to light when antibodies were found in human sera. They are all dominant characters and appear to have no effect on the MNSs antigens with which they segregate.

Mi^a. Vw(Gr). Mur. Hil (*see* Table 34.3)

These antigens belong to the complicated sub-system now usually called "Miltenburger." Two of them Gr (Graydon, 1946) and Mi^a (Levine *et al.*, 1951) had been discovered for some time before it was realised that they were related to the MNSs system. This came about after the discovery by Van der Hart *et al.* in 1954, that Vw a rare antigen was closely linked to the MNSs locus and that Vw was also related to Gr and Mi^a. In fact, it has been shown by Simmons *et al.*, 1959 that Vw and Gr are indistinguishable. Four different type sera have been identified each giving a different pattern of reactions; with these anti-sera four red cell phenotypes have been identified (Table 34.3) all of which are Mi^a positive and may be thought of as subgroups of Miltenburger. All four types of

Table 34.1

Rare Alleles at the MN or Ss Locus

Antigens	Characteristics	Occurrence	Antibodies
M^g	Anti-M and Anti-N negative	0 in 61,128 English 0 in 44,000 Boston 0·153% in Swiss	Anti-Mg fairly common
M^c	Intermediate between M and N. NM^c positive with anti-M_1 negative with anti-M^1	3 families	No specific antibody.
M_1	Variable reaction with anti-M	1 in 4 Negro M is M_1 1 in 20 White M is M_1	Anti-M_1 is a component of some human anti-M sera.
M^k	Absence of M, N, S, s and Mg. Weak reaction with a few rabbit anti-N	5 in 3,894 Swiss	Wk anti-M^k prepared in rabbits. No human anti-M^k found so far.
M^v	Positive with a rare "anti-N like" antibody	1 in 400M Whites 0 in 1,000M Negroes	Anti-M^v is human "anti-N" reacting with 1 in 400M.
N_2	Weak or negative with anti-N often associated with a positive direct anti-human globulin test	Very rare, 1 in 3,894 Swiss	No specific antibody.
T_m	Antigen variable in strength—usually with N	20% Whites 30% N.Y. Negroes	Anti-T_m fairly rare. (Reactions similar to those expected of an anti-N_1)
S_j	All S_j positives are also T_m positive	2% Whites 4% Negroes	Anti-S_j very rare.
S^u	Has no S or s	1% Negro, rare in Whites	Anti-U (reacts with all S+ or s+ and some S–s– cells).
S_2	Reacts with some anti-S sera	One family	No specific antibody.
M^z	NM^z negative with anti-M_1 positive with anti-M^1. Inherited as M^zs Produces M and N	One family	No specific antibody.
M^r	Produces M and N. M stronger than M^c or M^z. N reacts with all anti-N	A few families	No specific antibody.

antisera have caused hæmolytic disease of the newborn. Anti-Vw (Gr) is often found in the serum of patients with acquired hæmolytic anæmia and also in approximately 1 per cent of random individuals as an atypical cold antibody. Anti-Mi^a is also found

Table 34.2

Antigens Associated with MNSs

Antigens	Characteristics	Occurrence	Antibodies
Hu	Associated with N	7% Am. Negroes 22% W. Africans Rare Whites	Anti-Hu made in rabbits.
He	Associated variously with NS, Ns, MS and Ms according to ethnic origin	2·7% W. Africans 0 in 1,500 Whites	Anti-He made in rabbits.
Vr		3 in 12,000 Dutch	Anti-Vr.
Ri^a		3 in 17,013 English	Anti-Ri^a (one example in same serum as anti-St^a).
St^a	Variously aligned with NS, Ns, Ms	20 in 17,013 English 14 in 220 Japanese 6 in 414 Chinese	Anti-St^a (several found).
Mt^a	Aligned with Ns	28 in 11,907 Whites 3 in 318 Thais	Anti-Mt^a probably naturally occurring. Immune in rabbits.
Cl^a	Aligned with Ms in two families		Anti-Cl^a (found in 0·45% of blood donors).
Ny^a	Aligned with Ns in 12 families	10 in 5,931 Norwegians	Anti-Ny^a.
Sul	Aligned with Ns in one family	O in 4,935 mixed races	Anti-Sul.

Table 34.3

Miltenburger Phenotypes as Defined by the Four Main Types of Antisera (*note* all Phenotypes extremely rare)

Class	*Antisera* Vw(Gr)	Mi^a	Mur	Hil	*Phenotype*
I	+	+	−	−	Mi(a+)Vw+
II	−	+	−	−	Mi(a+)Vw−Mur−Hil−
III	−	+	+	+	Mi(a+)Vw−Mur+Hil+
IV	−	+	+	−	Mi(a+)Vw−Mur+Hil−

in patients with acquired hæmolytic anæmia but not, as yet, in the serum of normal, healthy donors.

The "N" of M Cells

Cross reactions between M and N and their practical importance have been mentioned in Chapter 16. Considerable additional knowledge about the cross-reactivity comes from a study of the rare variants. It will be remembered that the cross reactivity is due to the uptake of anti-N by M cells. Allen *et al.* (1960) attribute the cross reactivity to the production of some N antigen by the M gene. They observed that M, S–s–, U– cells do not react with anti-N and this observation was confirmed by biochemical methods. It is perhaps surprising that Mg in the homozygous MgMg type gives rise to even more "N"-ness that a normal M, while even the "silent" M^k shows some N activity.

It has been suggested that perhaps N is a basic substance upon which the M gene operates. This theory would fit many of the facts that if true would make Mm rather than MN the appropriate nomenclature for the system.

The Peculiarities of P

The discovery that the Tj^a antigen was part of P expanded this system in a clear and tidy fashion and a useful analogy with the A_1A_2 system was seen (Chapter 18). As so often happens with blood groups, complications arose with the finding, upon the necessity for crossmatching blood, of an antibody which agglutinated the red cells of 150 prospective donors (Matson *et al.*, 1959). The antibody was obviously detecting an antigen of high frequency and was therefore tested against a panel of rare cells including S^uS^u, "Bombay," Vel negative, Fy(a–b–), Yt(a–) and pp. All gave a positive reaction except pp and so the problem seemed solved with the finding of another example of anti-Tj^a (anti-P + P_1). But surprisingly, the red cells of the propositus did not give the expected negative reactions with anti-P + P_1 and anti-P_1 sera. Since an auto-immune condition was not involved, it seemed likely that the positive reaction of the cells of the propositus was due to a third antibody in the anti-P_1 and anti-P + P_1 sera and absorption tests proved this to be the case. For example when anti-P + P_1 was absorbed with P_1 cells until it would no longer react with these cells, it still reacted with the cells of the propositus. The extra antibody in the anti-P_1 and anti-P + P_1 sera was termed anti-P^K. Finally it was found that the serum of the propositus contained anti-P and not as at first assumed, anti-P + P_1. Absorption with P_2 cells failed to leave anti-P_1. It is now known that specific anti-P^K can be prepared from the serum of some p people by absorption with P_1 cells.

All P^K individuals have P^K and lack P; the majority have the antigen P_1 (phenotype $P_1{}^K$) but some are P_2 (phenotype $P_2{}^K$). P^K is not considered to be an allele at the P locus but to be the product of a precursor substance which is needed for the formation of the more familiar P antigens. As mentioned above this hints at a common pattern underlying most blood group systems and if true would bring the P system into line with the ABO and probably also Rh and Kell.

In 1965, Tippett *et al.* advanced the P system still further with work on the Luke phenotypes. The Luke antibody is like anti-P in failing to react with the cells of p and P^K people but in addition it further fails to react with the cells of about 2 per cent of P_1 and P_2 people. It seems that so far only three examples of this antibody have been found and these give graded reactions of +, weak and negative. The weak and negative reactions were significantly more common with P_2 than with P_1 cells and with A_1, either in group A or AB.

Table 34.4

The Reactions of P Phenotypes including P^K with the Various P Antibodies

Phenotype	Approx. frequency	Anti-P_1	Anti-P, P_1, P^K (Anti-Tj^a)	Anti-P	Anti-P^K
P_1	75%	+	+	+	−
P_2	25%	−	+	+	−
p	Very rare	−	−	− or w	−
$P_1{}^K$	Very rare	+	+	−	+
$P_2{}^K$	Very rare	−	+	−	+

Further Kell Phenotypes

In Chapter 17 six antibodies of the Kell system were described anti-K, anti-k, anti-Kp^a and anti-Kp^b, anti-Js^a and anti-Js^b. These are usually considered to be the products of three pairs of allelic genes Kk, Kp^aKp^b and Js^aJs^b.

In 1957, Chown *et al.* discovered a new phenotype negative with the four antisera known at that time. This was designated K−k−Kp(a–b–) or K_o for short. This rare type was discovered because the propositus had an antibody which reacted with all K+k+ samples (anti-Ku). Eleven such individuals are now known. All but two announced their existence by having antibodies, eight of these being anti-Ku and one anti-Kp^b. K_o is very rare, the phenotype frequency being about 0·00006 and the gene frequency about 0·008.

It will be remembered that the Sutter groups Js^a and Js^b were first considered to be an independent system and that it was the finding that two K−k−Kp(a–b–) persons were also Js(a–b–) which led to the family studies which showed that Sutter was part of Kell. There is more than one reason why persons may lack antigens corresponding to all three pairs of genes, for example in the Rh system some Rh null persons are thought to be homozygous for a gene complex—(*i.e.* having no Rh genes) while others arise because of a lack of basic substance suitable for conversion by normal Rh genes. So far we do not know which mechanism is operating in the Kell system or even if there may be some other explanation. There is even no decisive proof that the system is governed by three pairs of allelic genes, there is a possible alternative theory in which Js^a is considered to be an allele of K, Kp^a and k. This alternative theory has this disadvantage that it would mean that the antibodies, anti-k, anti-Kp^b and Js^b would have to be complex. That not all the gene combinations expected on a three allele system have been encountered is probably due to the fact that Js^a is almost confined to Negroes, while K and Kp^a are found in Whites. This fact, of course, makes Kell a very useful system, when a racial marker is needed.

Linkage studies on 3 families places the UL^a almost certainly within the Kell system but it is not yet known which part of the locus is responsible. No reactions have been found to relate UL^a to the K or Kp series. The relationship of UL^a to Js will be difficult to work out, as Js^a is almost confined to Negroes and UL^a to Finns.

Two individuals curious in their Kell types, give a clue to the genetic background of the system and suggest that it is built on the same lines as probably all blood group systems in requiring basic materials, the production of which is controlled by genes which are quite independent of the Kell locus.

The first of these, McLeod, was found by Allen *et al.*, 1961. The cells of the propositus reacted extremely weakly with anti-K^u, anti-k and anti-Kp^b. They were negative with anti-K and anti-Kp^a; their reaction was also unusually weak with anti-Js^b.

The second individual, Claas (van der Hart and van Loghem, 1965) was found to have an antibody which reacted with all cells with which it was tested including cells of type K−k−Kp(a–b–) Js(a–b–). The only negative reactions were the individuals own cells and the cells of McLeod. Claas cells behaved like those of McLeod. Extensive absorption and elution tests suggested that the Claas antibody was directed at the whole Kell complex of antigens. It is important in revealing the fact that K−k−Kp (a–b–) Js(a–b–) cells do have some kind of Kell type antigen. Perhaps the situation pertaining to McLeod and Claas is analogous to "Bombay" bloods which are believed to be hh; these two may be homozygous for the absence of a gene which is required for the production of a substance necessary for the expression of the various Kell genes. The analogy with the ABO system may be pressed further in that the trace of K, Kp^b and Js^b found can be compared with the finding of traces of the appropriate ABH antigen in "Bombay" types.

The Role of Xg^a in the Study of Human Genetics

The Xg blood group system has been outlined in Chapter 19. The following short account illustrates how this dominant X-linked character is being used both in studies of sex-chromosome abnormalities and in chromosome mapping.

Xg and Sex-chromosome Abnormalities, Sex chromosome abnormalities are usually due to a person having the wrong number of sex chromosomes and the accidents are of two kinds.

(1) Two X chromosomes, which should part at meiosis and each go into separate nuclei, stay together so that one daughter nucleus has two X's and the other none. This phenomenon is called non-disjunction.

(2) Sometimes an X or Y (or both) fails to reach the spindle poles at the anaphase of cell division and is thereby excluded from the newly derived nuclei. This is called anaphase lag and more often involves a Y chromosome.

Individuals exhibiting the syndromes of Klinefelter and Turner are examples of such abnormalities. Those demonstrating the Klinefelter syndrome are males with too many X chromosomes. They may be of the following types (*a*) XXY, (*b*) XXXY, (*c*) XXXXY, (*d*) XXYY, (*e*) XX males, (*f*) XXY mosaics.

Xg^a typing of such individuals may give information as to the origin of the extra X's and also at which of the meiotic divisions the accident has occurred. Two examples of family studies will illustrate these points.

1. Father Xg (a+)—mother Xg (a−) and Klinefelter XXY son Xg (a+). This Xg^a typing result shows that the extra X must be of paternal origin and that his father therefore must have some sperm carrying both X and Y. Moreover the types of the family show that the accident must have happened at the first meiotic division of the maturation of the sex cells, for it is only at this stage that there is the opportunity for non-disjunction to occur.
2. Father Xg (a+)—mother Xg (a+) or Xg (a−) and the Klinefelter XXY son Xg (a−). This family shows that both X's are of maternal origin (otherwise the son would be Xg (a+)) but they do not show whether the accident took place at the first or second meiotic division.

In the Turner syndrome there is the lack of an X; the individuals are females. Rarely, the syndrome is associated with the lack of the short arm of one X. In some of these families it can be shown from the results of Xg^a typing whether the single X is of paternal or maternal origin, *e.g.* father Xg (a+), mother Xg (a−), Turner daughter XO Xg (a+). In this case the single X must originate from the father. In fact it was such a family as this that provided the most convincing proof that the single X can be of paternal origin. It was generally believed that accidents did not happen to the maternal X.

X-Chromosome Mapping

Xg^a typing is being used extensively in the mapping of the relative position of genes on the X chromosomes.

It is our intention to do no more than outline the general principles. The interested reader who would like to delve more deeply into this subject and that of Xg and chromosome abnormalities discussed above, is referred to *Blood Groups in Man*, by Race and Sanger, the fountain head for these subjects.

The mapping of loci in the X chromosome has far outstripped the mapping of the autosomes for the simple reason that the linkage of characters with sex is comparatively easy to recognise and so are the sex chromosomes.

A great deal of work has already been done on Xg typing families with other X-linked characters, *e.g.* red–green colour blindness, glucose-6-phosphate deficiency, hæmophilia, retinitis pigmentosa.

Information about the distance between genes is derived from studying families in which the linkage between two characters can be followed through one or more generations. When two genes are on one chromosome pair and are fairly close to each other, the two characters they control will be seen travelling together through the generations but occasionally at meiosis crossing over will happen between the genes and the two characters will be found apart in some of the children. These children are termed recombinants. If for example 6 per cent of children are seen to be crossovers then the recombination frequency is said to be 0·06. This recombination can be taken as a direct index of the distance between genes on the chromosomes and this distance is called 6 centimorgans. Recombination frequencies greater than 0·15 have to have corrections for double cross-overs.

The study of suitable cross-over families has made possible a tentative map of the human X chromosome, the mathematics being far more complex (often needing a computer) than the above simple explanation of the basic principles suggests. The advent of the Xg^a blood group has increased the probable length of the X chromosome to 200 centimorgans and has added to knowledge of the relative positions of a number of genes along its length. These fall into two groups which are themselves too far apart for the distance between them to be measured at the present time. One group containing Xg itself also has the genes for ichthyosis and ocular albinism within measurable distance. The other group comprises the genes for deutan, G6PD, protan and hæmophilia.

As yet Less Complicated Systems

The systems Diego, Yt and Dombrock are discussed in Chapter 19 and so far are at a comparatively simple stage so that there is little we can add here. The next step for Diego and Yt will probably be the finding of a minus-minus group, *e.g.* Di(a–b–). It is unlikely that this will be found by direct search, and is more probable that in a direct matching problem a patient with an apparently 100 per cent positive frequency antibody which is not an auto-antibody will be found to be Di(a–b–) or Yt(a–b–). The Dombrock system still awaits the finding of the expected anti-Do^b. It is, however, just possible that some blood group systems really are as simple as these appear at present and that no further complications will arise.

Duffy, Kidd and Lutheran have been fairly adequately covered in Chapters 17 and 18 in that only two antibodies are known in each system anti-Fy^a and anti-Fy^b; anti-Jk^a and anti-Jk^b and anti-Lu^a and anti-Lu^b.

The main interest in these groups is in the minus–minus phenotypes. Fy(a–b–) while very common in Negroes is almost non-existent in Europeans. Family studies support the theory that the Fy(a–b) phenotype arises, at any rate in the main, not because of "suppressor" genes but as the result of a third allele Fy. It is possible that this allele is an amorph or that eventually an antibody may be found (in which case it would be called anti-Fy^c and the antigen Fy^c). Meanwhile the gene Fy is the most useful in distinguishing between Negro and White bloods as it has a frequency of over 90 per cent in West Africans, about 80 per cent in New York Negroes and only about 3 per cent or less in Europeans. There are also other anthropological differences related to the Duffy system, for instance the Fy(a–b–) phenotype is common in

Yemenite Jews while Japanese and Koreans have a very high frequency of Fy^a.

In the Kidd blood group system we again have the minus-minus phenotype but it is extremely rare. So far there is no real evidence as to whether it arises as the homozygous expression of a Jk gene (a third allele) or from some suppressor mechanism resulting in the nonavailability of basic material.

In this connection it is of interest to note that the very rare Lu(a–b–) phenotype has been shown to be of two kinds, one a dominant and one recessive in character. The first Lu(a–b–) found (Crawford *et al.*, 1961) was of the dominant character as was clearly shown by the family of the propositus. Perhaps the most likely explanation here is that a rare dominant factor at a locus independent of Lutheran converts basic substance which would normally be available for conversion to Lu^a and Lu^b to a new substance unsuitable for such conversion.

Later the recessive type of Lu(a–b–) was found (Darnborough *et al.*, 1963) when a patient with a high frequency antibody was found to be Lu(a–b–) and the antibody anti-Lu^a Lu^b.

The Lu(a–b–) story is further complicated by the fact that there is a close though unexplained connection between the dominant type and the Auberger blood group. In the families in which the Lu(a–b–) phenotype occurs persons who are not Lu(a–b–) are Au(a+) but the Lu(a–b–) persons are Au(a−) with only one exception.

The Blood Group antigen En^a

The first example of a rare antibody (anti-En^a) was described by Darnborough, Dunsford and Wallace (British Society of Hæmatology 1965) and a second example was found in Helsinki in 1968. A full account of the serological and physico-chemical studies is given by Furuhjelm *et al.*, 1969. The antigen En^a is a dominant character found in most people; its absence is very rare and so therefore is the corresponding antibody. En (a–) cells have several pecularities; their MN antigens are depressed and they behave towards incomplete Rh antibodies as do normal cells after treatment by enzymes. They are for example agglutinated, when suspended in saline, by incomplete antisera. The electrophoretic mobility of En (a–) cells is shown to be 40 per cent lower than that of normal cells and their sialic acid content is found to be markedly lower in comparison with normal cells. These facts almost certainly account for their behaviour with incomplete Rh antibodies and MN antisera.

BIBLIOGRAPHY

MNSs System

ALLEN, F. H., CORCORAN, PATRICIA A., KENTON, H. B., and BREARE, NANCY (1958) "M^g a new blood group antigen in the MNSs system." *Vox Sang.* **3,** 81.

ALLEN, F. H., CORCORAN, PATRICIA A., and ELLIS, F. R. (1960), "Some new observations on the MN system." *Vox Sang.*, **5,** 224.

GRAYDON, J. J. (1946), "A rare iso-hæmogglutinogen." *Med. J. Aust.*, **ii,** 9–10.

GREENWALT, T. J., SASAKI, T., SANGER, RUTH, SNEATH, JOAN, and RACE, R. R. (1954), "An allele of the S(s) blood group genes." *Proc. Nat. Acad. Sci., Wash.*, **40,** 1126.

HART, MIA V. D., BOSMAN, HÉLÈNE, and VAN LOGHEM, J. J. (1954), "Two rare human blood group antigens." *Vox Sang.*, **4,** 108.

IKIN, ELIZABETH W., and MOURANT, A. E. (1951), "A rare blood group antigen occurring in Negroes." *Brit. Med. J.*, **i,** 456.

LANDSTEINER, K., STRUTTON, W. R., and CHASE, M. W. (1934), "An agglutination reaction observed with some human bloods, chiefly among Negroes." *J. Immunol.*, **27,** 469.

LEVINE, P., STOCK, A. H., KUHMICHEL, A. B., and BRONIKOVSKY, N. (1951), "A new human blood group factor of rare incidence in the general population." *Proc. Soc. Exp. Biol., N.Y.* **77,** 402.

METAXAS, M. N., and METAXAS-BÜHLER, M. (1964), "M^k an apparently silent allele at the MN locus." *Nature, Lond.*, **202,** 1123.

METAXAS, M. N., METAXAS-BÜHLER, M., and ROMANSKI, J. (1966), "Studies on the blood group antigen M^g.1.Frequency of M^g in Switzerland and family studies." *Vox Sang.*, **11,** 157.

METAXAS, M. N., METAXAS-BÜHLER, M., and IKIN, E. W. (1968), "Complexities of the MN locus." *Vox Sang.*, **15,** 102.

SIMMONS, R. T., ALBREY, J. A., and MCCULLOCH, W. J. (1959), "The duplication of the Gr (Graydon) blood group by Vw (Verweyst)." *Vox Sang.*, **4,** 132.

WIENER, A. S., UNGER, L. J., and GORDON, EVE B. (1953), "Fatal hemolytic transfusion reaction caused by sensitisation to a new blood factor, U." *J. Amer. Med. Ass.*, **153,** 1444.

P System

MATSON, G. A., SWANSON, JANE, NOADES, JEAN, SANGER, RUTH, and RACE, R. R. (1959), "A 'new' Antigen and Antibody belonging to the P blood group system." *Am. J. hum. Gen.*, **11,** 26.

TIPPETT, PATRICIA, SANGER, RUTH, RACE, R. R., SWANSON, JANE, and BUSCH, SHIRLEY (1965), "An agglutinin associated with the P and the ABO blood group systems." *Vox Sang.*, **10,** 269.

Kell System

ALLEN, F. H., KRABBE SISSEL, M. R., and CORCORAN, PATRICIA A. (1961), "A new phenotype (McLeod) in the Kell blood group system." *Vox Sang.*, **6,** 555.

CHOWN, B., LEWIS, MARION, and KAITA, HIROKO (1957), "A 'new' Kell blood group phenotype." *Nature, Lond.*, **180,** 711.

CORCORAN, PATRICIA A., ALLEN, F. H., LEWIS, MARION, and CHOWN, B. (1961), "A new antibody, anti-Ku (anti-Peltz) in the Kell blood group system." *Transfusion, Philad.*, **1,** 181.

FURUJELM, U., NEVANLINNA, H. R., NURKKA, RIITA, GAVIN, JUNE, and SANGER, RUTH (1969), "Evidence that the Antigen UL^a is controlled from the Kell complex locus." *Vox Sang.*, **16,** 496.

HART, MIA VAN DER, and VAN LOGHEM, J. J. (1968), "A 'new' antibody associated with the Kell blood group system." *Vox Sang.*, **15,** 456.

STROUP, MARJORY, MACILROY, MIJA, WALKER, R., and AYDELOTTE, JANE V. (1965), "Evidence that Sutter belongs to the Kell blood group system." *Transfusion, Philad.*, **5**, 309.

Xg^a System

FRØLAND, A., SANGER, RUTH, and RACE, R. R. (1968), "Xg blood group studies on 76 patients with Klinefelters syndrome and on their parents." *J. med. Genet.*, **5**, 161.

MANN, J. D., CAHAN, A., GELB, A. G., FISHER, NATHALIE, HAMPER, JEAN, TIPPETT, PATRICIA, SANGER, RUTH, and RACE, R. R. (1962), "A sex-linked blood group." *Lancet*, **1**, 8.

RACE, R. R. (1965), "Contributions of blood groups to human genetics." *Proc. Roy. Soc. B*, **163**, 151.

RACE, R. R., and SANGER, RUTH. *Blood Groups in Man.* 5th ed., pp. 522–571.

SANGER, RUTH (1965), "Genes on the X chromosome." *Can. J. Genet., Cytol.*, **7**, 179.

Lutheran System

CRAWFORD, MARY N., GREENWALT, T. J., SASAKI, T., TIPPETT, PATRICIA, SANGER, RUTH, and RACE, R. R. (1961), "The phenotype Lu (a–b–) together with unconventional Kidd groups in one family." *Transfusion, Philad.*, **1**, 228.

DARNBOROUGH, J., FIRTH, R., GILES, CAROLYN M., GOLDSMITH, K. L. G., and CRAWFORD, MARY N. (1963), "A 'new' antibody anti-Lu^a Lu^b and two further examples of the genotype Lu (a–b–)." *Nature, Lond.*, **198**, 796.

En^a

DARNBOROUGH, J., DUNSFORD, I., and WALLACE, JOSEPHINE A. (1969), "The En^a Antigen-Antibody. A Genetical Modification of Human Red Cells Affecting their Blood Grouping Reactions." *Vox Sang.*, **17**, 241.

FURUHJELM, U., MYLLYLÄ, G., NEVANLINNA, H. R., NORDLING, S., PURKOLA, ANNA, GAVIN, JUNE, GOOCH, ANN, SANGER, RUTH, and TIPPETT, PATRICIA (1969), "The red cell phenotype En(a–) and anti-En^a; serological and physico chemical aspects." *Vox Sang.*, **17**, 256–278.

APPENDICES

Appendix I

REAGENTS

Pyrogen Free Distilled Water

It is essential that all distilled water used in the preparation of intra-venous solutions and also in the cleansing of apparatus should be pyrogen free. It should, therefore, always be freshly distilled when used. Satisfactory results are obtained from a Manesty still.

Technique No. A1.1. Pyrogen testing

The test is carried out on rabbits weighing not less than 1·5 kg and having a rectal temperature not exceeding 39·8°. One to three days before the test, a trial test is carried out, using 10 ml. per kg of body weight of a 0·9 per cent w/v solution of pyrogen free sodium chloride in water for injection. Animals which show an undue rise or fall in body temperature are not used.

The test is conducted with a room temperature within 3° of that of the rabbits' living quarters, or in which they have been kept for at least 18 hours. Food is withheld overnight and until the test is completed; water is not given during the test. Temperatures are recorded at regular intervals with a clinical thermometer inserted in the rectum to a depth of not less than 6 cm. and not more than 9 cm. The time intervals are not more than 30 minutes beginning at least 90 minutes before injection and continuing 3 hours after injection.

The mean initial temperature of the rabbit is the mean of temperatures taken before injection of the test material and the maximum is the highest recorded in the 3 hours after injection. The difference between the mean initial temperature and the maximum temperature is taken to be the rabbit's response. The test is first done on a group of three rabbits. The material passes the test if the summed response does not exceed 1·15° and fails if it exceeds 2·65°. If the value falls between these figures the test is repeated two or three times, if necessary. Further details of pyrogen testing can be found in the British Pharmacopoeia.

Technique No. A1.2. Preparation of isotonic saline

A 0·85 per cent solution of sodium chloride in distilled water is isotonic, *i.e.* of the same osmotic pressure as the contents of the human red cell. 8·5 g. dissolved in 1 litre of distilled water will probably be a convenient quantity. Saline should be freshly made but need not be sterilised.

Technique No. A1.3. Preparation of isotonic trisodium citrate

The isotonic solution of trisodium citrate is 3·8 per cent (*i.e.* 38 g. in 1 litre of distilled water).

Technique No. A1.4. Preparation of AB serum

This is obtained from group AB donors. Its main use is as a diluent for Rh antibodies and thus it must be free from other atypical antibodies. Tests are, therefore, carried out at 37°C, R.T. and 4°C by saline, albumin and papain indirect anti-human globulin techniques against A_1, A_2, B, and O cells. Not infrequently an identifiable atypical antibody, *e.g.* anti-A_1, is discovered which can then be removed by suitable absorption. The indirect anti-human globulin test at 4°C will detect the "cold incomplete" antibodies which are practically always present, and which can be removed by absorption with an equal volume of pooled group O red cells overnight at 4°C. If the AB serum is to be used in an enzyme technique it should be absorbed for 1 hour with a fifth of its volume of papainised group O cells.

Bovine Albumin

Bovine albumin is fraction V of the Cohn separation and is supplied by Armours as a 30 per cent solution. As it contains sodium azide it should not be frozen solid but stored at 4°C until required. It can be broken down to 20 per cent by the addition of one part of AB serum to two parts of the 30 per cent albumin.

Technique No. A1.5. Preparation of bromelin solution

The exact concentration of the bromelin solution is less critical than for trypsin or papain.

Using bromelin supplied by the Wallerstein Laboratories of New York, Myhre *et al.* reported that a 0·1 per cent by weight solution in saline which has a native pH of 6·0 to 6·5 was as efficient as bromelin in either acetate buffer at pH 4·5 or tris (hydroxy-methyl) aminomethane at pH 8·0. Alternatively a satisfactory bromelin solution can be prepared by making a 0·5 per cent solution by weight (in normal saline) of bromelin prepared for Rh testing by L. Light (Colnbrook, England).

Either solution will store satisfactorily for a week at 4°C, but is best used on the day of preparation. For convenience, therefore, it is as well to weigh out lots of 0·05 gr. of bromelin into a number of screw-capped bottles to one of which the appropriate quantity of saline can be added each day.

Technique No. A1.6. Preparation of trypsin solution

The trypsin solution can be prepared by dissolving 0·1 g. of pure crystalline trypsin in 10 ml. of N/$_{20}$ HCl. If kept at 4°C this stock solution will remain active for some months. As required, it is diluted with 0·1 M phosphate buffer, 1 in 10 v/v. This buffer, of pH 7·7, is prepared by mixing one part of M/$_{15}$ KH_2PO_4 with nine parts of M/$_{15}$ $Na_2HPO_4.2H_2O$. Eight grams of sodium chloride are added to each litre.

The buffered trypsin solution prepared by either method is then used for preparation of enzyme treated red cells as described in technique No. 10.4.

Technique No. A1.7. Löw's technique for the preparation of papain solution

Reagents. Purified, powdered papain (Merck, Savory & Moore, B.D.H., and Evans all supply suitable products).

M/$_{15}$ phosphate buffer (Sörensen) pH 5·4
M cysteine hydrochloride
M sodium hydroxide

The phosphate buffer consists of a mixture of M/$_{15}$ solutions of Na_2HPO_4 and KH_2PO_4. According to Sörensen's table they should be mixed in the proportions of 0·4 ml of the sodium salt to 9·6 ml. of the potassium salt. For each batch of reagent the pH should be checked and any small adjustment of the proportions made to give the required pH. Eight grams of sodium chloride are added to each litre of buffer.

Two grams of powdered papain are ground in a mortar with buffered saline (pH 5·4) and the suspension made up to 100 ml. and filtered. It is important that the solution should be clear; this is probably best effected by using a Seitz filter with a clarifying pad, alternatively filtration through fine grade filter paper using celite analytical filter-aid (John-Manville) is very satisfactory. Five millilitres of the molar solution of cysteine hydrochloride are neutralised with 5 ml. of the molar solution of sodium hydroxide. That the solutions have (as they should) exactly neutralised each other can be checked with a pH meter or with litmus paper; if not neutral the proportions are slightly adjusted until neutralisation is achieved. Ten millilitres of the neutralised solution are added to the 100 ml. of filtered papain solution, the whole made up to

200 ml. with buffered saline and incubated at 37°C for 1 hour. The solution is stored frozen solid at −20°C in convenient quantities. It will keep for some months frozen solid but will not tolerate thawing and refreezing.

M/15 solution of $Na_2HPO_4.2H_2O$ contains 11·93 g. per litre.
M/15 solution of KH_2PO_4 contains 9·07 g. per litre.
M solution of cysteine hydrochloride contains 157 g. per litre.
M solution of sodium hydroxide contains 40 g. per litre.

Technique No. A1.8. Preparation of ficin

Crude ficin is weighed out in 250 mg. amounts. The powder is stable indefinitely so it can be kept dry until needed. It must be handled with care and always weighed into stoppered containers as in sensitive individuals it is capable of causing sloughing of the mucous membranes. It is therefore recommended that mask and goggles are worn when handling the powder.

When needed, each 250 mg. is dissolved in 25 ml. of Hendry's buffer (pH 7·4). This is the stock solution. The buffer is designed to be isotonic with human red cells and is prepared by adding 19 ml. of a solution containing 2·34 g. $NaH_2PO_42H_2O$ per 100 ml. to 81 ml. of a solution containing 1·63 g. Na_2HPO_4 per 100 ml.

Anti-coagulant Solutions for the Preservation of Stored Blood for Transfusion

There are two important functions of the solution into which blood is taken for storage, first it must be an efficient anti-coagulant and secondly red cells stored in it for three to four weeks must survive well in the recipient's circulation.

The present solution, A.C.D., combines reasonably good storage with a good degree of anti-coagulant activity and a low caramelisation.

Technique No. A1.9. Preparation of A.C.D. (acid-citrate-dextrose)

Each M.R.C. bottle for the collection of 430 ml. of blood contains 120 ml. of A.C.D. containing 2 g. of disodium citrate and 3 g. of dextrose. A convenient quantity of this solution can be prepared by adding 800 ml. of a 15 per cent solution of anhydrous dextrose to 4 litres of a 2 per cent solution of disodium citrate ($Na_2H(C_6H_5O_7).H_2O$ m.wt. 254).

The solution is filtered through filter paper—Whatman No. 1—and then through a medium grade (3 or 4) cintered glass filter. It is then put into the bottles, using a simple mechanical apparatus to deliver exactly 120 ml. into each bottle; the cap is loosely screwed on and the bottle is ready for the autoclave (*see* Chapter 28).

Standard Cells

Careful selection of standard cells is of utmost importance. They must be chosen with a view to their sensitivity, specificity and availability.

Fresh Cells. Fresh cells are usually to be preferred to stored and can be used wherever suitable donors are readily available. Red cells are taken from an ear or finger prick into 3·8 per cent trisodium citrate. The tube is inverted frequently to prevent the blood from clotting on the dry surfaces. The cells are washed and can then be used for making saline or albumin suspensions. If wanted for the next day's work, they can be kept overnight in A.C.D. at 4°C.

Stored Cells. For the storage of small quantities of cells several methods are available. The simplest is to store the cells under their own unadulterated serum in a sterile clotted sample; in this medium they keep well for approximately a week. Alternatively the cells may be stored in A.C.D., or frozen solid in glycerol or liquid nitrogen.

A.C.D. can be used in small bottles (*e.g.* universal containers) for the storage of blood samples—blood being added to the solution in the ratio of four parts to one.

Technique No. A1.10. Storage of standard red cells in glycerol

Red cells have only a limited life even in the preservative solutions just described. If it is desired to keep them for several months they can be stored frozen solid at − 20°C in glycerol.

The concentration of glycerol in the red cell-glycerol mixture should be about 30 per cent w/v for efficient storage. This is achieved by adding an equal quantity of 40 per cent v/v glycerol in buffered tripotassium citrate to packed cells. The packed cells are obtained from blood which has been taken into A.C.D., centrifuged and the supernatant plasma removed; they are thus suspended in a minimal quantity of their own plasma plus A.C.D. Red cells stored in this way can be recovered into saline.

(*a*) **Preparation of the Standard Solutions.**

Buffered Tripotassium Citrate. This is a mixture of tripotassium citrate and phosphate buffer. It contains 3·25 per cent tripotassium citrate ($K_3C_6H_5O_7.H_2O$), 0·47 per cent potassium dihydrogen phosphate (KH_2PO_4) and 0·6 per cent dipotassium hydrogen phosphate (K_2HPO_4). In practice it is probably convenient to make up a litre of this stock solution which would, therefore, contain 32·5 g. citrate, 4·7 g. potassium dihydrogen phosphate and 6 g. of dipotassium hydrogen phosphate.

The "Laying-down" Solution. This is a 50 per cent w/v (approx.) or 40 per cent v/v which will give about a 30 per cent concentration of glycerol when mixed with an equal quantity of packed cells. 40 ml. of glycerol well mixed with 60 ml. of the buffered citrate is probably a convenient quantity.

The Recovery Solutions. These are 16, 8, 4, and 2 per cent w/v glycerol to buffered citrate.

Owing to the high viscosity of the glycerol it will be found best to make up the 16 per cent solution and then prepare the others by doubling dilution. 200 ml. of the 16 per cent can be prepared by adding 25·6 ml. of glycerol to 174·4 ml. of buffered tripotassium citrate. Care must be taken to ensure that the buffered citrate and glycerol are well mixed.

(*b*) **"Laying-down" Process.** The blood to be stored is taken into A.C.D. in the usual proportions (*i.e.* four parts of blood to one part of A.C.D.). The sample is centrifuged and the supernatant removed. An equal quantity of the 40 per cent v/v laying-down solution is added gradually to the packed cells mixing well so that none of the cells are subjected to excessive concentration of glycerol. The mixture is then frozen solid at − 20°C. If small quantities of the cells will be needed on several occasions the mixture can be divided into 1 ml. quantities before being frozen.

(*c*) **Recovery.** To recover the red cells the mixture is allowed to melt at room temperature, as much as is needed removed and the rest re-frozen. The sample is centrifuged, the supernatant fluid removed and the cells washed with each of the recovery solutions in turn (beginning with the 16 per cent and ending with the 2 per cent) followed by buffered tripotassium citrate and then twice with saline. A convenient method for the recovery of small quantities of red cells is to place them in a length of dialysis tubing, and dialyse against either saline or the buffered tripotassium citrate for 1 hour. The cells are then washed three times in saline. They can then be used in exactly the same ways as freshly bled cells.

Technique No. A1.11. Storage of red cells in liquid nitrogen

The blood to be stored is taken into either E.D.T.A. 1 mg./ml. or into A.C.D. in the normal proportions.

The blood should be frozen as quickly as possible and should not be more than two days' old if antigens are to store well.

Immediately before storage in liquid nitrogen, the blood is mixed with half its volume of 40 per cent sucrose. The sucrose is added gradually with mixing.

Freezing. A siliconed 50 ml. syringe is fitted with 2 in. plastic tubing and a needle from a transfusion "taking" set. It is then suspended over a 2 litre beaker which is lined with cotton-wool on sides and bottom. The beaker is filled with liquid nitrogen and the syringe fitted with the blood prepared as described above. The drop from the needle is controlled by a clip so that the blood forms discrete drops on entering the nitrogen which do not coalesce (a rate of 1–2 ml. per minute approximately).

The method can be modified for small or large quantities of blood, *e.g.* for large quantities a fenwal pack is convenient; its tubing fits into the socket of an Iver needle or over an olive mount needle.

Care should be taken to inspect the level of nitrogen in the beaker and the blood may require mixing a little to prevent sedimentation of cells.

The pellets of frozen blood are transferred with a cooled spoon to cardboard ointment boxes filled with liquid nitrogen before putting down in the liquid nitrogen container.

Recovery. The pellets are removed and placed in 1 per cent NaCl at 45°C. They quickly melt and thereafter the blood is washed in isotonic saline until the supernatant fluid shows no hæmolysis.

Choice of Standard Red Cells

Sensitivity of red cells will vary with different antigen content. It is best to use the most sensitive cells when testing unknown sera for antibodies and to use weakly reacting cells when controlling standard sera.

ABO. For ABO testing the required standard cells are A_1, A_2, B, and O. A_1 and A_2 cells must have been tested with at least two and preferably three anti-A_1 sera, and results must be clear cut, negative for A_2 and positive for A_1. It is possible to get a weak positive reaction which signifies a midway group between A_1 and A_2 (A_{int}); this group should not be used for standard cells. Having selected cells on the basis of their reactions with anti-A_1 sera, their strength is found by titration with a known anti-A serum in parallel with known A_1 and A_2 cells. This may show that the A which was negative with anti-A_1 is really an A_3 or weaker sub-group of A and not A_2 and is, therefore, not suitable for use. The sensitivity of B cells can be found in the same way by titration with anti-B serum, but this is not normally done since the variation is slight. It is not usually considered necessary to test the sensitivity of the group O cells. Both in selecting test cells and in interpreting results it must be remembered that any red cell has many blood group antigens, and anomalous results may arise because the serum contains an antibody belonging to another blood group system. Atypical Rh antibodies are among the most likely to be encountered and it is as well to select ABO standard red cells that are Rh negative; this is especially important when samples from pregnant women are being tested.

Rh. For Rh antibody screening a panel of four group O cells are required R_1R_1, R_2(R_2R_2 or R_2r), R_1R_2, and rr. These must all be established by sub-typing with at least two anti-C, anti-D, anti-E and anti-c sera, and, as in ABO testing, results must be unequivocal.

Sensitivity is again found by titrations of known anti-sera with known cells and with the cells under test, anti-C for R_1R_1, anti-E for R_2R_2 and R_2r, anti-c for rr, anti-D for R_1R_1, R_2R_2, R_2r and R_1R_2. Any cell which gives consistently low titres with several anti-sera of chosen specificity is obviously too insensitive for detecting antibodies in unknown sera.

For controls on anti-Rh sera, cells which have only a single dose of antigen should be used. These controls have been discussed in some detail in the Rh chapters especially with regard to using sera containing more than one specific antibody.

Other Blood Group Systems. Cells for other blood group systems must be chosen on the same principles and with as much care. The method used to select the cells must be the same as that by which they are to be used. In all cases it is essential to confirm the specificity of standard cells with more than one anti-serum. It is preferable to have the full typing for all known blood group systems of any standard cells used. For antibody detection a strong positive is needed while for control cells a weak positive and a negative are required. (*See also* procedure No. 3.)

Specific Anti-sera

These are dealt with in some detail in Chapters 3 and 13 for ABO and Rh and in the appropriate chapters for the other blood group systems. (*See also* procedure No. 2.)

Technique No. A1.12. Preparation of anti-human globulin serum (Coombs reagent)

The rabbit is the animal most commonly used for the production of anti-human globulin sera, although it is possible to immunise other species. Dunsford and Bowley, 1957; Ironside, 1968; have successfully immunised goats.

Not all strains of rabbit are equally good antibody producers. Hybrid species or brown rabbits if obtainable are often the most suitable.

Human group O serum pooled from several donors is used as a source of antigen. Groups A, B or AB, should be avoided, as it is undesirable to risk stimulating the animals to produce unwanted anti-A or anti-B antibodies. For a broad spectrum anti-globulin reagent* the gamma globulins are precipitated with a saturated solution of ammonium sulphate. A proportion of two parts serum to one of ammonium sulphate should be satisfactory. The resulting precipitate is carefully washed twice in 40 per cent ammonium sulphate, dissolved in a small quantity of Na_2HPo_4 and dialysed at 4°C against normal saline.

The separated globulin then has to be mixed with Freund's adjuvant. The material required can be obtained from Difco (Agents Baird and Tatlock) in complete and incomplete (without mycobacteria) forms.

It may also be made up as follows:

Bayol F (Esso Ltd.)	17 parts
Arlacel A (Honeywill and Stein Ltd.)	3 parts
Dried myc. butyricum (Ditco)	0·5 to 1·0 mg. per ml.

Equal volumes of adjuvant and 1 g./100 ml. antigen solution are emulsified together. This process is greatly facilitated by using a homogeniser, as the final product should be of the consistency of stiff toothpaste and should be completely emulsified. A drop placed in water should not spread. There is great variation possible in the schedule of injections, and they should be subjected to trial and error.

The first injection is usually 1–2 ml. emulsion intramuscularly into each leg (4 injections). After two weeks or later, a second similar injection into each shoulder. About one week after this there can be a short intravenous course of 1 ml. of 1 per cent aqueous solution of antigen without adjuvant. These injections can be given every two days for about ten days. The animals must be carefully watched for signs of anaphylaxis as indicated by respiratory distress. If this occurs the injections must be stopped. Small test bleeds are made before a larger quantity, 60–80 ml. by

* There are several methods for the preparation of more specific antisera, *e.g.* anti-IgG, anti-β_1, C, etc. For technical details and references *see* Mollison (1967).

ear is taken. After 2–6 months' test a further intravenous course (without adjuvant) may be tried.

Absorption of Unwanted Antibodies. The serum is freed of antibodies for human red cell antigens by absorbing with group O and group AB red cells. The cells used for the absorption must be very carefully washed in a large excess of saline, approximately one part of cells to ten parts of saline. At least six washings are necessary to free the cells completely of serum globulin. The serum can be absorbed with a mixture of O and AB red cells, or alternatively with the group O cells and then with the group AB cells. The absorptions are carried out at 4°C using equal parts of serum and cells and allowing the mixture to stand for 2 hours. A second or even a third absorption may be needed.

Removal of Unwanted Agglutinins by Heating. An alternative method of freeing the sera of unwanted agglutinins is by heating the serum at 70°C. This destroys the saline agglutinins but leaves the anti-human globulin antibodies virtually unimpaired (there is sometimes a loss of the anti-non-IgG fraction). The serum is diluted with an equal part of normal saline (to minimise the risk of coagulation) and heated for 20 minutes at 70°C.

Whichever method has been used the serum is now ready for standardisation.

Technique No. A1.13. Standardisation of anti-human globulin (Coombs reagent)

The absorbed and/or heated reagent is tested for residual "anti-man" agglutinins. This is done by making serial dilutions of the serum and testing them with washed group AB cells on an opalescent tile as for the actual anti-human globulin test (technique No. 23). If the absorption has been successful there will be little or no reaction above a dilution of 1 in 4 or 1 in 8 before 10 minutes; after this time there may be a reaction in higher dilutions but this should not occur at dilutions greater than 1 in 64. The titre should be read at 2, 5, 10, and 15 minutes, the results and the time being carefully recorded.

Once the rabbit serum has been successfully absorbed it is then titrated for its ability to react with sensitised red cells. Rabbits differ in the type of anti-human globulin that they produce, nearly all of them produce antibodies against the IgG and non-IgG (IgA and IgM) fractions of the globulin but the proportion of each of the antibodies will vary from serum to serum and often from immunisation to immunisation of the same rabbit. The routine laboratory will in the main require a reagent having a high titre of anti-IgG-globulin which will, therefore, react well with "warm" antibodies, in particular anti-Rh.

Sera which can only be used at less than a 1 in 30 dilution are considered to be inadequate, an average reagent can be used

	Neat*	$\frac{1}{10}$	$\frac{1}{20}$	$\frac{1}{40}$	$\frac{1}{60}$	$\frac{1}{80}$	$\frac{1}{100}$	$\frac{1}{200}$	$\frac{1}{300}$	$\frac{1}{400}$	$\frac{1}{500}$
Ml. of serum .		0·2									
" " . $\frac{1}{10}$.			0·5	0·25	0·15	0·1	0·2				
" " . $\frac{1}{100}$.								0·5	0·3	0.25	0·2
Saline . .		1·8	0·5	0·75	0·75	0·7	1·8	0·5	0·6	0·75	0·8
Total ml. . .		2·0	1·0	1·00	0·90	0·8	2·0	1·0	0·9	1·00	1·0

* Often omitted as rather wasteful of the reagent.

diluted about 1 in 60 to 1 in 100 and good reagents may work well (especially for instance for the testing of cells for D^u) at dilutions of 1 in 200 or 1 in 500 or even higher. Doubling dilutions are close together at the lower end of the range which provides no useful information and too widely spaced in the 100 to 500 range;

Table A1.1

The Standardisation of an Anti-human Globulin Rabbit Serum

	Dilutions of anti-human globulin serum											
	Neat	$\frac{1}{10}$	$\frac{1}{20}$	$\frac{1}{40}$	$\frac{1}{60}$	$\frac{1}{80}$	$\frac{1}{100}$	$\frac{1}{200}$	$\frac{1}{300}$	$\frac{1}{400}$	$\frac{1}{500}$	Time, min.
(1) O D positive cells strongly sensitised	±	2+	2+	4+	5+	5+	5+	5+	4+	4+	3+	2–5
(2) O D positive cells moderately sensitised . . .	3+	4+	4+	5+	5+	5+	5+	4+	3+	3+	2+	2–5
(3) O D positive cells weakly sensitised	3+	4+	4+	4+	4+	4+	4+	3+	2+	—	—	2–5
(4) O D positive cells unsensitised . .	+	±	—	—	—	—	—	—	—	—	—	15
(5) O D negative cells	+	+	—	—	—	—	—	—	—	—	—	15
(6) A_1B D negative cells . . .	3+	+	—	—	—	—	—	—	—	—	—	15
(7) O cells sensitised with cold antibody	5+	5+	5+	4+	4+	2+	—	—	—	—	—	5

a more profitable series of dilutions are given below together with a chart for their preparation.

The extra quantity of the $\frac{1}{10}$ and $\frac{1}{100}$ dilutions is used for the making up of the dilutions $\frac{1}{20}$ to $\frac{1}{100}$ and $\frac{1}{200}$ to $\frac{1}{500}$ respectively. Each dilution is tested with the following:

Group O Rh positive cells: (1) strongly (2) moderately and

(3) weakly sensitised with Rh antibodies (this can probably be done by using a single anti-Rh serum neat, 1 in 10 and 1 in 100 for sensitising the cells); (4) the same cells unsensitised; (5) O Rh negative cells incubated with the same anti-Rh serum; (6) group A_1B Rh negative unsensitised cells and (7) cells sensitised with "cold" type antibody. (Cells from a clotted sample stored at 4°C will usually be found to be coated with a cold auto-antibody.)

Specimen results are shown in Table A1.1. (Note the prozone with the strongly sensitised Rh positive cells.) On the basis of these results the serum could be used at $\frac{1}{60}$, at which dilution it will detect both the "warm" and the "cold" types of antibody and $\frac{1}{200}$ for the detecting of the "warm" type only. At this last dilution it would be very useful for testing cells for the presence of D^u with incomplete anti-D as it will not detect any sensitisation with "cold" antibody—in particular the incomplete "cold" auto-antibody which would otherwise give a false positive reaction.

BIBLIOGRAPHY

MOLLISON, P. L. (1967), *Blood Transfusion in Clinical Medicine.* (Fourth Edition), 422–447.

Appendix II—A Practical Guide to Laboratory Procedure

"I never knew you played the banjo. . . ." "Not exactly," replied George, "but it is very easy, they tell me—and I've got the instruction book."

Jerome K. Jerome, THREE MEN IN A BOAT

Procedure No. 1. Routine Procedure for all Investigations

(1) Decide upon tests required. If sample is inadequate, decide which tests shall have priority.

(2) Assemble all apparatus needed, including blocks filled with tubes in the pattern required for each test.

(3) Clearly label the block with the name of the test to be performed and the names of the samples to be tested.

(4) Run in all diluents and all standard sera, rinsing pipette very carefully between each different fluid.

(5) Run unknown sera in all serum grouping, antibody testing and titration tests—there is no need to rinse the pipette between each type of test but it must, of course, be rinsed very carefully between each unknown serum.

(5*a*) Check contents.

(6) Make red cell suspensions in saline (and where appropriate in albumin) from the first unknown sample and without rinsing pipette run it into every test.

(7) Run standard cells into the appropriate tests and into the controls of the cell typing tests.

(7*a*) Check tubes.

(8) Incubate tests for required time at appropriate temperature.

(9) Read and record controls and then read and record tests. Results must be entered as they are obtained.

If this basic procedure is followed, each reagent and unknown serum or red cell suspension is handled only once in the whole manipulation, thereby reducing to a minimum the time taken and the risk of errors.

Procedure No. 2. Selection and Preparation of Typing Sera

(1) Titrate to test strength and avidity of serum, by techniques which are likely to be used routinely.

(2) Select suitable sera according to the criteria laid down in Table A.2.1.

(3) Confirm the specificity of the antiserum by testing against a panel of standard cells.

(4) Remove unwanted antibodies either by absorption with appropriate red cells or by dilution.

(5) Test absorbed serum for successful removal of unwanted antibodies.

(6) Sterilise serum by Seitz filtration.

(7) Re-titrate and standardise for use.

(8) Bottle in suitable quantities.

(9) Check sterility.

Table A2.1

Criteria for the Selection of Anti-sera

Type of anti-serum	Type of red cell against which it should be titrated	Minimum titre acceptable with each type of red cell*	Avidity	Remarks
Anti-A	A_1	512	V to ++ at 64	
	A_2B	16	3 macroscopic readings	
	A_3B (if available)	4	1 macroscopic reading	
Anti-B	B	256	++ to + at 64	
Group O ($\alpha\beta$)	A_1	512	V to ++ at 64	
	B	256	++ to + at 64	
	A_3 and A_4 (if available)	4		
Anti-A_1 (α_1)	A_1	16	2 macroscopic readings	
	A_2	–		Titre with $A_2 > 2$ serum needs re-absorption.
Anti-M	M	32	3 macroscopic readings	
	MN	16	2 macroscopic readings	
	N	–		Titre with $N > 2$ serum needs re-absorption.
Anti-N	N	32	3 macroscopic readings	
	MN	16	2 macroscopic readings	
	M	–		Titre with $M > 2$ serum needs re-absorption.
Anti-S	S positive	Any	V to ++ using neat serum	If possible these should be titrated against known "single" or "double dose" cells
Anti-K	K positive	Any		
Anti-Fy^a	Fy^a positive	Any		
Anti-Lu^a	Lu^a positive	Any		
Anti-Jk^a	Jk^a positive	Any		

Table A2.1 (*contd.*)

Type of anti-serum	Type of red cell against which it should be titrated	Minimum titre acceptable with each type of red cell*	Avidity	Remarks
Anti-P_1	P_1 strong	16	2 macroscopic readings	
	P_1 weak	2		
Anti-Le^a	Le^a positive	Any		
Anti-Le^b	Le^b positive	Any		
Anti-C	R′r	16	2 macroscopic readings	
	R_1R_1	32	3 macroscopic readings	
Anti-D	R_1r	64	4 macroscopic readings	
Anti-E	R_2r	16	2 macroscopic readings	
	R_2R_2	32	3 macroscopic readings	
Anti-CD	R′r	16	2 macroscopic readings	
	R_2r	64	4 macroscopic readings	
Anti-DE	R″r	16	2 macroscopic readings	
	R_1r	64	4 macroscopic readings	
Anti-c	R_1r	16	2 macroscopic readings	
	rr	32	3 macroscopic readings	
Anti-e	R_2r	Any		

* Variation in titre demanded is mainly due to rarity of anti-sera. Where "any" titre has to be accepted, negative results must be interpreted with caution.

Procedure No. 3. Testing of Red Cell Samples for a Number of Blood Group Systems

(1) Arrange precipitin tubes in blocks to cover the whole investigation, including controls on each anti-serum used.

(2) Run each anti-serum into all tubes in which it is required.

(3) Run out the packed washed test cells into any tubes for indirect anti-human globulin test first, before making up a 2 per cent suspension of the cells for the other tests.

(4) Handle one sample at a time and place red cells into all the appropriate tubes before picking up another sample.

It is an advantage to use as controls red cells typed for as many blood group systems as possible, so that a few standards will provide controls for all the anti-sera used. The control cells for each anti-serum are shown in Table A.2.2.

Table A2.2

Control Cells for the Various Blood Group Typing Sera

Anti-serum	Control cells	
	Positive	Negative
Anti-A	A	B and O
Anti-B	B	A and O
O serum ($\alpha\beta$)	A and B	O
Anti-A_1	A_1	A_2
Anti-M	M and MN	N
Anti-N	N and MN	M
Anti-S	S positive*	S negative
Anti-K	K positive*	K negative
Anti-Fy^a	Fy^a positive*	Fy^a negative
Anti-Lu^a	Lu^a positive*	Lu^a negative
Anti-Jk^a	Jk^a positive*	Jk^a negative
Anti-P_1	P_1 strong and P_1 weak	P_1 negative
Anti-Le^a	Le^a positive	Le(a− b+) and Le(a− b−)
Anti-Le^b	Le^b positive	Le(a+ b−) and Le(a− b−)

For controls on Rh anti-sera *see* Table 21.
* Known single and double dose cells if available.

Procedure No. 4. Identification of Antibodies

This procedure should be followed when the results of serum ABO grouping (technique No. 3.1 or 3.2) and/or routine Rh antibody testing suggest the presence of atypical antibodies.

(1) Examine routine antibody and grouping results and determine if possible from these or by further testing against appropriate red cells at room temperature and 37°C whether the atypical antibody is of the "cold" or "warm" type.

(2) If the antibody is a cold agglutinin reacting with A_1 cells, test for presence of anti-A_1 with known standard A_1 and A_2 red cells, and test patient's cells with anti-A_1 (technique No. 6.2 or 6.5).

(3) If suspected to be a cold antibody other than anti-A_1, test by saline technique at room temperature against a panel of chosen red cells of group O similar to those recommended for technique No. 21.1.

(4) Record results in the manner shown in Table 21.1 and interpret results with the help of Chapter 21.

(5) If the atypical antibody is of the "warm" type with a pattern of reaction in routine antibody tests suggesting that it might be one of the Rh antibodies, plan confirmatory tests accordingly.

(6) If not an Rh antibody, carry out technique No. 21.1.

(7) If a mixture of antibodies is suspected, consult Chapter 21.

Procedure No. 5. Serological Testing of Donors

(1) At donor session group donor by slide technique.

(2) In the laboratory perform the following tests on the clotted blood in the pilot tube corresponding to each bottle:

a. ABO grouping, technique No. 3.1 or 3.2.

b. Rh typing, technique No. 9.2 or 9.3.
(c) Syphilis test, technique No. 28.2a or 3.
(3) Test red cells of D negative donors by technique No. 12.1, followed by techniques Nos. 12.2–4 if required.
(4) Test serum of D negative donors with R_1R_2 (CDe.cDE) red cells by techniques 10.2 and/or 10.4 or 5.
Any antibody detected should be identified by procedure No. 4 and other anomalies by procedure No. 13.

Procedure No. 6. Direct Matching Procedure

(1) ABO group patient—technique No. 3.1 or 3.2.
(2) Rh type patient—technique No. 9.2 or 9.3.
(3) Test serum for antibodies—techniques Nos. 10.1–6.
(4) Identify any antibody found—procedure No. 4.
(5) For non-emergency direct matching, perform technique No. 22.4.
(6) For direct matching in varying degrees of emergency, *see* Table 23.2 and techniques No. 23.5 and 6.

Procedure No. 7. Investigation of Suspected Hæmolytic Transfusion Reaction

Samples needed	Tests to perform
Pre-transfusion sample.	1. ABO grouping, technique No. 3.1 or 3.2. 2. Rh typing, technique No. 9.2 or 9.3. 3. Full antibody tests: (*a*) saline—technique No. 10.1. (*b*) albumin—technique No. 10.2. (*c*) indirect anti-human globulin—technique No. 10.3a. (*d*) trypsin—technique No. 10.4 or papain—technique No. 10.5. 4. Repeat direct match, using cells from each bottle given (technique No. 22.4).
Samples of bottles given or started.	1. ABO grouping, technique No. 3.1. 2. Rh typing, technique No. 9.2 or 9.3. 3. Antibody tests as No. 3 above.
Post-transfusion sample.	1. Examine 2 per cent cell suspension in saline. 2. Perform direct anti-human globulin test (technique No. 10.3b). 3. ABO grouping, technique No. 3.1. 4. Rh typing, technique No. 9.2 or 9.3. } Examine carefully for "mixed blood" (3 and 4).

Procedure No. 7 (*contd.*)

Samples needed	Tests to perform
Post-transfusion sample.	5. Perform antibody tests on serum, techniques as 3. 6. Titrate antibodies present by appropriate techniques. 7. Perform Schumm's test (technique No. 24.1). 8. Estimate serum bilirubin (technique No. 24.2 or 24.5 or 24.6).
10th day post-transfusion sample.	1. Titrate antibody responsible for reaction. 2. If necessary, examine cells by Ashby technique to estimate cell survival—technique No. 24.4.
Post-transfusion sample of urine.	1. Examine for red cell casts. 2. Examine for urobilinogen or urobilin, technique No. 24.3.

Procedure No. 8. Ante-natal and Post-natal Testing (*see* page 261–273)

Samples at first attendance at clinic	Tests to perform
All ante-natal cases.	ABO grouping, technique No. 3.2. Rh typing (D), technique No. 9.1. or 9.2. Antibody screening, technique No. 10.2 and 10.4 or 10.5.
All cases divided into *Class* (1) Rh positives with no antibody and normal obstetric history.	No further samples.
Class (2) Rh positives with bad obstetric history.	Test serum for atypical antibodies technique No. 21.1, request samples at 32nd week, delivery and 10 days post-partum.
Class (4) Rh negatives, normal history.	On present sample further Rh tests, technique No. 12.1–12.4, request samples at delivery, and 10 days post-partum.
Class (5) Rh negative, with bad history.	Request samples monthly from 28th week, and at delivery and 10 days post-partum.
Classes (3) *and* (6) Women with atypical antibodies (3) Rh positive (6) Rh negative	Identify and titrate antibody. If too weak for conclusive identification, re-test monthly, otherwise re-test fortnightly from 28th week and at delivery and 10 days. Test husband.

Procedure No. 8 (*contd.*)

Delivery Samples	Tests to perform
Rh negative women with no antibodies and Rh positive women with bad obstetric history.	Full antibody test. Maternal serum *v.* infant's red cells by saline, albumin and indirect anti-human globulin tests (techniques Nos. 10.1, 10.2, 10.3a and 10.5b.)
Infant's Sample	ABO grouping, technique No. 3.2. Rh typing, technique No. 9.1 or 9.2. Direct anti-human globulin, technique No. 10.3b.
Women with antibodies.	As above for both maternal and infant's samples. Also titrate antibody in maternal and cord serum. Fully test infant for the blood group system to which maternal antibody belongs (*e.g.* if antibody is anti-E, Rh sub-type baby).
Women with no causative antibody found but baby is clinically a suspected case of hæmolytic disease.	See procedure No. 9.
10*th Day Samples* Rh negative women, etc. Women with antibodies.	Full antibody test. Titrate with purpose of obtaining donation for use as typing serum if titre adequate.
Husband's Sample (only tested where wife has antibodies or bad obstetric history)	
If maternal antibody belongs to Rh system (or no antibody has so far been found but obstetric history bad).	ABO grouping, technique No. 3.2. Rh typing and sub-typing, techniques Nos. 9.3 and 12.5. Test with wife's serum, techniques Nos. 10.1, 10.2, 10.3a and 10.5b.
If maternal antibody has other specificity.	ABO grouping, technique No. 3.2. Rh typing, technique No. 9.3. Test for the antigens of the system to which maternal antibody belongs. Test with wife's serum by techniques Nos. 10.1, 10.2, 10.3a, and 10.5b.

Procedure No. 9. Procedure in a Case Suspected on Clinical Grounds to be Hæmolytic Disease but where no Ante-natal Serological Testing has been Done

1. Perform direct anti-human globulin test on infant's red cells, technique No. 25.1. If this is positive, the clinical diagnosis is confirmed, but proceed as below. If direct anti-human globulin is negative, the clinical diagnosis may still be correct, particularly if the disease is due to an ABO incompatibility between maternal serum and infant's red cells; the investigation should be continued as below, sections 2–4, after which, if no causative antibody has been detected, the clinical findings should be reviewed. If no alternative diagnosis seems possible, a full antibody investigation as indicated in technique No. 21.1 should be made.

2. ABO grouping (technique No. 3.1) and Rh typing (technique No. 9.2 or 9.3) or mother and infant.

3. Test maternal serum for antibodies with R_1R_1, R_2R_2 or R_2r, and rr red cells by techniques Nos. 10.1–5.

4. Test maternal serum against infant's red cells by techniques Nos. 10.1–5. If an atypical antibody is found, follow procedure No. 4. If no atypical antibody is found, and there is an ABO incompatibility between maternal serum and infant's red cells, investigate by procedure No. 10.

Procedure No. 10. Demonstration of Immune Anti-A and Anti-B Antibodies

1. Titrate anti-A and/or anti-B of:
   (*a*) the pre-immunisation sample,
   (*b*) post-immunisation sample taken at approximately 4 days,
   (*c*) post-immunisation sample taken at approximately 10–15 days,

or in the case of stimulation due to pregnancy, compare the titres at progressive stages during pregnancy, and at delivery and 10 days after delivery. For titration method *see* technique No. 4.2 or 4.4.

2. Test for incomplete antibodies after heating serum or after neutralisation of the complete antibody with group specific substance.

3. Titrate any hæmolysin present—technique No. 5.1.

4. Enhancement. Compare titre in saline with titre in fresh, normal human serum.

5. Titrate with A_x cells.

6. Test with A_p positive pig cells for hæmolysis.

7. Test for IgG type antibody by technique No. 25.5a or 25.6.

Procedure No. 11. Serological Investigation of a Suspected Case of acquired Hæmolytic Anæmia

1. Perform direct anti-human globulin test (technique No. 10.3b) on patient's cells, using several anti-human globulin sera, at least one chosen for good reactivity with cold type antibody. If test negative, the case is probably of the congenital type. If positive, it is of the acquired, auto-immune type and a full serological investigation must be made.

2. Consult Chapter 26.

Procedure No. 12. Paternity Tests

Samples needed are:

5–10 ml. of clotted blood from each adult and
10–20 drops of clotted blood from baby.

Preferably these should be taken by the serologist who will do the tests. In addition, the individuals tested must offer some proof of their identity. Samples sent by post should be registered and accompanied by a certificate which identifies them.

The typing techniques that should be done in all cases are as follows:

(1) ABO grouping, technique No. 3.1 or 3.2.
(2) Full Rh sub-typing, techniques Nos. 9.3 and 12.5.
(3) MN typing, technique No. 16.1 or 16.2.
Include anti-S (if available), technique No. 16.3.

In most cases, particularly for the estimation of a probability of paternity, it is profitable to include typing with anti-K (technique No. 17.1), anti-Fy^a (technique No. 17.2), anti-Lu^a (technique No. 18.1) and anti-Jk^a (technique No. 17.3 or 17.4), Gm^a (technique No. 31.1) and haptoglobins (technique No. 31.3).

For typing of red cells for a number of blood group systems *see* procedure No. 3.

Procedure No. 13. Investigation of Anomalies

Repeat tests, using same reagents, and test with additional reagents of the same specificity. If anomaly still present, perform appropriate procedures; *i.e.* if anomaly occurs in typing tests, determine sub-type, *e.g.* A_3, D^u, C^w, etc.; if anomaly appears to be due to an antibody, identify (procedure No. 4).

Other causes of anomalous results may be poly-, pan-, auto-, or pseudo-agglutination.

Appendix III—Glossary

" 'When I use a word,' Humpty Dumpty said in a rather scornful tone, 'it means just what I choose it to mean—neither more nor less.' "

Lewis Carroll, THROUGH THE LOOKING GLASS

Absorption. Removal of antibodies from a serum by adsorption on to red cells. Hence, absorbed serum—a serum from which antibodies have been so removed.

Acquired antigen. Antigen not genetically determined and sometimes transient.

Adsorption. The attachment of one substance to the surface of another, in particular the attachment of antibody to specific receptors on the red cell surface.

Agglutinates. Clumps of agglutinated cells.

Agglutination. The clumping of red cells by agglutinins.

Agglutinin. An antibody which causes agglutination of red cells in a saline medium by virtue of reacting with the specific agglutinogen.

Auto-agglutinin. An agglutinin which reacts with the red cells of the individual in whose serum it is found; it usually agglutinates the red cells of most other individuals also.

Atypical agglutinin. One which is occasionally present in the serum of some individuals whose red cells lack the corresponding antigen.

Cold agglutinin. An agglutinin whose optimum temperature of reactivity is in the cold, whose potency decreases rapidly with increase of temperature, and whose reaction at 37°C is negative (except in rare circumstances).

Hetero-agglutinin. An agglutinin directed against antigens found in another species, cf. iso-agglutinin.

Iso-agglutinin. An agglutinin directed against antigens found in the same species, cf. hetero-agglutinin.

Normal or typical agglutinin. An agglutinin which is regularly present in the serum of all individuals whose cells lack the corresponding antigen.

Pan-agglutinin. An agglutinin which agglutinates the red cells of all individuals, irrespective of blood group.

Agglutinoid. One type of incomplete antibody.

Agglutinogen. Any substance which, acting as an antigen, stimulates the production of agglutinins.

Albumin. *See* Bovine Albumin.

Allele, allellomorph, or allelic gene. One of two or more genes which determine alternative characters in inheritance being located at the same locus on homologous chromosomes.

Allotypes. A set of allelomorphic characters *e.g.* serum allotypes.

Amino acid. Any one of a class of organic compounds containing the amino (NH_2) group and the carboxyl (COOH) group. Amino acids form the chief structure of proteins.

Anæmia. A condition in which the blood is deficient either in quantity or in quality.

Anamnestic response. The redevelopment of antibodies on the introduction of an antigen different in specificity from the one which provided the initial stimulus.

Antibody. An antibody is a substance which appears in the plasma or body fluids as a result of stimulation by an antigen and which will react specifically with that antigen in some observable way.

Anticoagulant. A substance which prevents coagulation or clotting of the blood.

Antigen. Any substance which, when introduced parenterally into an individual who himself lacks the substance, stimulates the production of an antibody, and which when mixed with the antibody, reacts with it in some observable way.

Antigenicity. Potency as an antigen.

Anti-human globulin. Coombs reagent. An antibody produced in an animal (often a rabbit) in response to the injection of human globulin.

Aqueous. Watery—hence aqueous extract, an extract made with water.

Atypical antibody. An antibody which occurs as an irregular feature of the serum, *e.g.* anti-D.

Auto-antibody. An antibody which reacts with the red cells of the individual in whose serum it is found; usually reacts upon the red cells of most other individuals also. *See* Auto-agglutinin.

Autosome. Any chromosome other than a sex chromosome.

Avidity of an antiserum. Power of agglutinating red cells rapidly and strongly.

Bilirubin. A red pigment found in the bile and present in the serum.

Blocking. The coating of a red cell receptor by an incomplete antibody in such a way as to render it partially or completely inagglutinable by agglutinins of the same specificity—hence, blocking antibody.

Blood group. One of a number of types into which blood may be classified according to particular antigens possessed by the red cells—hence blood grouping.

Blood group substance. *See* Group specific substance.

Bovine albumin. The Fraction V of the Cohn separation of bovine plasma (Cohn, E. J. *et al.*, 1946).

Buffer. Any substance or substances in solution which resist changes in pH.

Chromosome. One of a number of more or less rod-shaped, dark staining bodies situated in the nucleus of a cell. It is only distinguishable at the time of cell division. It is made up of a series of genes in linear arrangement.

Cis position. Being on the same chromosome and within the same cistron.

Cistron. A collection of genes situated so close together that they can have conjoint expression effects only when in the cis position.

Closely-linked genes. Genes in close proximity on a chromosome so that they are inherited together, usually without cross-overs occurring.

Co-dominant genes. Two or more allelic genes, each capable of expressing itself in single dose.

Cold agglutinin. *See* Agglutinin.

Compatible blood. Blood, the red cells of which are not sensitised or agglutinated by the recipient's serum.

Complement. A complex of substances present in normal serum which cause lysis of red cells sensitised by hæmolysins. Heating the serum at 56°C for $\frac{1}{2}$ hour destroys the thermolabile components which are necessary for hæmolysis.

Complete antibody. Agglutinin.

Conglutination. The clumping of sensitised red cells by a substance conglutinin, present in normal bovine sera, in the presence of complement. It is sometimes erroneously applied to the clumping effect of human serum or bovine albumin on cells sensitised by incomplete Rh antibodies, which is independent of complement.

Crossing over. The segregation of linked genes.

Cryptagglutinoid. A type of incomplete antibody.

Dominant gene. One which gives rise to its corresponding character, whether present in "double dose" (in the homozygote) or in "single dose" (in the heterozygote).

Dosage. A quantitative difference in the strength of the antigen in the homozygote and the heterozygote.

Electrophoresis (of serum). The separation of serum proteins according to their rate of travel when an electric current is passed through a buffer solution. The supporting medium can be a Whitman paper, or starch or agar gels.

Eluate. In serology, denotes an antibody solution made by recovery into a fluid medium of antibodies that have been taken up by red cells. Saline is usually the fluid selected and the splitting off of antibodies from the red cells is effected by raising the temperature of the sensitised cells to 56°C.

Elution. The process of making an eluate.

Enzyme. *See* Proteolytic enzyme.

Erythrocyte. Red cell.

Experimental error. The maximum variation in results given by any technique in the hands of an expert.

Factor. Gene. Sometimes also applied to the product of a gene.

Fertilisation. The fusion of the male and female sex cells to form the zygote.

Gamete. A sex cell.

Gastric mucin. Gluco proteins occurring in the stomach, often rich in blood group substances.

Gene. One of a number of portions of chromatin material strung in linear arrangement along a chromosome and controlling the development of an inherited characteristic.

Genotype. A group of individuals having the same genetic make-up with regard to particular alleles, *e.g.* AO.

Globulin. A class of proteins to which antibodies belong. They can be separated by electrophoresis into α, β and γ fractions (*see also* Immunoglobulins).

Group specific substance. A term applied to an antigen or hapten which possesses blood group specificity.

Hæmoglobin. The oxygen-carrying red pigment of the red blood cells; esp. hæmoglobin estimation; the quantitative assessment of the hæmoglobin content of red cells.

Hæmolysin. An antibody which causes hæmolysis of red cells, in the presence of complement.

Hæmolysis. The breaking-down of the red cell envelope with the liberation of hæmoglobin.

Hæmolytic. Causing, or marked by, hæmolysis.

Hæmolytic anæmia. Anæmia caused by excessive destruction of red cells.

Hæmolytic disease of the newborn. The modern name for erythroblastosis fœtalis. A disease of the fœtus or newborn which is caused by a maternal antibody attacking the fœtal red cells and probably also the tissues.

Hæmolytic transfusion reaction. A reaction due to an increased rate of destruction of red cells *in vivo* following transfusion.

Hapten. A substance which will combine specifically with the corresponding antibody but will not stimulate the formation of antibodies *in vivo*. Haptens are often polysaccharides, *e.g.* group specific substances A and B as isolated from saliva and pseudomucinous ovarian cysts.

Heparin. An anti-coagulant.

Hetero-agglutinin. *See* Agglutinin.

Heterophile antibody. Antibody produced by the so-called heterophile or Forssman antigen which is present in the organs of some animals, *e.g.* guinea-pig, horse, dog, cat, and absent from others, *e.g.* man, rabbit, ox, sheep.

Heterophile antigen. Forssman antigen distributed as above. Has a close antigenic relationship to the human group A antigen.

Heterospecific pregnancy. A pregnancy in which the maternal serum contains an anti-A or anti-B antibody incompatible with the fœtal red cells, *e.g.* O mother, A fœtus.

Heterozygous. Having unlike alleles on the corresponding loci of a pair of chromosomes.

Homologous chromosome. One of a pair of identical chromosomes.

Homologous blood. Blood of the same group. Is usually restricted to mean of the same ABO group.

Homologous serum jaundice. Jaundice caused by a virus contained in transfused compatible human plasma.

Homozygous. Having like alleles on the corresponding loci of a pair of chromosomes.

Hydrops fœtalis. One form of hæmolytic disease of the fœtus (or newborn) in which the fœtal tissues retain abnormal quantities of fluid.

Hyper immunisation. Immunisation to an unusually high degree—hence hyper immunity, hyper immune antibody, etc.

Hypertonic solution. A solution of greater osmotic pressure than blood.

Hypotonic solution. A solution of less osmotic pressure than blood.

Icterus. Jaundice.

Icterus gravis neonatorum. Severe jaundice of the newborn—one of the manifestations of hæmolytic disease of the newborn.

Immunisation. The process by which antibodies are produced in response to antigenic stimulus—hence immune antibody and immune response.

Immuno-electrophoresis. The identification of proteins separated by agar gel electrophoresis by means of lines of precipitation formed against specific antisera diffusing through the agar.

Immunoglobulins. The name given to antibody containing globulins. They can be fractionated as follows: 1 IgG(γG). By definition is that fraction of gamma globulin contained in fraction 1 of the DEAE column. Contains most incomplete antibodies and some agglutinins. 2 IgA(γA). Contains some antibodies. 3 IgM(γM). The fraction containing macroglobulins—most agglutinins and "papain" type antibodies.

Inactivation of serum. The heating of serum at 56°C for 30 minutes to destroy the heat labile fractions of complement.

Incompatible. Not compatible.

Incomplete antibody. Any antibody which sensitises red cells suspended in saline but fails to agglutinate them.

Incubate. To place tests in an apparatus which will keep them at a constant temperature.

Inhibition. The prevention of the normal reaction between an antigen and its corresponding antibody, usually because an antigen of the same specificity but from another source is present in the system—hence to inhibit.

Inhibition technique. A test which can be either qualitative or quantitative, devised for the detection of group specific substances by means of their inhibiting effect on the corresponding antibody.

Irregular. Atypical.

Iso-agglutinin. *See* Agglutinin.

Isotonic solution. A solution having the same osmotic pressure as blood.

Karyotype. Group of individuals with the same chromosome number and similar linear arrangement of genes in homologous chromosomes; chromosome complement of such a group.

Kernicterus. Damage and pigmentation of the brain nuclei, particularly of the basal ganglia, associated with severe neonatal jaundice.

Linked genes. Genes situated on the same chromosome. *See also* Closely linked genes.

Locus. The position on a chromosome occupied by a gene.

Lysis. The breakdown of cells.

Meiosis. The cell division which produces mature sex cells with half the number of chromosomes possessed by the original cells.

Mitosis. Cell division which produces daughter cells with the same number of chromosomes as the original cells. All cell division, with the exception of that to produce mature sex cells, is mitotic.

Modifying gene. A gene which modifies the expression of another gene.

Mosaic. A mixture of characters produced by a cross-over occurring within the confines of a gene.

Mutation. A change in a gene between one generation and the next. Allelomorphs are thought to have arisen as the result of mutations. Mutation is very rare in man.

Naturally-occurring antibodies. *See* Agglutinin (typical).

Non-secretor. An individual who does not secrete the appropriate A, B, or H group specific substances in his body fluids.

Normal saline. Isotonic saline.

Nucleus. The deeply staining body contained within a cell, forming the essential part. It contains the chromosomes.

Ovum. The female gamete or sex cell.

Pan-agglutinable cells. Red cells which are agglutinated by all human sera irrespective of blood group.

Panel of cells. A set of standard red cells specially selected to detect and identify blood group antibodies.

Phenotype. A group of individuals who when tested with a particular set of antisera are found to belong to the same type or sub-type, but who may not necessarily all be of the same genotype, *e.g.* group A, which includes the genotypes AO and AA.

Plasma. The fluid portion of unclotted blood.

Poly-agglutinable red cells. Cells that are agglutinated by most but not all human sera regardless of blood group.

Polysaccharide. One of a group of complex carbohydrates of large molecular size.

Position effect. The effect which blood group antigens have upon each other by virtue of the relative position of their genes on the chromosome pair, *e.g.* the different effect of E upon D in the genotypes R_2r (cDE.cde) and R_0R'' (cDe.cdE).

Potency. Strength, particularly strength of antiserum.

Precipitin. An antibody which reacts with its corresponding antigen to form a precipitate.

Proteolytic enzyme. An organic compound which specifically effects the digestion of protein, *e.g.* trypsin.

Protocol. The original record made of the results of a test.

Prozone phenomenon. In an antigen-antibody system, a negative reaction obtained with low dilutions of the antibody, although a positive reaction is obtained with higher dilutions of the same antibody. Only rarely encountered in blood group serology.

Pseudo-agglutination. Clumping of red cells by other agents than antibodies. The cells are not distorted or damaged.

Pseudomucinous ovarian cyst fluid. A fluid from certain ovarian cysts which is rich in blood group substances.

Putative. Reputed, supposed—hence putative father, the reputed father of a particular child.

Pyrogen. A substance capable of causing rise of temperature when injected into an animal. Distilled water pyrogens are filtrable, thermostable products probably of bacterial origin, and tend to cause a severe rigor if injected intravenously.

Recessive gene. A gene which only gives rise to its corresponding character when present in "double dose" (in the homozygote).

Recombination. The re-arrangement of genes at gametogenesis so that offspring have new combinations which differ from those of either parent.

Rouleaux formation. A form of pseudo-agglutination in which the red cells give the appearance of piles of coins.

Screening. Preliminary testing.

Secretor. An individual who secretes the appropriate A, B, and H substances in the body fluids.

Sensitisation of red cells. Red cells are said to be sensitised when they have antibody specifically attached to their receptors but are not agglutinated.

Sensitisation of individuals. Stimulation of an individual by an antigen which renders him liable to form antibodies.

Serum. The fluid portion of clotted blood.

Siblings. Children of the same parents.

Somatic cells. Body cells as opposed to sex cells.

Specificity. The special affinity between an antigen and its corresponding antibody.

Sperm. The male gamete or sex cell.

Suppressor gene. A modifying gene which will completely or partially suppress the expression of another gene.

Thermal amplitude. The temperature range within which an antibody reacts.

Titrate. To make a series of dilutions. To determine the strength of an antigen or antibody by making a series of dilutions and testing their strength against the corresponding antibody or antigen—hence titration.

Titre or titration value. A numerical evaluation of the strength of an antiserum, usually expressed as the reciprocal of the highest dilution at which it reacts with the corresponding antigen by a given technique.

Trans position. Being on opposite chromosomes and may or may not be within the same cistron.

Variant. Different type, usually applied to the rarer forms.

Warm antibody. An antibody reacting better at 37°C than at lower temperatures.

Wash. To free red cells from the liquid in which they were suspended (usually serum or plasma) by successive centrifuging in large volumes of saline.

Zygote. A fertilised egg cell

Appendix IV—Serum Fractionation

SERUM can be fractionated either on DEAE cellulose or by sephadex filtration. The first method gives pure IgG, reasonably pure IgA and is not quite so satisfactory for IgM. The sephadex method on the other hand where the IgM is the first fraction obtained gives a good yield or pure IgM but is not so satisfactory for the other fractions. Both the methods are described therefore.

Technique No. A.IV.1. Fractionation of a serum using DEAE cellulose

DEAE cellulose (Whatman DE11) is washed with Sorensens phosphate buffer 0·02 M at ph 8·0. It is then packed into a suitable sized column *e.g.* 1 × 12 cm and at least 500 ml of buffer allowed to run through the column to bring the DEAE cellulose into equilibrium with the buffer; for a large column a correspondingly larger volume of buffer has to be used.

The serum fractionated is dialysed for eighteen hours against a large volume of the buffer. The serum is carefully layered on top of the buffer; many people recommend a pad of filter paper above the DEAE to ensure a level surface but we have not found this essential. Buffer is then run through the column at a steady rate and the effluent collected. In practice about 30 ml of buffer are needed to elute 0·5 ml of serum from a 1 × 12 cm column. This is concentrated to a suitable volume for testing (*i.e.* about 2 ml) by dialysing against polyethylene glycol and then dialysed for 2 hrs at room temperature against normal saline. The second fraction is eluted with Sorensens phosphate buffer and 0·08 M at pH 6·5 and contains IgA usually a trace of IgG, albumin and other serum constituents. IgM can then be eluted with 0·2 M buffer at pH 5·0. These second and third fractions are concentrated and dialysed against normal saline as for the first, before being tested.

Technique No. A.IV.2. Fractionation of a serum by Sephadex G.200

Materials:

Buffer solutions (Stock)

1. 0·2 M tris (hydroxymethyl) amino-methane (24·2 gm per litre).
2. 2 N HCl.
3. 0·42 M NaCl (24·68 gm per litre).

Working solution

500 ml 0·2 tris with 26·8 ml 2 N HCl. Make up to 1 litre with 0·42 M NaCl. This gives 0·1 M tris HCl buffer (ph 8) in 0·2 M salt. Sephadex. G.200 and G.25.

Column: A convenient column is 30 × 70 cm. It is usual to allow 200 ml column volume to 0·5 ml serum and 1 gm Sephadex for 100 ml column volume.

Method: The Sephadex is soaked for 48 hours in buffer solution prior to use and the fine particles are poured off and discarded. One gm of G.25 Sephadex in 50 ml working buffer is allowed to settle at the bottom of the column and about 8 gm of G.200 Sephadex in 500 ml buffer is packed in above. Plenty of buffer is run through the column and it is allowed to settle overnight before use. At the same time a convenient amount of the serum to be fractionated (*e.g.* 2 ml) is dialysed against the working buffer solution overnight. The whole contents of the dialysis sac is then introduced on to the top of the column. For the optimum results it is best to introduce the dialysed serum on to the column through a nylon sieve very gently by means of a syringe with a rubber nozzle. The top of the column is then closed by means of a screw cap with a central perforation which allows for a connection with the buffer solution which is clamped about 12 inches above the level of the top of the column. Buffer solution is allowed to pass down through the column under the positive pressure thus produced. The drops issuing from the nozzle at the base of the column are collected by means of a fraction collector. The automatic slow rotation of the collector allows for the collection of a predetermined number of fractions per hour (*e.g.* 4). The number of fractions collected will depend on the capacity of the fraction collector and the size of the cell used in the spectrophotometer. A certain amount of trial and error is necessary to find the optimum rate of collection and number of fractions to collect. The process usually takes about 24 hours.

At the end of the separation, the tubes may be gently shaken when frothing will indicate the presence of protein. An accurate estimation of the protein concentration is made by measuring the optical density at 280 mμ on the spectrophotometer. A graph is plotted which will show the protein peaks. The fractions are then pooled around the peaks. They have to be concentrated before they are tested for antibody activity. This can be done most satisfactorily by pressure dialysis. The dialysis tubing containing the best material is suspended in a loose coil in a flask which is evacuated thus causing fluid to be expressed through the wall of the tubing. The volume should be reduced to about 2 ml.

The first peak from Sephadex G.200 separation contains pure IgM immunoglobulin in contrast to peak 1 from the DEAE column which is pure IgG. Sephadex separation is more suitable than DEAE separation for the isolation of IgM because the IgM peak from DEAE is liable to be contaminated with globulin from the preceding IgG and IgA peaks. However, Sephadex G.200 is unsuitable for the preparation of IgA.

Appendix V

BLOOD TRANSFUSION APPARATUS

THIS appendix contains the description of the blood bottle, taking and giving sets re-introduced from our first edition (1957). This is for the benefit of those, in some parts of the world, who still use a similar apparatus, although it has become obsolete elsewhere.

Although details may be different (e.g. gas mantle filters are probably no longer used), the assembly, cleansing and maintenance of such equipment, is essentially unaltered.

The Blood Bottle

This is a glass bottle capacity 540 ml.; the one in general use in this country being the M.R.C. bottle (*see* Plate 13(b)). It will stand much hard wear, usually being satisfactory up to ten to twelve autoclavings. Bottles are discarded if there is a slight fluorescence in the autoclaved fluid, this being due to scaling of the inner glaze. Bottles can be washed by hand or in a variety of bottle washing machines. If the bottle washer is not equipped with rotary brushes the bottles must be cleaned with jets of solutions under pressure. The machine in use at the Blood Transfusion Centre, Sutton, has a moving belt by which the bottles are carried over jets of fluid which cleanse them both inside and out. The sequence is warm tap water, detergent (the one at present in use and giving satisfactory results is Mertonite grade 304), several rinses of warm tap water and finally steam under pressure. The bottles are stacked upside down in crates as they come from the machine and are dry within a few minutes at room temperature. The circuit is accomplished by one bottle in 3½–4 minutes, the machine being capable of handling 750–800 bottles per hour.

The bottles have aluminium screw caps with rubber wads. The wads are discarded after use and replaced with new ones. The caps themselves are cleansed by soaking, scrubbing, boiling in distilled water for 10 minutes, rinsing, draining, and rinsing with distilled water. They are dried in a hot air oven (temperature 70–80°C).

The bottles have 120 ml. of ACD (*see* Ap. I) added to each or, if they are "dry" bottles for the preparation of serum, 3–4 ml. of saline. The caps with the rubber wads are loosely screwed down

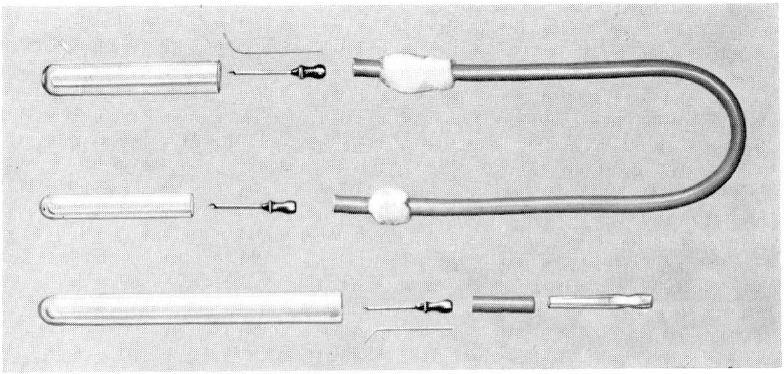

PLATE 13(*a*). Component parts of taking set, including airlet.

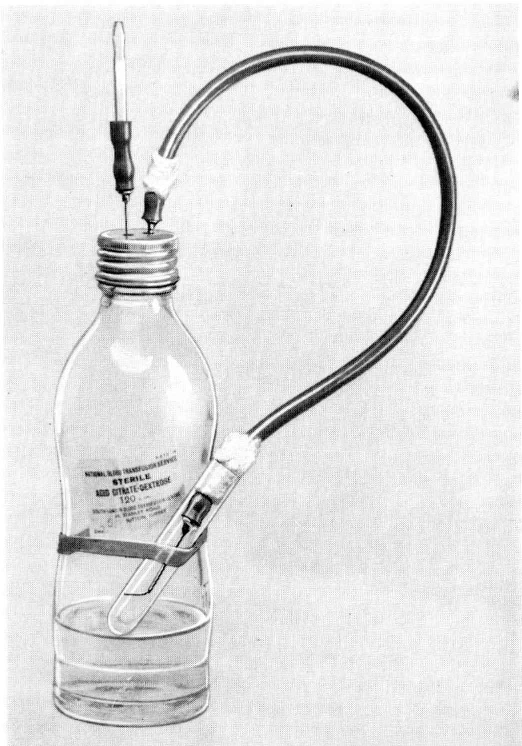

PLATE 13(*b*) Blood bottle with taking set in position.

[*To face p.* 446

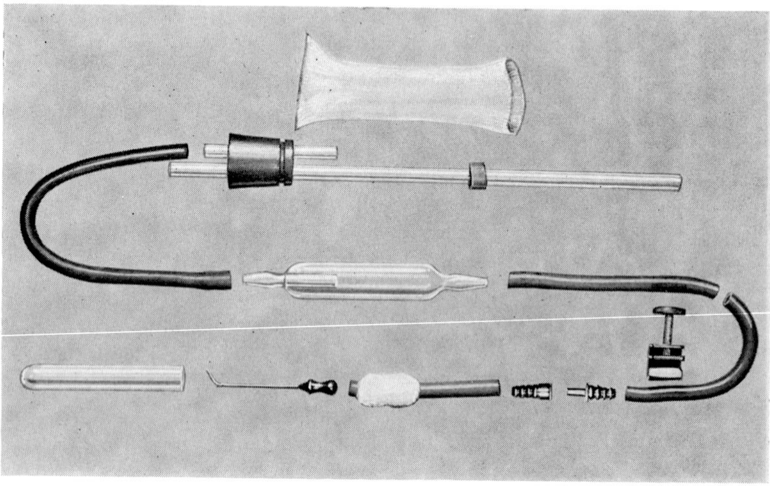

PLATE 13(*c*) Component parts of giving set.

The illustration shows: the ridged rubber bung pierced by the long air inlet and short blood outlet tubes: the gas mantle filter, shown separately, is attached to the ridged bung and the rubber collar; the "short" length (5–7 in.) of rubber tubing connects the blood outlet tube to one end of the drip chamber, while to the other end is attached 36–40 in. of rubber tubing, only part of which is shown: male adaptor, female adaptor, rubber tubing with cotton wool plug, intravenous needle with stillette, and covering glass test tube. The screw clip, which regulates the flow of blood, is placed in a convenient position on the long length of tubing just prior to the insertion of the apparatus in the bottle of blood.

and covered with small brown paper bags. The bottles are then autoclaved at 20 lb. for 30 minutes and the autoclave is left overnight before opening.

Next morning the caps are screwed tight, the bottles inspected for vacuum—any found being released—and the paper bags secured with elastic bands. The bottles are examined for flaking and labelled with the date of sterilisation (*see* Plate 13(b)).

Taking Apparatus

Plate 13(a) shows the component parts of a taking set including airlet and Plate 13(b) the assembled bottle with taking set in position ready for use.

The size of needle used is 19/10 (14 S.G.). The airlet needle and the needle that goes into the bottle are blunt; the intravenous needle is sharpened to give a medium bevel and also at the sides to give a cutting edge, a stillette being placed in the needle to protect the point. The rubber tubing is grade 6819 supplied by William Warne (this particular grade is extremely efficient and will withstand about ten to twelve autoclavings). The tubes that enclose the needles are firmly plugged with non-absorbent cotton wool, while the airlet must be plugged loosely; if the airlet is too tightly plugged then pressure would build up in the bottle with the risk of a back flow of air into the patient and possible air embolism.

The taking apparatus is autoclaved at 20 lb. pressure for 30 minutes. The airlets, each in a plugged test tube, are packed into wire baskets; the taking sets are wrapped in brown paper in bundles of twenty-five.

Following sterilisation they are dried while in the autoclave, firstly *in vacuo* for 30 minutes and then in a current of hot dry air. They are inspected and packed in suitable containers for transfer to the blood-taking sessions.

The Giving Set

Plate 13(c) shows the component parts of the giving set. New gas mantle filters* are used at each assembly but the other component parts can be cleansed and re-used. The adaptors are Luer fitting and are tied in with a rayon cotton. The same quality rubber tubing is used as for the taking set. The needle size is 15/10 (16 S.G.). The assembled set is wrapped in cellophane and placed in a tin with a brown card lining; the tin is loosely closed and the whole is autoclaved at 20 lb. for 30 minutes. These sets also are dried for 30 minutes *in vacuo* and 30 minutes with a stream of

* Metal filters usually used now.

hot dry air while still in the autoclave. They are then removed from the autoclave and the tin carefully sealed. Only apparatus from tins with unbroken seals may be used for a transfusion.

After use the giving set is soaked overnight, dismantled and the various parts cleansed, dried and reassembled.

Cleansing and Maintenance of Component Parts of Giving and Taking Apparatus

Rubber Tubing

New rubber tubing is cut into 40 inch lengths and rinsed through with a stream of tap water. It is then boiled for 10 minutes in distilled water, rewashed with tap water, drained, rinsed in distilled water, drained and dried in hot air oven at 70°–80°C (several hours are needed to dry completely).

These 40 inch lengths are used for the long section of the giving set. After each use they are soaked overnight, washed as before and dried. A short length (about ½ inch) is cut from the end so that a good fit is obtained. The minimum length suitable for a giving set is 36 inch so that after being used four times the tubing is too short and is, therefore, cut in half and used for the taking set. Here again the same cleansing and shortening procedure is followed and when the tubing is reduced to 15 inch it is cut in half for the short length in the giving set between gas mantle filter and drip chamber. If after this the tubing is still in good condition it can be used on the giving needle or on sample needles.

Needles

The intravenous needles are cleaned and resharpened after use. The needles having soaked overnight in tap water are attached to a tap and rinsed through with a strong jet, probed with wire, re-rinsed, boiled for 10 minutes in distilled water, washed again on the tap, drained rinsed in distilled water and dried. They are then resharpened to a medium bevel, the sides of the needle being given a cutting edge. This is done on a grindstone of constitution 37C.400.N 11 V.*

This produces a very good sharp needle which does not need further polishing.

After sharpening, the needles are soaked in trichlorethylene overnight (or for minimum of 2 hours) to remove the grease and any small attached particles, drained and polished with a soft

* Key to coding: 37C = Abrasive, Crystolan. 400 = grain size, very small N = grade, medium hardness. 11 = structure, wide spacing. V = bond, vitrified.

dry cloth and using a large rubber bulb rinsed through vigorously several times with industrial spirit. They are then inspected and the protecting stillette inserted.

Needles can be resharpened about ten to twelve times before having to be discarded.

Glass Parts. *e.g.*, **Tubing. Drip Chambers. etc,**

After the initial overnight soaking all glass parts are rinsed in tap water, boiled in distilled water with preferably one of the new detergents (a good quality soap flake or soap powder can be substituted if preferred) for 10 minutes, they are then rinsed in tap water, drained, rinsed in distilled water, drained again and dried in a hot air oven.

Adaptors

Adaptors are cleansed in exactly the same way as needles except that they do not of course need the sharpening and grease removing processes.

The Apparatus for Plasma-aspiration, and Preparation of Packed Cells

This is soaked after use and each part subjected to the appropriate cleansing process as described for the giving and taking apparatus. The apparatus is sterilised, packed into dressing drums with a layer of lint between each complete outfit. The drums are autoclaved at 20 lb. for 30 minutes with the holes open; the holes are shut when the drum is removed from the autoclave.

Syringes

Syringes are cleansed in the same manner as other glass and/or metal fittings. They are wrapped in lint and dry sterilised at 160°C for 1 hour. Syringe needles are cleansed as for other intravenous needles if used for taking blood—if merely used for local anæsthetics they are rinsed in tap water, followed by distilled water, touched up on a dry stone and rewashed in tap and distilled water. They are sterilised in the hot air oven as for syringes.

Sample Needles

It is preferable and more convenient to take intravenous blood samples not with a syringe but by gravity through a sample needle. This is a S.G. 19 needle with a short length of rubber tubing attached. The whole is sterilised in a plugged test tube by autoclaving for 30 minutes at 20 lb. pressure.

Dressings

Two types of dressing are commonly used. The first, a small ball of cotton wool, is used in cleansing the skin. The second is a small pressure pad, made of cotton wool covered with gauze, and is used to cover the venepuncture, being taped or bandaged firmly into position and not removed until the day following venesection. These dressings are autoclaved at 20 lb. pressure for 30 minutes and dried while still in the autoclave for 30 minutes *in vacuo* and 30 minutes in a current of hot air.

Sterility Checks

(1) Check on Autoclave Efficiency by Means of Agricultural Spores

Spores of a prolific, hardy agricultural organism (*e.g.*, a form of B subtilis) are used. For the test a piece of lint which has had a small quantity of broth culture of the organism dried on to it is enclosed in a sealed envelope. Envelopes are placed inside M.R.C. blood bottles, giving set tins, dressing drums, etc., in each part of the autoclave. After autoclaving for 30 minutes at 20 lb. pressure the contents of each envelope are added to 15 ml. of enriched broth and incubated; any growth necessitates an immediate overhaul of the autoclave. Autoclaves should be checked weekly by this method.

(2) Additional Tests on Actual Equipment

Once a week a representative selection of citrate bottles is cultured. The number tested will depend upon the size of the autoclave but it will approximate 10 per cent of an autoclave loading and will be selected from various positions within the autoclave. From each bottle selected two cultures are made each using an inoculum of 2–3 ml. of citrate to 15 ml. of enriched broth, one culture is kept at room temperature and the other incubated at 37°C. They are examined for any growth daily for 7 days. Samples of snippings of rubber tubing from both giving and taking sets, pressure pads, needles, etc., can all be tested by dropping them in 15 ml. of enriched broth and proceeding as above.

Sterility Tests on Bottles Containing Blood

These check not only the sterilisation of all apparatus but also the efficiency of the skin sterilisation and the taking of the blood generally.

It is our practice to culture every bottle which for any reason is not completely filled with blood (this represents about 0·2 per cent of bottles used). Three samples are taken each of 2–3 ml. in 15 ml. of enriched broth, they are incubated at 4°C, room temperature, and 37°C respectively and examined daily up to seven days for any growth. The same tests are also made on a selection of bottles returned unopened from hospitals, those whose plasma appears unsuitable for pooling being chosen for culturing.

Both the sterility checks and the hospital reports on cases who receive transfusion suggest that the techniques of sterilisation, venesection, etc., are good and that the infection rate of bottles of blood taken with this apparatus by the method recommended is very low indeed.

Appendix VI—Numerical Index of Techniques

INDEX

825
770

Stages in the production of ABH

STAGE I	STAGE II	STAGE III	STAGE IV
genes unknown	Lewis genes	Hh genes	Secretor genes

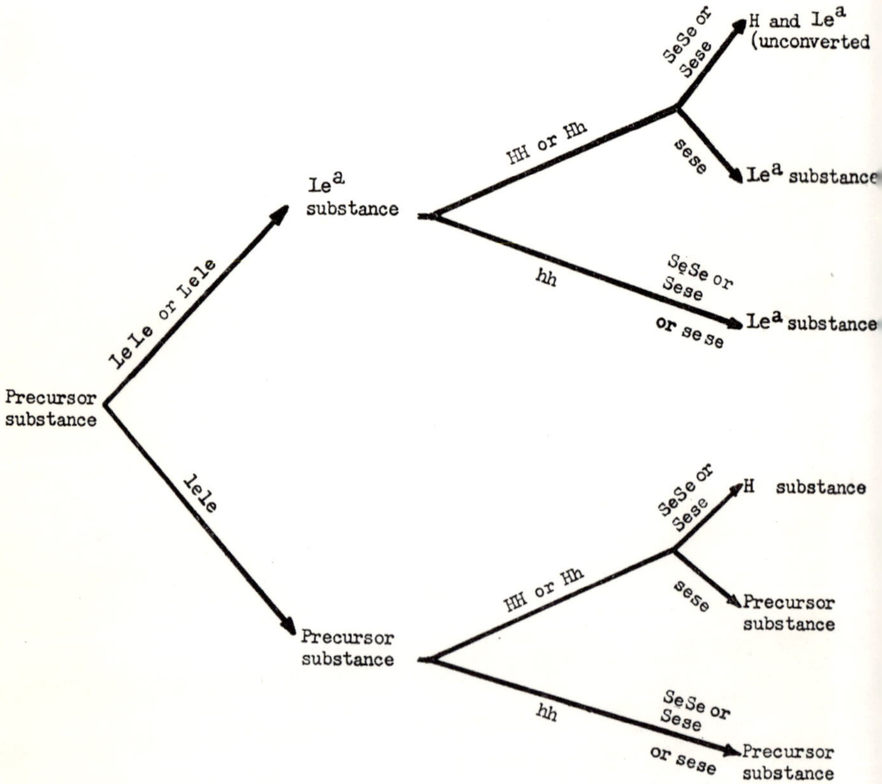